AF332950

OPERATIVE UROLOGY

A Comprehensive Guide

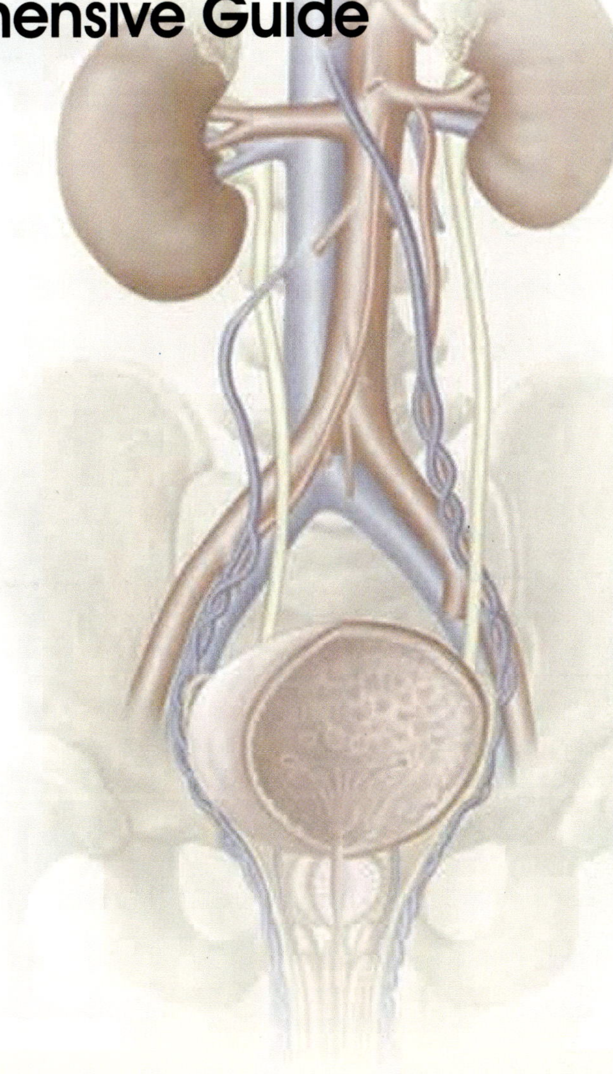

OPERATIVE UROLOGY
A Comprehensive Guide

Chief Editor

Arvind P Ganpule
Vice-Chairman
Department of Urology
Chief, Division of Laparoscopic Urology and Robotic Surgery
Muljibhai Patel Urological Hospital (MPUH)
Nadiad, Gujarat, India

Associate Editors

Abhishek Singh
Senior Consultant Urologist
Department of Urology
Muljibhai Patel Urological Hospital (MPUH)
Nadiad, Gujarat, India

Rohan Batra
Consultant Urologist
Department of Urology
Muljibhai Patel Urological Hospital (MPUH)
Nadiad, Gujarat, India

Assistant Editor

Akshay Nathani
Consultant Urologist
Department of Urology
Muljibhai Patel Urological Hospital (MPUH)
Nadiad, Gujarat, India

Foreword

Ravindra B Sabnis

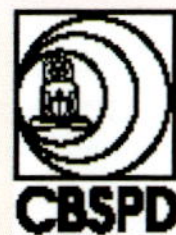

CBS Publishers & Distributors Pvt Ltd

New Delhi • Bengaluru • Chennai • Kochi • Kolkata • Lucknow • Mumbai
Hyderabad • Jharkhand • Nagpur • Patna • Pune • Uttarakhand

OPERATIVE UROLOGY
A Comprehensive Guide

ISBN: 978-93-5466-753-4

Copyright © Editors and Publisher

First Edition: 2025

Published by Satish Kumar Jain and produced by Varun Jain for

CBS Publishers & Distributors Pvt Ltd
4819/XI Prahlad Street, 24 Ansari Road, Daryaganj, New Delhi 110 002, India
Ph: 011-23266838, 23289259

Website: www.cbspd.com
e-mail: delhi@cbspd.com

Corporate Office: 204 FIE, Industrial Area, Patparganj, Delhi 110 092, India
Ph: 011-4934 4934   Fax: 011-4934 4935   e-mail: publishing@cbspd.com; publicity@cbspd.com

Branches

- **Bengaluru:** Seema House 2975, 17th Cross, KR Road, Banasankari 2nd Stage, Bengaluru 560 070, Karnataka, India
  Ph: +91-80-26771678/79   Fax: +91-80-26771680   e-mail: bangalore@cbspd.com
- **Chennai:** 7, Subbaraya Street, Shenoy Nagar, Chennai 600 030, Tamil Nadu, India
  Ph: +91-44-26680620, 26681266   Fax: +91-44-42032115   e-mail: chennai@cbspd.com
- **Kochi:** 42/1325, 1326, Power House Road, Opp KSEB, Power House, Ernakulum Kochi 682 018, Kerala, India
  Ph: +91-484-4059061-65,67   Fax: +91-484-4059065   e-mail: kochi@cbspd.com
- **Kolkata:** 147, Hind Ceramics Compound, 1st Floor, Nilgunj Road, Belghoria, Kolkata 700 056, West Bengal, India
  Ph: +91-33-25633055/56   e-mail: kolkata@cbspd.com
- **Lucknow:** Basement, Khushnuma Complex, 7 Meerabai Marg (behind Jawahar Bhawan), Lucknow 226 001, UP, India
  Ph: +910522-4000032   e-mail: tiwari.lucknow@cbspd.com
- **Mumbai:** PWD Shed, Gala no 25/26, Ramchandra Bhatt Marg, Next to JJ Hospital Gate no. 2, Opp. Union Bank of India, Noorbaug, Mumbai 400 009, Maharashtra, India
  Ph: +91-22-66661880/89   e-mail: mumbai@cbspd.com

Representatives

• **Hyderabad**	0-9885175004	• **Jharkhand**	0-9811541605	• **Nagpur**	0-8692091830
• **Patna**	0-9334159340	• **Pune**	0-9664372571	• **Uttarakhand**	0-9716462459

Printed at Magic International Pvt. Ltd.

Contributors

Abhishek Singh
Senior Consultant Urologist
Department of Urology
Muljibhai Patel Urological Hospital
Nadiad, Gujarat, India

Akshay Nathani
Consultant Urologist
Department of Urology
Muljibhai Patel Urological Hospital
Nadiad, Gujarat, India

Aruj Shah
Resident Urology
Department of Urology
Muljibhai Patel Urological Hospital
Nadiad, Gujarat, India

Arvind P Ganpule
Vice-Chairman
Department of Urology
Chief, Division of Laparoscopic Urology and
Robotic Surgery
Muljibhai Patel Urological Hospital
Nadiad, Gujarat, India

Ashwin Sunil Tamhankar
Consultant Uro-oncologist
Department of Uro-oncology
Apollo Hospital, Navi Mumbai
Mumbai, India

Chandramohan Vaddi
Director and Consultant Urologist
Preeti Hospitals
Hyderabad, Telangana, India

Gagan Gautam
Vice-Chairman
Uro-oncology and Robotic Surgery
Urology and Andrology
Kidney and Urology Institute
Medanta—The Medicity
Gurugram, Haryana, India

KR Seetharam Bhat
Assistant Professor
Department of Urology
State University of New York Upstate Medical
University, New York, United States

Nagaraja VH
Uro-oncologist
Ex-Consulant
HCG Cancer Hospital
Bengaluru, Karnataka, India

Nitesh Kumar
Consultant Urologist
Sri Kripa Urocare and Ford Hospital
Patna, Bihar, India

Pavan Jain
Consultant Urologist
Zydus Hospital
Anand, Gujarat, India

Puneet Ahluwalia
Director and Head
Uro-Oncology and Robotic Surgery
Urology and Andrology
Kidney and Urology Institute
Medanta—The Medicity
Gurugram, Haryana, India

Raghunath S Krishnappa
Director and Consultant Uro-oncologist
HCG Hospital
Bengaluru, Karnataka, India

Raisa Shetty
Resident Urology
Department of Urology
Muljibhai Patel Urological Hospital
Nadiad, Gujarat, India

Rajesh Kukreja
Consultant Urologist
Urocare Hospital
Indore, Madhya Pradesh, India

Ravindra B Sabnis
Chairman and Head
Department of Urology
Muljibhai Patel Urological Hospital
Nadiad, Gujarat, India
President
Urological Society of India, 2022–2023

Rohan Batra
Consultant Urologist
Department of Urology
Muljibhai Patel Urological Hospital
Nadiad, Gujarat, India

Srivatsa N
Consultant
Uro-Oncologist and Robotic Surgeon
Sri Shankara Cancer Hospital
and Research Centre
Bengaluru, Karnataka, India

Sudharsan Balaji
Consultant Urologist
Apollo Hospital
Thiruvallur, Tamil Nadu, India

Surya Prakash Ojha
Department of Urooncology
Max Institute of Cancer Care
Max Superspeciality Hospital
Saket, New Delhi, India

Tejus C
Consultant Urologist
Sparsh Hospital
Bengaluru, Karnataka, India

V Mohan Kumar
Consultant Urologist
Manipal Hospital
Bengaluru, Karnataka, India

Vijay Victor
Resident in Urology
Department of Urologist
Muljibhai Patel Urological Hospital
Nadiad, Gujarat, India

Vineet Malhotra
Consultant Urologist and Andrologist
VNA Hospital
New Delhi, India

Foreword

Urology is a speciality which is rapidly advancing. New imaging modalities, procedures, instruments and energy sources have come in the vogue in the last few years. Several methods and procedures which were the treatment of choice have become obsolete and are not practised nowadays. Naturally, it becomes imperative for the trainee and consultants in urology to be updated about the developments.

"Nothing is constant, change is the rule". This is so true for medical science. The timing of publication of this book is apt and suitable, as we are at a cusp of evolution in medical science with the explosion of technique and technology. Urology is fast developing its subspecialities.

The editors of this book have very nicely brought out the technical points in various urologic procedures for trainees and consultants to imbibe the principles. They have dived deep into the nitty-gritty of the technicalities. This book discusses in detail everything from basics to advances in endourology, laparoscopy and procedures such as AV fistula constructions. These topics are very nicely complemented by figures and diagrams, for clarity of the concepts. The addition of QR-coded videos has added a unique feature wherein the readers get the opportunity to learn the technique in a step-by-step manner while watching the videos.

I am sure, this book would help one and all to enhance their skills and reach them to the next level. I congratulate all the editors and contributors for their efforts which are very obvious and hope this would make a useful read for one and all.

Ravindra B Sabnis
Chairman and Head
Department of Urology
Muljibhai Patel Urological Hospital
Nadiad, Gujarat, India
President
Urological Society of India, 2022–2023

Preface

The adage, *See one, do one and teach one*, remains the Achilles' heel of surgical training and teaching alike. As surgeons, we need to be properly trained in technique of a given procedure. In the good olden days, the teaching used to be done with the help of didactic talks, ward rounds and then onsite/in theatre surgical training by the mentor/teacher or the proctor. The onslaught of social media has changed the way we perceive and imbibe teaching. The easily available information is like a weapon, the trainee has the potential to learn good as well as bad techniques through these platforms.

Given this paradigm shift that we are witnessing from broad specialities to subspecialities, I feel publication of this book is timely and apt for young consultants and postgraduates alike.

With this background in mind, we have decided to provide the readers an abridged version of the monogram in urology volumes already published 6 years back. In this edition, we have tried to provide the readers a book which focuses on various techniques in different aspects of laparoscopic urology. The book is divided into four sections on laparoscopic urology, endourology, general urology and miscellaneous topics. The basics are discussed threadbare. The book aims only on technical aspects important to the trainees and young consultants alike. The value-added addition of the book is QR-coded videos which have voice overs and the techniques are discussed in a step-by-step manner.

Last but not the least, I would like to put on record, if it was not for the enthusiasm of Mr Verma and Mr Gala, this book would not have seen the light of the day. I would like to thank Mr SK Jain (CMD), Mr Varun Jain (Director) and Mr YN Arjuna (Senior Vice-President) of CBS Publishers and Distributors and their team members, Dr Ashu Singh and Mrs Ritu Chawla for their support and guidance, and also for being so vigilant to ensure the book maintains the required standards.

I would be unfair if I do not acknowledge the support of all my contributors and associate/assistant editors.

Hope this makes an excellent reading for all.

Arvind P Ganpule
Chief Editor

Contents of Videos

Contents

Section 1: TIPS AND TRICKS IN LAPAROSCOPIC UROLOGY

Section 2: TIPS AND TRICKS IN ENDOUROLOGY

Section 3: PRACTICAL TIPS AND TRICKS IN GENERAL UROLOGY

Part 1: AV FISTULA

Part 2: BASICS IN ROBOTIC INSTRUMENTATION, DOCKING AND PORT PLACEMENT

Part 3: PARTIAL PENECTOMY AND VEIL

Section 4: MISCELLANEOUS

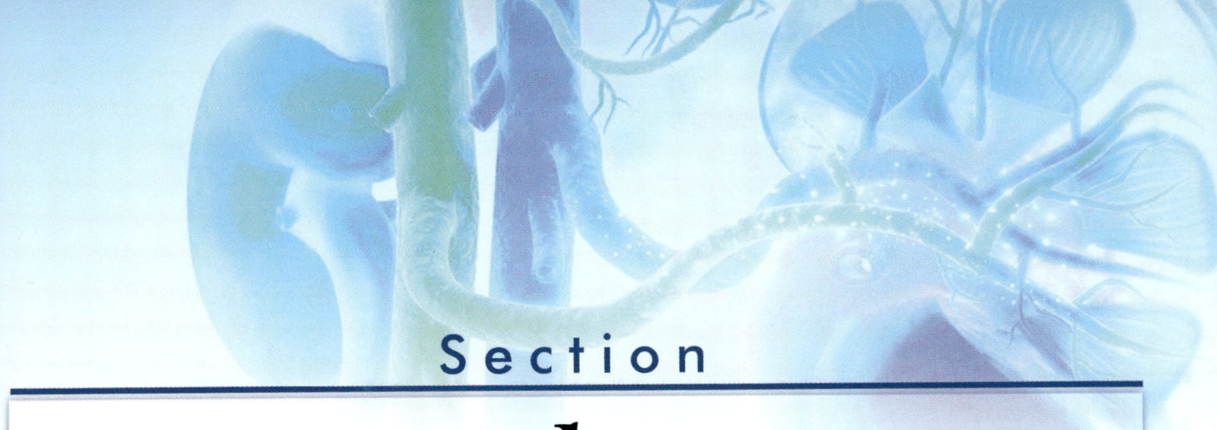

Tips and Tricks in Laparoscopic Urology

CHAPTERS

1

Ergonomics in Laparoscopic Surgery

Abhishek Singh, Arvind P Ganpule, Sudharsan Balaji, V Mohan Kumar

INTRODUCTION

Laparoscopic surgery has slowly and steadily evolved over the last century. It all probably started in the year of 1902 when Georg Kelling, a German surgeon, was working on minimally invasive techniques to stop gastrointestinal (GI) bleeding. Kelling proposed that creating a pneumoperitoneum and raising the intra-abdominal pressure could stop GI bleeding, he named this procedure Luft-tamponade (air-tamponade). In an endeavor to observe the effect of air-tamponade on the visceral organs, Kelling introduced the Nitze cysto-scope through the abdominal wall of a dog and visualized the visceral organs. This was the genesis of laparoscopic surgery and it was named Coelioscopy.[1]

The first human laparoscopic observations were made by Hans Christian Jacobaeus, who was an internist from Stockholm Sweden. Jacobaeus introduced a trocar with a trap valve, in the abdominal cavity of the patients having ascites and after evacuation of the fluid, he created pneumoperitoneum and laparoscopy was again done using a cysto-scope.[2]

In early 1980s Semm's demonstrated laparoscopic appendectomy, influenced by his work Erich Mühe on 12th September 1985 did the first laparoscopic cholecystectomy.

He was a surgeon ahead of time, he had the tenacity to fight the German Medical and so-cial system to prove his rationale. Today, it may seem the most predictive evolution but in the 1980s, Mühe's work was not very well received by the surgical community.[3]

Development of Laparoscopy in the Field of Urology

Laparoscopic surgery in the field of urology was relatively late to develop. Cortesi et al demonstrated first diagnostic use of laparoscopy in a case of undescended testis in 1976.[4] But, it was only in the year 1990 that Dr Ralph Clayman demonstrated laparo-scopic nephrectomy.[5] Around the same time Schuessler, et al demonstrated first pelvic lymphadenectomy and later on he went onto describe laparoscopic radical prostatectomy.[6] In 1990, 1st laparoscopic varicocele surgery was also demonstrated. Laparoscopic donor nephrectomy was demonstrated by Ratner et al in 1995 and now progressively has become a very commonly done procedure.[7]

The development of laparoscopic urology was very slow, by 1990 it was already about 50 years since laparoscopy had come into existence and still there were not many surgeons around the world who were perfor-ming urological procedures laparoscopically.

Urological laparoscopic surgery developed late as it had a steep learning curve, two-dimensional vision was difficult to adapt, there was loss of haptic sensation, surgeons believed that very few urological surgical procedures could be done laparoscopically and lastly it was thought that urological laparoscopic procedures are much more complex as compared to gynecological and general surgical procedures.

Why do Urological Laparoscopic Surgery?

- *Magnificent visualization:* If there is one reason that a surgeon should start doing laparoscopic surgery, it is the magnificent visualization that laparoscopy offers. During the 1980s, major advances took place in the camera systems. By late 1990s and early 2000s, high definition (HD) camera systems became available. HD systems had higher resolution than standard definition systems, in general, they have a video image of greater than 480 vertical scan lines. After HD systems came the full HD systems with progressive scan which had 1080 vertical lines. These vertical lines are a measure of the clarity, the screen or the camera is going to offer. Now we have 4k systems available, these systems have a resolution of 2 times the vertical and 2 times the horizontal resolution of a full HD system (1080p). Further to this, quantum laser emitting diode (Q LED) and 8k technologies have already hit the television market and soon will be incorporated into medical grade monitors and cameras. The vision that laparoscopic surgery offers is only getting better with technology and surgeon has started to see anatomical details better than before.

  Many open surgeons who have started doing laparoscopy confess that they had never seen anatomical details like it is seen in laparoscopic surgery. To site a few examples, the two layers of Gerota's fascia or the course of lumbar vein on left side and the distinction between the retroperitoneal and gerotal fat are much better appreciated in laparoscopic vision.

- *Dramatic postoperative recovery:* The postoperative recovery after surgery is dramatic in patients undergoing laparoscopic surgery. The patients are ambulatory early, most of them ambulate by the evening of the surgery and allowed orally 8 hours after the surgery. Objectively, postoperative recovery has been studied in randomized controlled trails by measuring the levels of acute phase reactants like C-reactive protein (CRP), interleukin-6 (IL-6), HLA-DR expression on monocytes, level of growth hormone and cortisol levels. It is seen that the rise in these acute phase reactants is less in laparoscopic surgery when compared to open surgery, supporting accelerated recovery of patients post-laparoscopic surgery.[8] The above also proves that immune response to laparoscopic surgery is much less when compared to open surgery.[8]

- *Significant reduction in pain and decreased analgesic use:* Laparoscopic surgery induced pain is less in intensity than the pain caused by open surgery. The visual analog scale pain scores for the patients are significantly less. Though the pain is less it is different in character as compared to open surgical pain. It can be classified as visceral pain which is vague abdominal pain occurring predominantly in the first 24 hours of the surgery, second type of pain is parietal pain which arises from the incision site which also subside in the 1st 24 hours and the third type of pain is the shoulder pain which arises due to irritation of the diaphragm by CO_2, this pain is maximum on the 2nd day and decreases in intensity as the days pass by.[9]

- *Lesser wound related and infectious complications:* Laparoscopic surgery is associated with a lower risk of surgical site infection.[10] As the wounds are smaller the incidence of infection is also less. Not only the superficial and deep wound infection occur with decreased severity and incidence, also the rate of infection in the deep organ spaces decreases with the use of laparoscopic surgery.[10] Incidence of deep organ space infection decreases in laparoscopic surgery as the abdominal contents are not exposed to the external environment.

- *Reduction in postoperative adhesions:* As the surgical incision is small in laparoscopic surgery, smaller raw areas are created, which in turn leads to a lesser adhesion. Although adhesion can occur at the port site.

- *Video imaging allows active participation of the mentors, trainees and theater technicians:* Laparoscopic surgery is team work and the video imaging system helps the whole team to be involved in the procedure. It makes mentoring possible and allows the team to be prepared for the next surgical steps. If the surgeon is going away at any surgical step, he can be guided by other team members.

Starting a Urological Laparoscopic Program

- Strong leadership support is required to set up a laparoscopic program.[11] As the program is equipment driven, procurement of the instruments is a major task, this is done by the people in leadership position. In an individual practice this role is done by the operating surgeon. In a corporate or government organization, it is the administration which does it.

- The chief surgeon is the center piece of the project; he should initially train himself by attending training program and short fellowship courses. Deterrent here is the cost of training and travelling, which has to be borne by individual surgeon in a stand-alone practice. Detailed description of the surgical procedure should be read, anatomy understood and teaching video watched. Simulation based training helps in developing laparoscopic skills, surgeon should start by doing simple exercises in dry lab, if facilities are not available office endotrainers are commercially available, they can be bought and training started. Cost may be deterring factor; this can be overcome by using low cost endotrainer which surgeon can himself developed (described later in text). Dry laboratory training is followed by wet laboratory simulations and finally the surgeon should embark on the real-time situation.

- *Developing a dedicated laparoscopic team (Fig. 1.1):* Laparoscopic surgery is team work, surgeon is only as good as his team. The team consist of a chief surgeon, camera driver (ideally should be a surgeon), anesthesiologist, scrub nurse, circulating nurse and theater electronic technician who can manage all the electronic and other equipment (camera, light source, insufflator) which are used in laparoscopic surgery.

- *Inviting a proctor and sequential training:* The program should be started by inviting a proctor to mentor cases. He or she can be

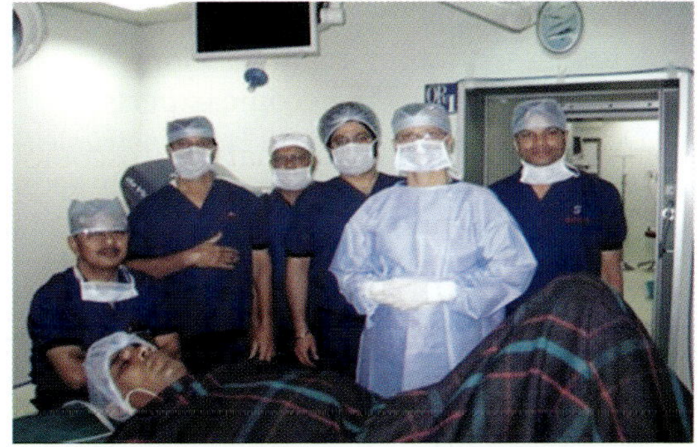

Fig. 1.1: A dedicated laparoscopy team

Table 1.1: List of basic laparoscopic instruments

Basic instrumentation

• Scissors	• Laparoscopic cart
• Hook	• Television monitor
• Suction and irrigation	• Color video chip camera
• *Grasping forceps:* Maryland, right angled, bowel holding, toothed grasper	• High intensity light source
• *Diathermy:* Monopolar and bipolar	• High flow CO_2 insufflator
• Harmonic scalpel	• *Laparoscope:* 0 and 30°
• Port closure device	• Clip applicator: 5 mm/11 mm
• Specimen retrieval bag	• *Trocars:* 12 mm and 5 mm

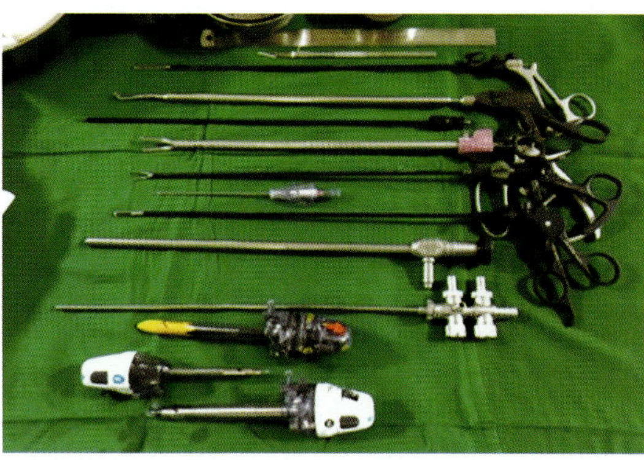

Fig. 1.2: A basic laparoscopic instrument trolley

Table 1.2: Criteria of patient selection for laparoscopic surgery for a novice

Patient selection

- Upper tract—preferable
- Should have no history of:
  - COPD
  - *Obesity:* BMI >30
  - Extensive prior abdominal or pelvic surgery
  - Pelvic fibrosis
  - Organomegaly
  - Ascites: Benign etiology
  - Hernia
  - Iliac or aortic aneurysm

an expert urological laparoscopic surgeon, if unavailable one can consider inviting and experienced laparoscopic general surgeon. Sequential training by observing a few cases, then assisting a few and finally doing a few steps of the surgery and then migrating to do the whole procedure. This basic Halstedian model along with simulation based training will go a long way in training surgeons to become experts.

- *Developing familiarity with basic instrumentation (**Table 1.1 and Fig. 1.2**):* Surgeon should be familiar with the instruments and know correction of basic malfunction. This will remove the frustration barrier and help in development of the program.
- *Initial case selection (**Table 1.2**):* Initial cases that an urologist does should be carefully selected, a well-done case will help the

surgeon develop confidence and will go a long way in determining his learning curve. Initially one should start with a beginner-friendly case, in urologic laparoscopy, beginner-friendly case will be an upper tract extirpative surgery in a perimenopause female, with a body mass index of about 25–27. The patient should not have any comorbid illness like chronic obstructive airway disease and vascular malformations of great vessels. Patient should not be suffering from pelvic fibrosis, diseases which may ascites, hernias and any organomegaly.

Components of a Laparoscopic Operating Room (OR) Set up (Figs 1.3 to 1.5)

Components of OR set up include imaging systems, insufflators, hemostatic generators

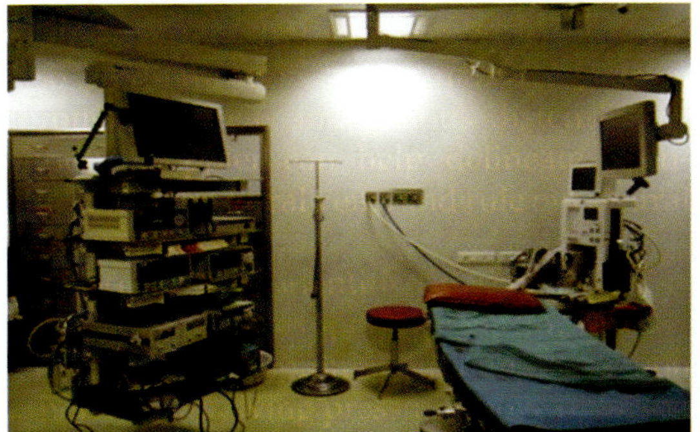

Fig. 1.3: Components of OR set up

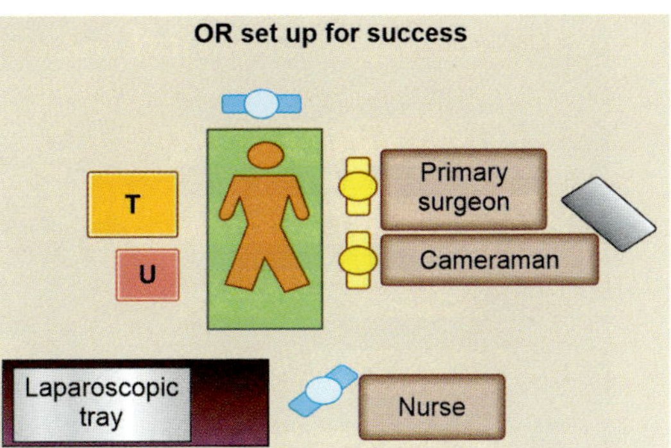

Fig. 1.4: OR set up for right upper tract laparoscopic procedure

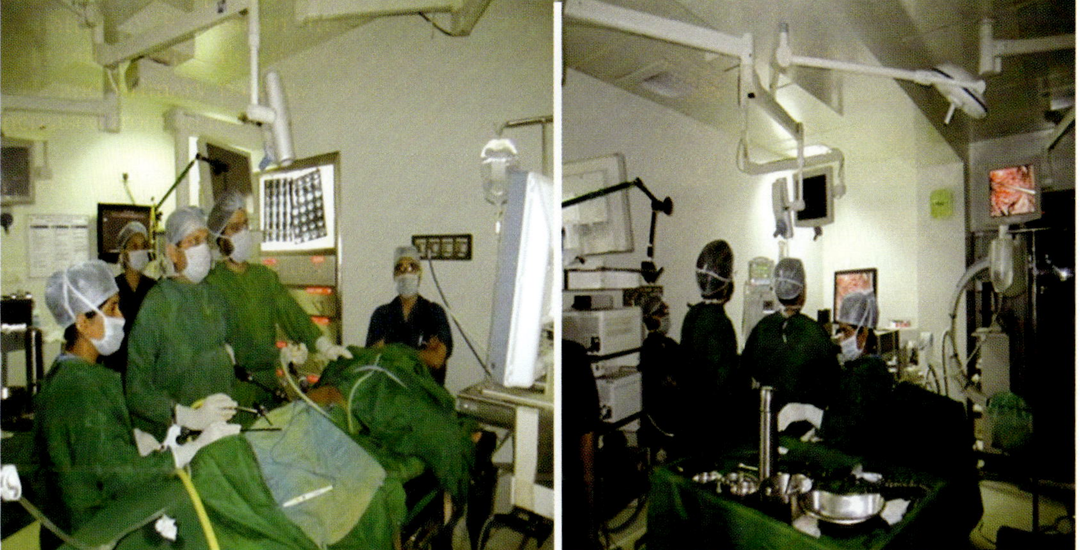

Fig. 1.5: OR set up for left upper tract laparoscopic procedure

and instrumentation. For carrying out a surgical procedure there should be a smooth interaction between the various components and the surgical team.

General principles of laparoscopic or room set up:

- The OR room should have a vision cart, which should ideally be hanging from a boom. Vision cart has the monitor and below the monitor are 3–4 shelves which house the insufflator, camera unit, light source, electrosurgical units and other hemostatic generators **(Fig. 1.3)**.
- There should be at least 2 monitors on opposite sides of the OR table. The surgeon should be optically correct and the one monitor should be in front of the surgeon.
- Insufflator should be just below or along the side of the monitor, during initial cases if the surgeon has to turn to look at

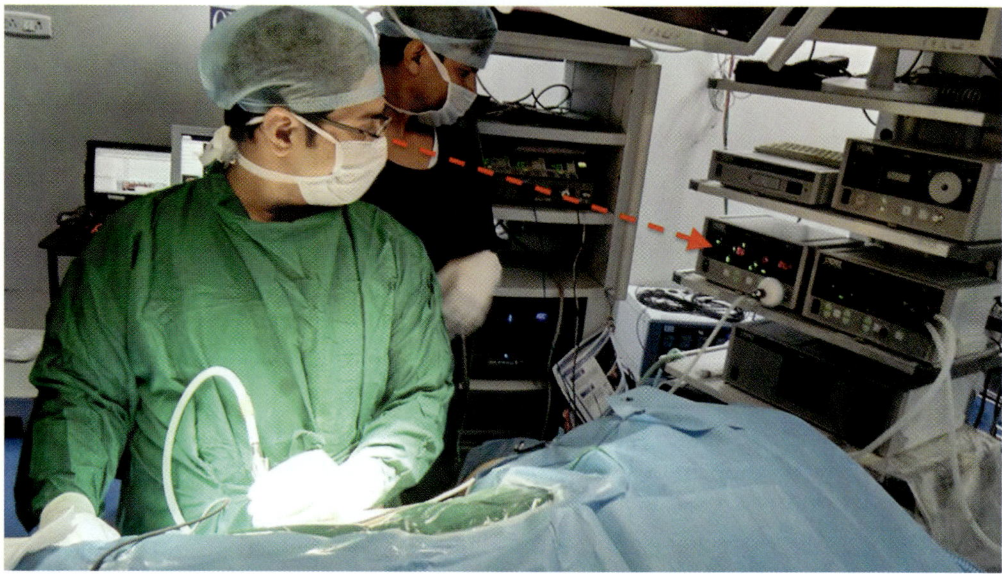

Fig. 1.6: Inappropriate positioning of insufflator

the quadromanometric indicator it will be anxiety provoking and also surgeon may not be able to appreciate the uniform distension of abdomen and other signs of appropriate intraperitoneal insufflation **(Fig. 1.6)**.

- The vision cart should be placed in front of the surgeon to make him optically correct.
- All the tubes and cable should be tangle free; this will help in free movement of all the instruments and make the surgery seamless **(Fig. 1.7)**.
- Specially designed drapes and custom made bags can be used to position the instruments, telescope and working elements of the hemostatic generators. The commercially available drapes are disposable, but have multiple pockets where instruments can be placed. If not available bags made of cloth can be designed and used by pinning these bags to the drapes, they can be re-sterilized and used **(Fig. 1.7)**.
- *Positioning of the personnel in the laparoscopic OR (**Fig. 1.5**):* For an initial upper tact procedure the anesthesiologist is at the head and the camera driver stands cranial to the surgeon and the staff nurse will stand caudal to the surgeon. The 1st assistant should stand opposite to the operating surgeon and will visualize the procedure on the screen which is behind the operating surgeon. The circulating nurse stands behind the operating surgeon and the scrub nurse. For the right-sided upper tract surgeries, the camera driver may move caudal to the surgeon when the surgeon is working in the area of upper pole of the right kidney. The camera driver and surgeon should adjust to each other's body habitus so that minimal restriction of instrument movement occurs **(Fig. 1.8)**. If there is a height discrepancy between the operating surgeon and the camera driver, the camera driver can sit down on an operating chair **(Fig. 1.9)**. Other way around a tall surgeon can sit down and a shorter assistant can drive camera while standing. There may be situations like doing a single port surgery where both may have to sit.

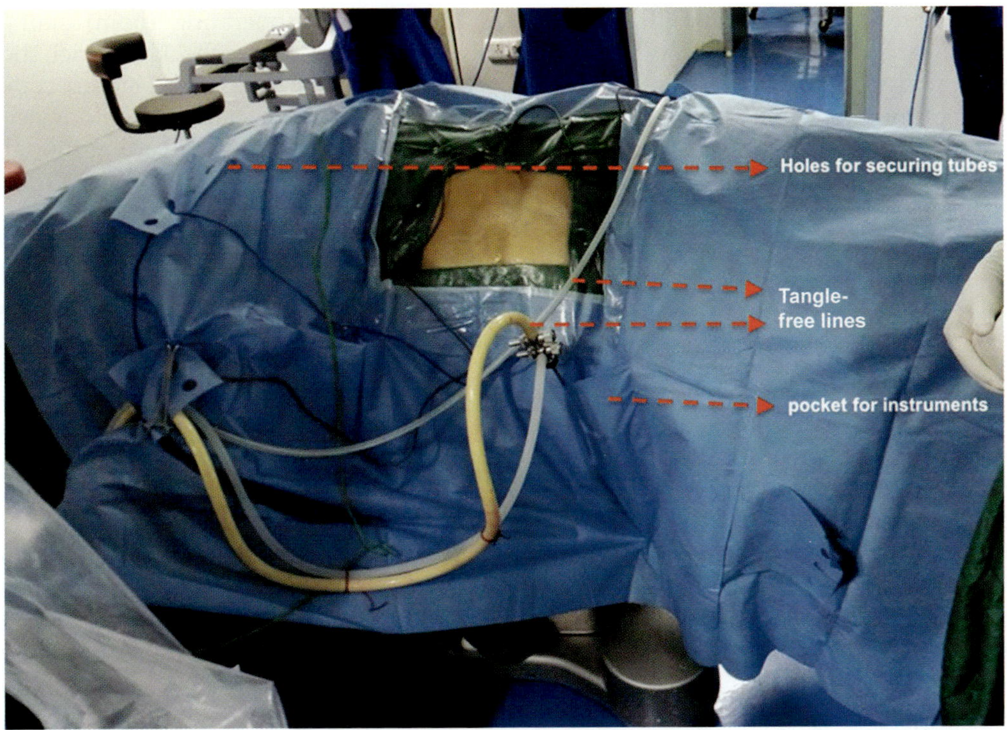

Fig. 1.7: Inappropriate positioning of insufflator

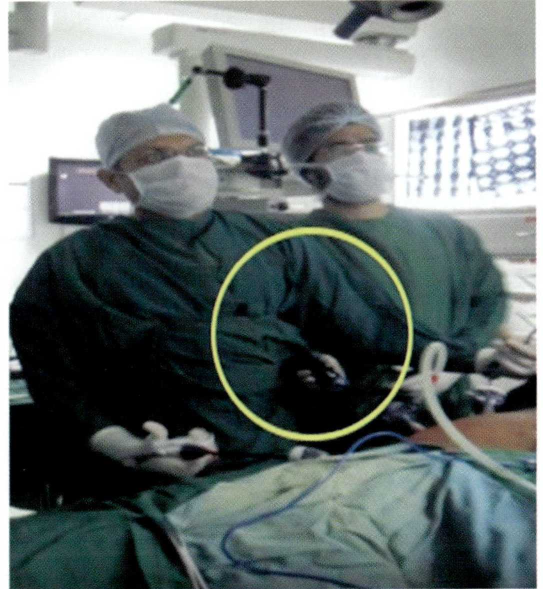

Fig. 1.8: Appropriate positioning of camera driver and surgeon

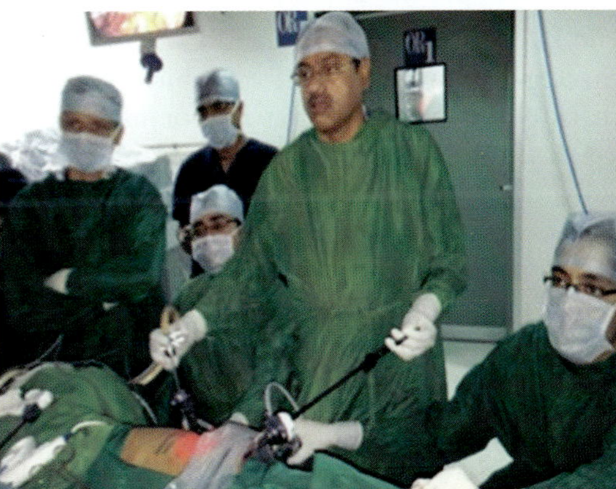

Fig. 1.9: Appropriate camera driver sitting and driving the camera and surgeon is standing and operating

Urological Surgeries can be Done Laparoscopically

- Surgeries which are accepted as standard of care when done laparoscopically:
  - Adrenalectomy for benign pathology

- Radical nephrectomy for T1–T3a renal cell carcinoma
- Simple nephrectomy for benign disease
- Nephroureterectomy for transitional cell carcinoma
- Dismembered pyeloplasty in adults
- Pelvic lymphadenectomy

Note: Excluding severe inflammatory conditions such as XGP

- Surgeries which are being done routinely at many centers laparoscopically:
  - Partial nephrectomy
  - Radical prostatectomy
  - Living donor nephrectomy
- Surgeries which are only done at centers of excellence:
  - Radical cystectomy and urinary diversion
  - Adrenalectomy for adrenal cortical carcinoma
  - Adrenalectomy for masses greater than 6 cm
  - Retroperitoneal lymph node dissection.

Laparoscopic OR Checklist

The famous book by Dr Atul Gawande "The checklist Menifesto" led to the birth of WHO checklist. In his book, the author talks about the errors in medicine, and they are basically either errors of ignorance which are due to lack of knowledge or there are errors of ineptitude, these errors occur due to lack for appropriate application of the existing knowledge. Modern medicine is all about errors of ineptitude and these sorts of errors can be corrected using checklist.

Laparoscopic surgical checklist that can be used by novice surgeon
- Irrigation aspiration working: Yes/No
- Electrosurgical unit working: Yes/No
- CO_2 tank full and extra CO_2 tank available: Yes/No
- Camera is white balanced and light source is working: Yes/No
- Insufflation is checked for flow and response to kinking of tubing: Yes/No
- Veress needle is checked for flow and proper tip retraction: Yes/No

All the OR (operating room) staff and surgeon should make a checklist which should be pasted on the wall of the laparoscopic or next to the WHO checklist and before incision in all the cases, a ritual of reading though all the checklist items should be done.

Important Pillars of Laparoscopic Surgeries

Laparoscopic surgery stands on the shoulder of excellence in open surgery, because it was the open surgery that gave the surgeons a detailed insight into the human anatomy. But, when this interface of minimally invasive surgery was developed, it required more than only knowledge of surgery. The pillars of laparoscopic surgery are:
- Ergonomics
- Task analysis
- Psycho-engineering

Ergonomics in Laparoscopic Surgery

The word ergonomics come from the Greek words "ergon" meaning work and "nomos" meaning laws of nature. By definition ergonomics is a scientific study of people at work, considering the equipment design, workplace layout, the working environment, safety, productivity and training. In simpler terms, it is designing a working interface between man and the machine to improve task performance. The above can be done by creating working environment that fits the worker's needs. Ergonomics can be universal or specific, and sensorial and physical.

Universal ergonomics include creating a well-ventilated room with appropriate temperature and specific ergonomics include maneuvers like adjusting the height of the operating table to surgeon's height.

Sensorial ergonomics are issues like improving vision, with use of better camera and optical systems precision and dexterity will improve. Physical ergonomics include positioning of surgeon's hands, neck, back in a relaxed position to generate maximum surgical performance.

Factors Unrelated to Human Skill Which Affect the Efficiency in Laparoscopic Surgery

- *Decoupling of the visual and motor axis:* In open surgery vision and the motor movements are in the same axis and they get decoupled in laparoscopic surgery. Humans have to train for this decoupling.
- *Loss of tactile feedback:* There is loss of haptics and the laparoscopic instruments replace the human fingers.
- *Changed visual orientation:* The anatomy that an open surgeon was used to seeing outside-in, will now be oriented inside-out. The surgeon has to compensate for the same.
- *The loss of depth perception (Table 1.3):* Initially surgeon will not be able to make out whether the structures are near or far as laparoscopy offers monocular vision which leads to loss of depth perception.
- *Loss of peripheral vision:* Monocular vision is responsible for loss of peripheral vision.
- Relatively static posture during major part of the procedure gives rise to fatigue and ergonomically speaking, contributes to the inefficiency.

Equipment Related Challenges in Laparoscopic Surgery

- 2D vision
- Loss of peripheral vision
- Laparoscopic instruments have only 4 of freedom of movement, which are rotation, up/down angulations, left/right angulations, in/out movement. The robotic endo-wrist technology has 7 of freedom movement as it can flip back on itself.
- Laparoscopic instruments work on reduced efficiency.
- The instrument movements are counter-intuitive, which means that the instrument tip moves to right when the handle is moved to left.

Comparison of open and laparoscopic surgery is given in **Table 1.4**.

Ergonomical considerations for laparoscopic instruments (Figs 1.10 to 1.12).

- The instruments should be held at the level of the elbow of the operating surgeon. This will keep the shoulders relaxed.
- *Manipulation angle:* Manipulation angle is the angle formed by the tip of two working instruments. Ideally the manipulation angle should be 60°. If the manipulation angle increases to >75°, there will be abduction of shoulder and fatigue will occur after a period of time.[12]

Manasnayakorn et al in an experimental set up studied the manipulation angle. Ten different surgeons were asked to do a 5 cm porcine enterotomy closure in a wet lab using different ports which corresponded to different manipulation angle ranging from 45° to 90°. The muscle workload was studied using an electromyography electrode. It was concluded that when

Table 1.3: Comparing open and laparoscopic surgeon

Open vs laparoscopic surgeon	
• Fast	• Slow and steady
• Hand is as good as eye	• Stop when you do not see
• Dissection precedes	• Hemostasis precedes
• Ergonomics optional	• Ergonomics vital

Table 1.4: Comparison of open and laparoscopic surgery

Potential problematic areas	
Open	**Laparoscopy**
• High degree of freedom	• 2D vision
• Surgeons work in-line with visual axis	• Loss of depth perception to some extent
• Three-dimensional direct vision	• Fulcrum effect with tremor enhancement
• Direct tactile feedback	• Only 4° of freedom
	• View is not under the control of operating surgeon

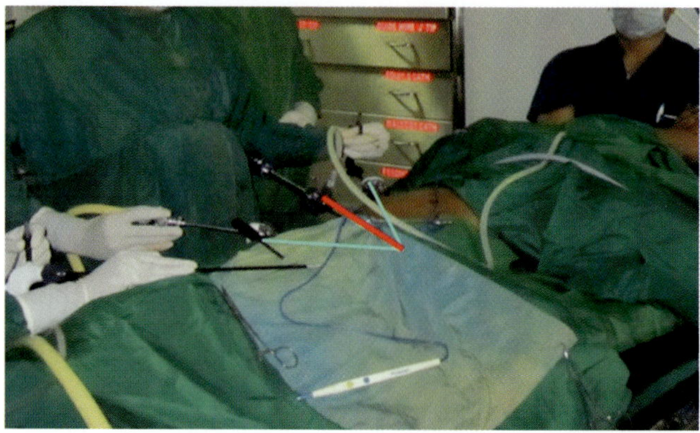

Fig. 1.10: Manipulation and azimuth angles

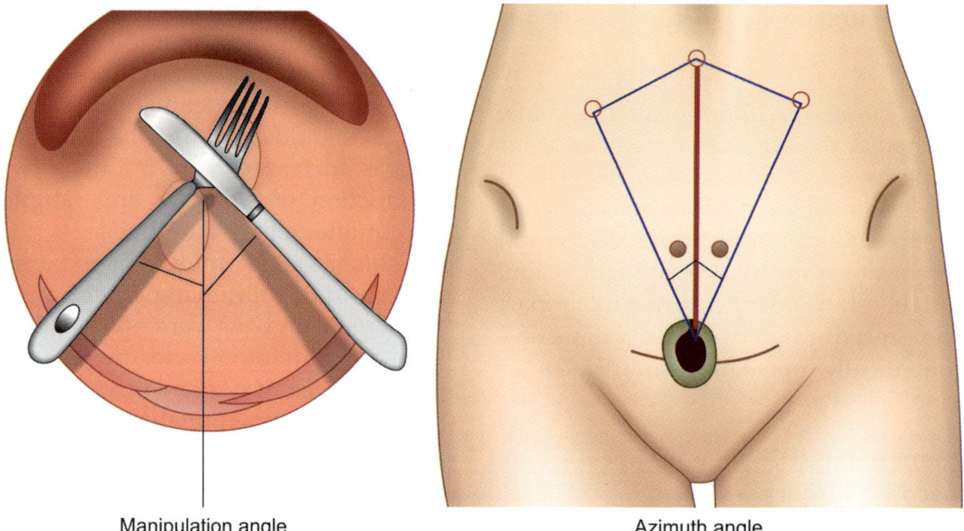

Fig. 1.11: Schematic representation of manipulation and azimuth angles

the manipulation angle is between 45° to 60° the workload on deltoid, trapezius and forearm muscle was least with best outcome which was measured as leak pressures of anastomosis, execution time and error score.[12]

- *Azimuth angle:* Azimuth angle is the angle formed between the single working instrument and the laparoscope. This angle should ideally be 30°, if this angle is less than 15° or greater than 45°, there will instrument fighting and a lot of strain on the upper limbs. Task efficiency is better if both the azimuth angles are equal.[13]

- *Elevation angle:* It is the angle formed between the instrument and the body of the patient. Ideally it should be 30°, whenever it increases to greater than 60°. Shoulder becomes abducted and fatigue occurs. Also, if the elevation angle decreases to 15°, shoulders will have excessive adduction and movement of the instrument will be difficult.

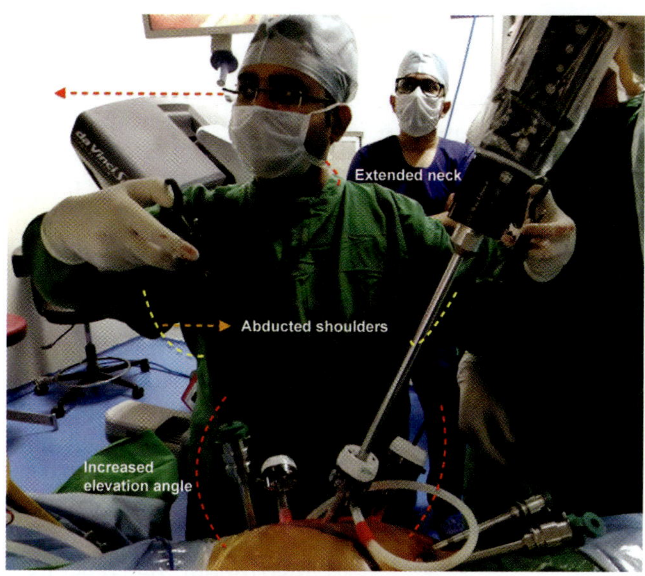

Fig. 1.12: Elevation angle

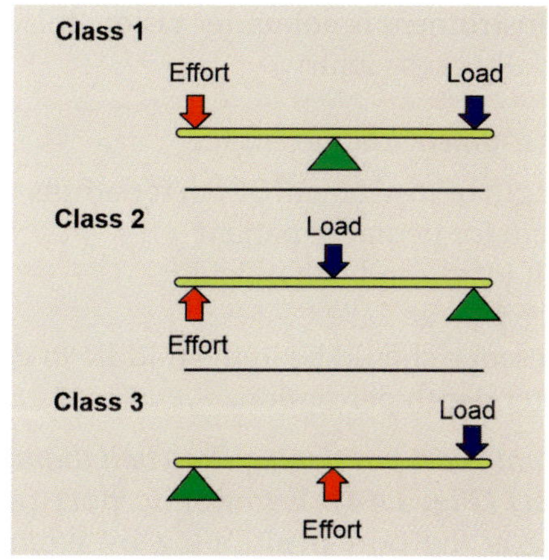

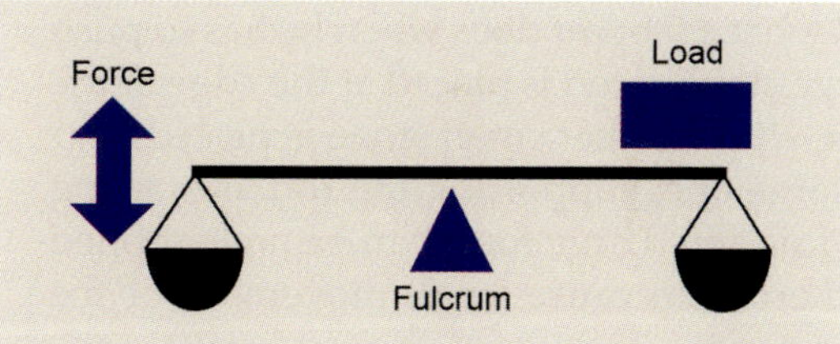

Fig. 1.13: Fulcrum effect

The elevation angle increases when the target organ is too near the port and decreases when the target organ is too far.

*Mechanism of working of laparoscopic instruments and its ergonomical implication (**Fig. 1.13**):* If the long laparoscopic instrument is used to perform an open surgery, surgeon will surely not be able to operate. This is because the instrument will tend to wobble and there will be minimal control. Laparoscopic instruments behave like levers and abdominal wall is a fulcrum on which this lever moves, therefore, it is possible to do laparoscopic surgery. The portion of the instrument inside the abdominal wall is called the force arm and the portion outside is called the load arm.

Laparoscopic Instruments as Type 1 Lever

Ideally the length of the load arm and the force arm should be the same, this will lead to 1:1 transmission of movement and tip of the instrument will move only as much as the handle moves. Most of the adult instruments are 36 cm in length; so, ideally always 18 cm should be inside. Whenever this happens instruments behave like type 1 lever and there is an exactly equal and opposite transmission of force at the two ends. This may not be always possible; therefore, it is practical to have 18–24 cm of a 36 cm instrument inside the abdominal cavity.

Laparoscopic Instruments as Type 2 Lever

If more than two-thirds of the working length of the instrument are outside, the laparoscopic instrument behaves like type 2 lever. Large movements outside will lead to smaller movement inside. Force is magnified and the movement is rectified (large movement outside leads to smaller movements inside). This what a laborer does when he has to push a large stone, a rod is placed at the edge of the stone with another small stone is placed near the large one, supporting the rod and acting as a fulcrum. Large force can be now applied on the rod to cause small movement of the large stone.

Ergonomically speaking whenever instrument behaves like a type 2 lever, the port is very near the target organ. This leads to another problem, that is, it causes increase in the elevation angle beyond 60°, leading to fatigue. In cases where metal ports are being used and the instrument behaves like type 2 lever, direct coupling of the electric current may occur as the metal tip of the operating instrument is very close to the metal port.

Laparoscopic Instruments as Type 3 Lever

When greater than two-thirds the length of the working instrument are inside the abdomen, the instrument behaves like a type 3 lever. Small movement outside gets transmitted as large movements inside, force gets rectified and movement gets magnified. Type 3 lever behavior of a working instrument is seen when the ports are placed far away from the target organ. When a surgeon is working on the upper pole of the kidney, typically the instrument behaves like a type 3 lever, overshooting of the tip of the instrument may occur, which may lead to the instrument tip to go out of field of vision and injure the spleen or diaphragm on the left side. Diving board used by swimmers is an example of type 3 lever, where the swimmer jumps from the tip of the board and his movement get amplified with minimal force. When working instrument behaves like type 3 lever, the elevation angle decreases leading to fatigue of shoulders. Also, majority of the long length of the instrument is not under vision, this can potentially cause injury.

Ideal Instrument Characteristics

- Length of instrument 36 cm for adults and 28 cm for pediatric patient
- Half inside and half outside
- Type 1 lever
- Telescope should be in the middle to get a better depth perception.

Ergonomic port positioning (baseball diamond concept) (Fig. 1.14): Ergonomic port positioning is the port positioning by which a surgeon can achieve ideal working instrument characteristics. If all the ports are ergonomically placed, then the instruments behave like a type 1 lever, the manipulation angle is 60° and telescope is in the middle of the working instruments.

For ergonomic port positioning, baseball diamond concept should be followed. The concept states that 1st determine the target area, for a nephrectomy renal hilum is the target area, for a pyeloplasty pelviureteric

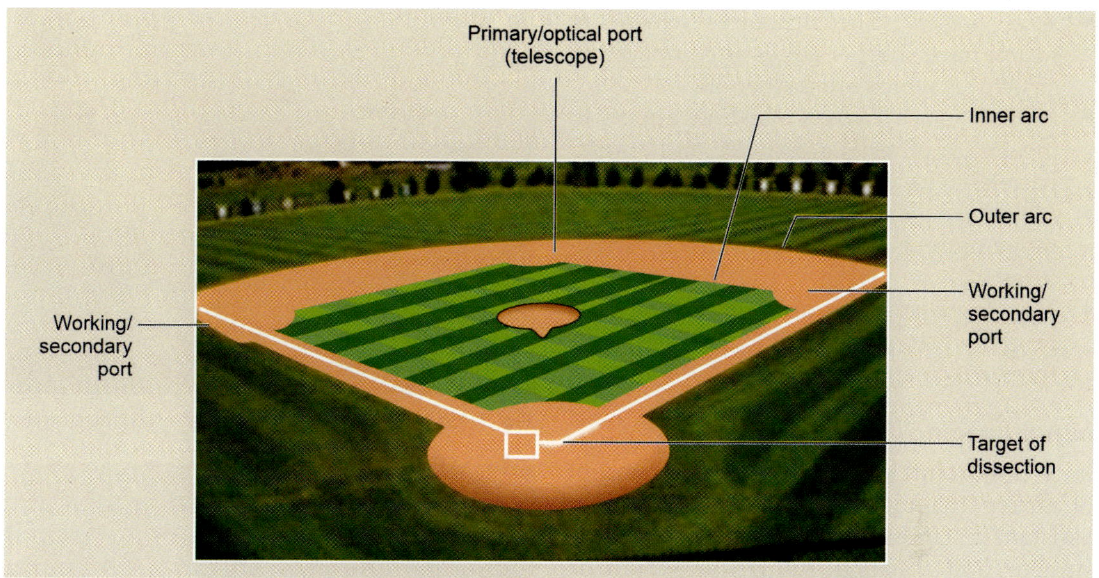

Fig. 1.14: Ergonomic port positioning using baseball diamond concept

junction is the target. After marking the target, two arcs are drawn, 18 cm and 24 cm away from the target area, all the working ports should be between these two arcs for the instrument to behave like type 1 lever.

In real-time situation after marking the target area and drawing two arcs, the camera port is placed in straight line with the target organ, now the right and left ports are placed between the two arcs in such a way that the instruments when placed from these ports form an angle of 60° with each other. 'Triangle law' states that the distance of the working ports from the camera depends on the length of the instrument used. If a pediatric instrument of 28 cm length is used, the distance of the working port from the camera port should be 5 cm to make manipulation angle of 60°, this distance is 7.5 cm when standard 36 cm adult instruments are used and becomes 10 cm when 45 cm bariatric instruments are used.

In real time the above can be achieved in an adult by making a diamond with your both index fingers and thumb. The tip of both the index fingers should be placed at the target organ, the confluence of both the thumbs will give us the camera position and the working ports will be in at the level of anatomical snuffbox. The distance from tip of the thumb to the snuffbox is roughly 7.5 cm.

Depth Cues

As laparoscopes are monocular scope there is a loss of depth perception. Placing camera between both the working instruments gives a better depth perception. Surgeon progressively learns to understand these depth cues and hence is able to say which structure is deep and which one near.

- *Occlusion:* The structure in front will occlude the one behind and cast a shadow, therefore, one may be able to conclude that the structure which is occluding is nearer as compared to the structure which is being occluded.

- *Relative size:* The structures closer to camera appear bigger and the structures which are farther off appear smaller.

- *Ariel gradient:* The structures which are nearer have sharper edges as compared to structures which are farther off.
- *Linear parallax:* Two parallel lines appear to meet each other at a distance and appear parallel to each other at a closer distance.
- *Motion parallax:* Structures near appear to move more as compared to deeper structures.
- *Texture gradient:* Nearer structures appear bright when compared to deeper structures which appear dark.

Mirror Imaging (Fig. 1.15)

It is important to understand the concept of mirror imaging in laparoscopy. When an assistant is standing opposite to the operating surgeon and assisting, though he would be seeing the same image as the surgeon all his movements will be opposite to the surgeon's movement as seen on the screen.

Summary of instrument characteristics • Head should be straight, in axis of trunk, without rotation or extension of the cervical spine. • Shoulders in relaxed and in neutral position. • Arms should be along the side of the body • Elbows should be bent to 70° to 90° • Forearms in horizontal or in a slightly descending axis • Hands pronated • Hands and fingers lightly grip the handles/ handpiece • Gaze should be down • Neck slightly flexed and in straight line with the monitor.

Ergonomic posture of operating surgeon is shown in **Fig. 1.16**.

Co-axial Alignment (Fig. 1.17)

It is an important ergonomic consideration in laparoscopic surgery, the surgeon, target organ and the monitor should be in the same line. The monitor should be slightly lower than the eye level of the surgeon, so that the surgeon has a 15°–20° downward gaze.

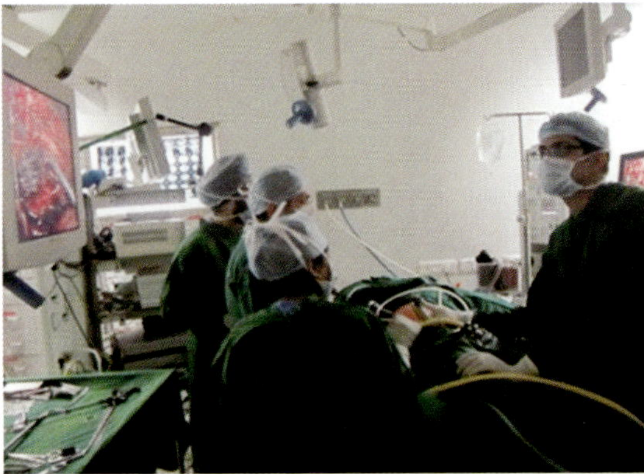

Fig. 1.15: Mirror imaging for the 1st assistant surgeon

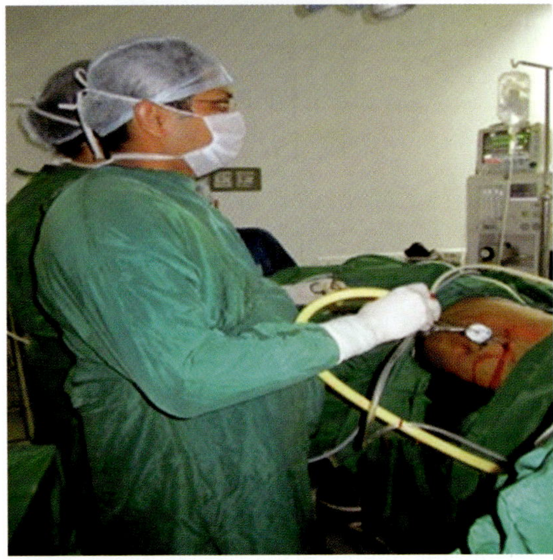

Fig. 1.16: Ergonomic posture of operating surgeon

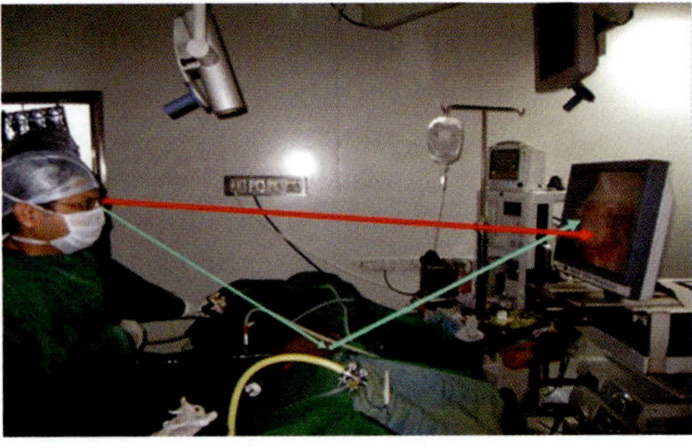

Fig. 1.17: Co-axial alignment

Downward gaze keeps the sternocleido-mastoid muscle relaxed and prevents its fatigue. This will also keep the eye in resting position preventing the oculomotor fatigue.

Position of the Monitor in Relation to the Surgeon

The monitor should be placed at a distance of 5 times the length of the diagonal of the monitor, for a 21-inch monitor the surgeon should be standing 105 inches away from the monitor. At this distance image formation occurs on macula of retina which has maximum acuity of vision and color perception. When the image is placed near it is large for macula and when away it is small for macula.

Operating Room Considerations in Ergonomics

- *Height of OT table:* Height of the operating table should be calculated by the formula $0.49° \times$ height of the surgeon. Laparoscopic OT table must be able to reach up to 24 cm from ground. The patient should be roughly at the level of waist of the surgeon.
- OT lights should have an illumination of 20 lacs, dark light leads to poor visualization and bright light causes optical illusions.

Task Analysis

- Stepwise description of any task
- Components
  - Procedural steps
  - Executional steps
- Scientific sequential arrangement of steps

Task analysis is stepwise description of any task and the task is restructured into its component steps, each of these steps is arranged in a sequence for the task to be finished.

Task analysis is a learning tool and can be used by a novice surgeon for further training.

Psychoengineering

It is one of the pillars on which laparoscopic surgery stands. All the surgeons should be familiar with their machines. They should know the basic management of troubleshooting. For example, if the pneumoperitoneum is not being maintained, the gas tubing may be kinked, inlet valve of the port may be closed or CO_2 cylinder may be empty. Anticipating these troubles may save the day for any surgeon. A laparoscopic surgeon should not be temperamental, should be polite to the entire team, this will help form a better team and the member will work with more commitment.

Training in Laparoscopic Surgery

In this section of the chapter, we will try to understand:
- Ingredients of a surgery
- Learning curve
- How to use dry and wet lab to best of our advantage?
- Do you have a mentor?
- Top professionals have coaches, do we?

Learning a Laparoscopic Motor Skill

Learning a laparoscopic motor skill should start in a dry lab using basic simulation models, after this the trainee can proceed to wet lab on animal models.

Fitts and Posner have described 3 phases of learning a new motor skill:[14,15]

- *Cognitive phase:* In this phase student tries to learn a task and he is tentative, takes small steps at a time and all the steps are intellectualized. This can be seen when a novice starts practicing motor skill in a dry lab on an endo trainer. If the task given to him is transferring bead from one bowl to other, he will slowly hold the instrument, tentatively grasp the bead and slowly move it to the other bowl.
- *Integrative phase:* It is a phase where the information that the trainee has about the task has been converted into purposeful movements. The trainee is still thinking about the task but is able to finish the task with fluidity. If we consider the above

example of bead transfer, the trainee is now able to hold the bead in his instrument and fluidly transfer it from one bowl to other the movement is slow but purposeful and continuously being thought about. Here the trainee is gradually developing hand eye co-ordination, dexterity and depth perception.

- *Stage of automation:* This is a stage of learning where the movements become precise and quick, and are extremely purposeful. Considering the example of bead transfer, the trainee will quickly be able to grasp the bead in non-dominant hand and transfer it to the dominant hand and then into the bowl. As he does the task he is not continuously thinking about the task, it starts to come to him naturally.

Factors Affecting Training in Laparoscopic Surgery

Whenever training programs are started, it is extremely important to understand whether they are effective or not. Also, what are the steps needed to improve training.

1. *Effective feedback:* Feedback is very important to know if one is doing the right thing. Feedback can intrinsic or extrinsic. Intrinsic feedback is what a trainee gives to himself, it is like talking to oneself. After training for a few hours one realizes the depth cues, like what is near is bigger and brighter, remembering this fact in one's mind is intrinsic feedback.[16] Extrinsic feedback is the one which is given by a mentor, it can be a summative feedback given at the end of the training or it can be concurrent feedback which is given as your performing training.[17] It has been found that summative feedback is more effective in training students as they are able to concentrate better once the task is over.

2. *Deliberate practice:* Goal directed learning and practice helps in better training. Deliberate practice is mindful practice of a particular step of surgery. "It is like, when cricketer Virat Kohli gets out to a hook shot, he will keep practicing the hook shot till perfects it".

   If a surgeon has struggled to reflect the colon off the kidney in one case, he should revisit the video of the surgery and practice the component steps like precision, hand-eye co-ordination and dexterity. This mindful training leads to transference of the motor skill to the operating room.[18] Question which remains to be answered is how much should one practice and for how long? Broadly speaking practice should be distributed over period of time, not extending to more than 45 min to 1 hour in a session, but should extend over longer period of months to a year.[19,20] Aim of deliberate practice is to reach the stage of automation.[21]

3. *Concept of a pre-trained novice:* The term pre-trained novice was coined by Gallagher, pre-trained novice is a trainee who has reached a stage of automation in a simulated environment.[22] This trainee when starts operating a case, he does not have to be bothered about concentrating on dexterity, hand-eye co-ordination, etc. he starts to pay attention to anatomical details and avoiding complications. The problem with this learning model is that we do not know how much time does an index individual take to get to the stage of automation. Certain academic institutions have based it on the number of hours, a trainee has spent in lab doing exercises, but rather it should be proficiency bases and assessed by a mentor.[23,24]

4. *Graded sequential practice:* While practising motor skills, a surgeon should start with easier exercises and progressively graduate to more difficult ones. It has been demonstrated in studies that, with increasing level

of difficulties in simulation models the motor skills improve.[25]

5. *Cognitive learning:* Surgery is not only about learning a motor skill, this skill should blend with excellent anatomical, physiological and pathological knowledge. In cognitive training, apart from the motor skills the trainee is also taught anatomical details and pathological basis of the surgery. This knowledge helps him apply his motor skill better and leads to faster and more efficient training.[26]

Simulators in Laparoscopic Surgery

- *Mechanical simulators:* They can be either a commercially available box trainer or a home-made endotrainer. Home-made endotrainer is equally effective in training but are not validated.
- *Animal-based simulation models:* They can be made to train in particular skill or also a particular procedure. They can be cadaveric animate models or living animal models. A few animal models available are:
    - Porcine nephrectomy model
    - Porcine partial nephrectomy model
    - Chicken pyeloplasty model
    - Chicken model for urethrovesical anastomosis.

- *Virtual reality training models:* These models are like video games; these are computer generated programs which create situations on a screen and motor action are carried out to complete the tasks.[27]

Constructing an office endotrainer:[28] (Muljibhai Patel Urological Hospital's Office Endotrainer) **(Figs 1.18 to 1.20)**.

Design Construct

A wooden frame 20 inches in length by 15 inches in breath is made **(Fig. 1.18)**. In the center of the frame, two half-inch wooden bars, 15 inches in length are nailed vertically, 2 inches apart **(Fig. 1.18)**. At the base of the above two vertical bars a third, half an inch wooden bar, 4 inches in length is nailed horizontally. Lateral to the vertical bars on both sides, whole of wooden frame is fitted by a 6 mm thin wooden sheet. Multiple holes of 15 mm are cut out on the wooden sheets and are covered by a rubber cork, which is a bottle cap of 100 ml saline/contrast bottles **(Fig. 1.18)**. These corks act like ports. The whole assembly is mounted on 4 wooden rods, the two rods in front are 9 inches in height and the rear two rods are 5 inches in height **(Fig. 1.19)**. All these four rods are screwed on hinges and are

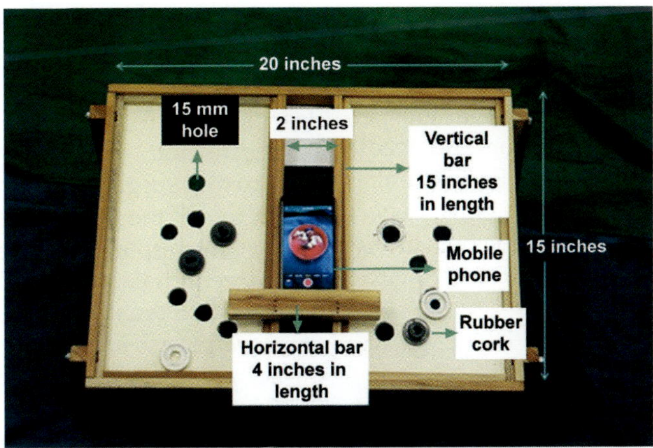

Fig. 1.18: Endotrainer design

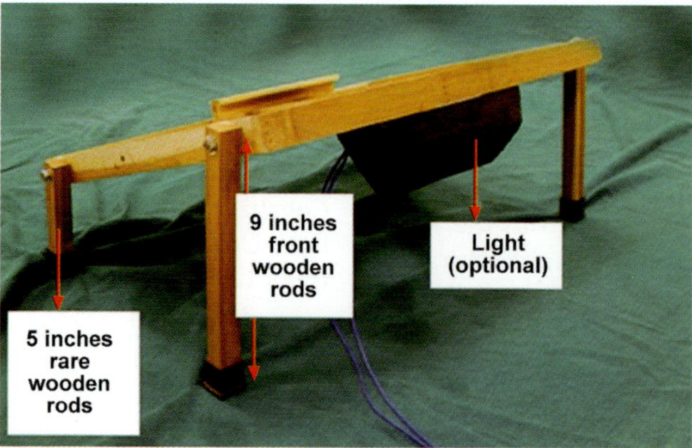

Fig. 1.19: Endotrainer design

foldable. It takes about an hour for a carpenter to make this device and cost of construction of device was 700 rupees. An additional light can be fitted under the frame **(Fig. 1.19)**, but on most occasions a well-lit room provides adequate light as the device is open by the sides.

Using this Device

This device is simple to use, a mobile phone or a tablet is used as a screen with this device. The device is vertically placed on the two vertical bars of the wooden frame and rests on the horizontal bar. The device is put on camera mode and then the desired exercise is carried out. The room light of a well-illuminated room is good enough for vision; the light mode off mobile phone or tablet can also be used.

Conventional laparoscopic or laparoscopic training instruments like Maryland grasper, bowel grasper, laparoscopic scissors and needle holder are used with the device. Endo-training material like suturing mat, beads, glove fingers and needles can be used for carrying out various exercises like bead holding and transfer, circle cutting and suturing **(Fig. 1.20)**.

Advantages

- Device is simple to construct and low cost.
- It is sleek and can be used as an office endotrainer, which will be very helpful for busy surgeons wanting to learn laparoscopy as it can be kept in their office.
- Vision is good as most of the mobile phones and tablets have high quality cameras. One can zoom in and out.
- Multiple holes on both sides act as multiple ports, has an ergonomical advantage.

Disadvantages

- Surgeon looks in same axis as the device though the exercise in question is not visible to him.
- Surgeon may take some time to adapt to the device.

Ingredients of Laparoscopic Surgery

As we try to learn laparoscopic surgery we must know what are the key ingredients of learning laparoscopy.

- *Anatomical knowledge in general:* While starting surgery, it is of utmost importance to know the basic anatomy. For example, in any upper tract urological procedure, surgeon has to know the relation of renal artery to renal vein.
- *Laparoscopic anatomical knowledge:* Laparoscopic anatomy is different from open surgical anatomy. The anatomy does not change but the orientation and the perspective changes. To site an example, in

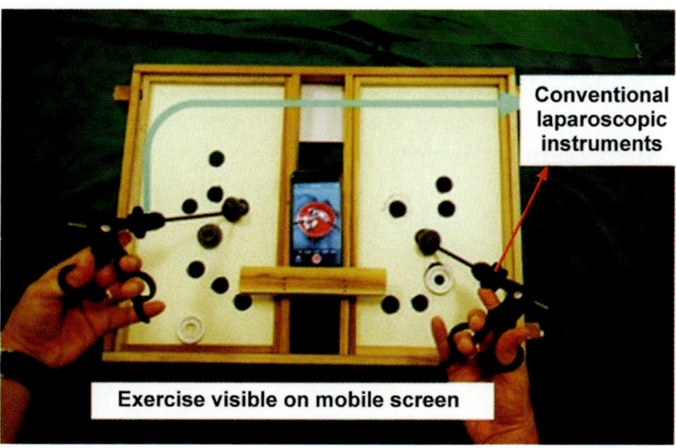

Fig. 1.20: Use of an office endotrainer

laparoscopic surgery it is easier to find the renal artery from the lower margin of the renal vein, even when the artery is at the upper border of the renal vein.

- *Radiological information:* Radiological information acts like global positioning system in laparoscopic surgery. It tells the operating surgeon the details of all the landmarks and where can one find them intraoperatively. Also, the surgeon can be well prepared for the anatomical variations.
- *Procedural steps:* Each procedure is divided into procedural steps. Like for a nephrectomy, procedural step will be port placement, bowel reflection, lifting the ureterogonadal packet, identification of renal vein, dissecting the upper pole, identification of aorta and renal artery, dissection of artery followed by vein, clipping of vessel, ureteral clipping and separating the specimen all around.
- *Executional steps:* Each procedural step is further divided into smaller steps known as executional steps. Let us consider an example of lifting ureterogonadal packet during laparoscopic nephrectomy. This procedural step is divided into the following executional steps:

- Identifying the ureterogonadal packet
- Identifying Gerota's fascia
- Opening the Gerota's fascia
- Lifting the packet—at a point where gonadal and ureter cross
- Keeping the psoas sheath with psoas muscle
- Do not dissect in-between gonadal vein and ureter, keep tissue on ureter.
- *Extent of dissection:* Carinal—renal vein, caudal—crossing over the iliac artery and lateral—up to lateral abdominal wall

- *Component movements involving the executional steps:* Component movements should be individually practiced to execute a step.
Skill sets required to complete an executional step.
For example: Lifting ureterogonadal packet:
- Why do it? As it helps exposing the renal hilum.
- Identification of ureter is done by anatomical knowledge, by the acronym, water flows under the bridge and by peristalsis.
- Opening of the Gerota's fascia requires ambidexterity, traction, countertraction.
- Lifting of the packet at the point where gonadal and ureter cross is done using

suction and a dissector alternately making a to and fro motion ambidextrously.
- Keeping the psoas muscle sheath with psoas is done using suction as a dissector and depth perception is critical for this step.

Keys to Learning Laparoscopy
- Deconstruct the skill to component parts
  - Know your anatomy very well
  - Learn the steps of a laparoscopic procedure
- Practice component parts
  - Hand-eye co-ordination, ambidexterity
  - Depth perception
  - Cutting and suturing
- Practice to the point of failure
- Immerse yourself in the process

Learning Curve of Laparoscopic Surgery (Fig. 1.21)

Malcom Gladwell in his book the outliers said that it takes 10,000 hours to master a skill.[29] When he said this, he meant that for somebody to become world class athlete or musician it requires 10,000 hours, it is not that we need 10,000 hours to learn a new skill. Skill acquisition will start as early as 20 hours of training. While learning, the trainee should deconstruct the skill into smaller part. Always one should learn enough to self-correct and remove all the distraction barriers. Frustration barriers can be removed by repetitive practice. The learning curve will have a slow beginning followed by a steep acceleration and finally a plateau.

Top Athletes and Singers have Coaches, should we Surgeons also have them?
This is a very intriguing question that Dr Atul Gawande asked in his article published in the New Yorker.[30] When all the top professions have coaches why do not we surgeons have them, in a profession which requires error elimination to the level of sigma six.

He described in this article that when he invited a mentor to observe him for a parathyroid surgery, how a summative feedback given by the mentor improved his performance. Small errors like improperly directed headlight when directed properly could make surgery easier.

I had a similar personal experience in the gym (AS) one day, when I saw two young men train, one of them would train his latissimus dorsi muscle and the other one would train his forearm muscles almost everyday. I happened

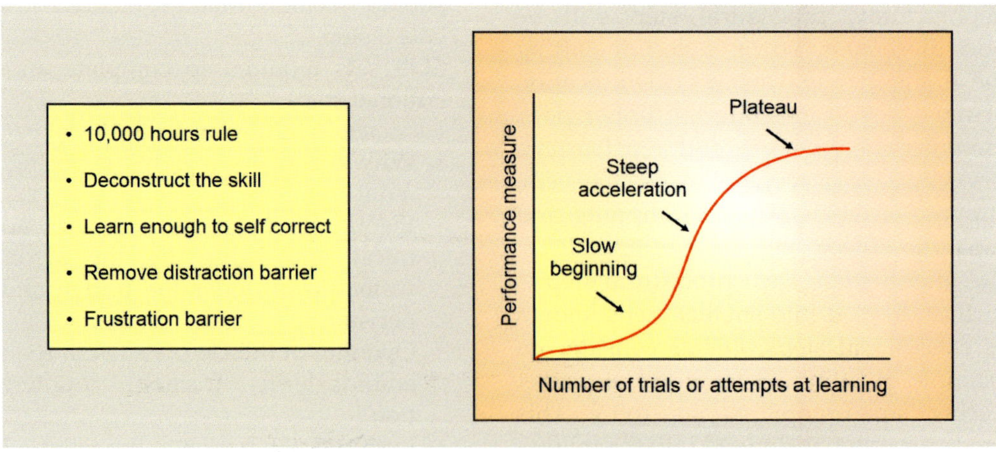

Fig. 1.21: The learning curve

to ask them the reason for this training, the first bloke replied that "I am a bowler and I need strong wings to bowl faster" and the second one said "I am a batsman and play for a local T20 league, I need strong forearms so that I could hit the ball out of the park". After listening to both of them I wondered, "I also use my shoulders everyday for performing laparoscopic surgery, which is technically very demanding, yet I had never thought of training my deltoid muscles".

REFERENCES

1. Litynski GS. Laparoscopy: The Early Attempts: Spotlighting Georg Kelling and Hans Christian Jacobaeus. JSLS: Journal of the Society of Laparoendoscopic Surgeons 1997 Jan;1(1):83.
2. Jacobaeus HC. Ueber die oglichkeit die Zystosk opiebeiUntersuchungseroserHonlungenanzuwenden. unchen Med Wchenschr. 1910;57:2090–2092.
3. Walker Reynolds J. The first laparoscopic cholecystectomy. JSLS: Journal of the Society of Laparoendoscopic Surgeons 2001 Jan;5(1):89.
4. Cortesi N, Ferrari P, Zambarda E, Manenti A, Baldini A, Morano FP. Diagnosis of bilateral abdominal cryptorchidism by laparoscopy. Endoscopy 1976;33:8.
5. Clayman RV, Kavoussi LR, Soper NJ, Dierks SM, Meretyk S, Darcy MD, Roemer FD, Pingleton ED, Thomson PG, Long SR. Laparoscopic nephrectomy: initial case report. The Journal of urology 2017 Feb 28;197(2):S182–86.
6. Schuessler WW, Schulam PG, Clayman RV, Kavoussi LR. Laparoscopic radical prostatectomy: initial short-term experience. Urology 1997 Dec 1;50(6):854–7.
7. Ratner LE, Montgomery RA, Kavoussi LR. Laparoscopic live donor nephrectomy: a review of first 5 years. Urol Clin North Am 2001;28: 709–19.
8. Veenhof AA, Vlug MS, van der Pas MH, Sietses C, van der Peet DL, De Lange-De Klerk ES, Bonjer HJ, Bemelman WA, Cuesta MA. Surgical stress response and postoperative immune function after laparoscopy or open surgery with fast track or standard perioperative care: a randomized trial. Annals of surgery 2012 Feb 1;255(2):216–21.
9. Kum CK, Wong CW, Goh PM, Ti TK. Comparative study of pain level and analgesic requirement after laparoscopic and open cholecystectomy. Surgical Laparoscopy, Endoscopy and Percutaneous Techniques 1994 Apr 1;4(2):139–41.
10. Richards C, Edwards J, Culver D, Emori TG, Tolson J, Gaynes R, National Nosocomial Infections Surveillance (NNIS) System. Does using a laparoscopic approach to cholecystectomy decrease the risk of surgical site infection? Annals of surgery 2003 Mar;237(3):358.
11. Gyedu A, Bingener J, Dally C, Oppong J, Price R, Reid-Lombardo K. Starting a Laparoscopic Surgery Programme in the Second Largest Teaching Hospital in Ghana. East African medical journal 2014;91(4):133–37.
12. Manasnayakorn S, Cuschieri A, Hanna GB. Ideal manipulation angle and instrument length in hand-assisted laparoscopic surgery. Surgical endoscopy 2008 Apr 1;22(4):924–29.
13. Supe AN, Kulkarni GV, Supe PA. Ergonomics in laparoscopic surgery. Journal of minimal access surgery 2010 Apr;6(2):31.
14. Anastakis DJ, Regehr G, Reznick RK, Cusimano M, Murnaghan J, Brown M, Hutchison C. Assessment of technical skills transfer from the bench training model to the human model. The American Journal of Surgery 1999 Feb 28;177(2): 167–70.
15. Rowan AN. Is justification of animal research necessary? JAMA 1993;269:1114.
16. Stefanidis D, Heniford BT. The formula for a successful laparoscopic skills curriculum [discussion in Arch Surg 2009;144(1):82.] Arch Surg 2009; 144(1):77–82.
17. Xeroulis GJ, Park J, Moulton CA, Reznick RK, LeBlanc V, Dubrowski A. Teaching suturing and knot-tying skills to medical students: a randomized controlled study comparing computer-based video instruction and (concurrent and summary) expert feedback. Surgery. 2007 Apr 30;141(4):442–49.
18. Ericsson KA. Deliberate practice and the acquisition and maintenance of expert performance in medicine and related domains. Acad Med. 2004;79(10 suppl):S70–81.
19. Moulton CA, Dubrowski A, MacRae H, Graham B, Grober E, Reznick R. Teaching surgical skills: What kind of practice makes perfect? A randomized controlled trial. Annals of surgery. 2006;244(3):400–9.

20. Mackay S, Morgan P, Datta V, Chang A, Darzi A. Practice distribution in procedural skills training. Surgical Endoscopy and Other Interventional Techniques. 2002;16(6):957–61.

21. van Dongen KW, Ahlberg G, Bonavina L, et al. European consensus on a competency-based virtual reality training program for basic endoscopic surgical psychomotor skills. Surg Endosc 2011;25(1):166–71.

22. Gallagher AG, Ritter EM, Champion H, et al. Virtual reality simulation for the operating room: proficiency-based training as a paradigm shift in surgical skills training. Ann Surg 2005; 241(2): 364–72.

23. Korndorffer JR, Dunne JB, Sierra R, Stefanidis D, Touchard CL, Scott DJ. Simulator training for laparoscopic suturing using performance goals translates to the operating room. Journal of the American College of Surgeons. 2005 Jul 31;201(1): 23–29.

24. Ahlberg G, Enochsson L, Gallagher AG, Hedman L, Hogman C, McClusky DA, Ramel S, Smith CD, Arvidsson D. Proficiency-based virtual reality training significantly reduces the error rate for residents during their first 10 laparoscopic cholecystectomies. The American journal of surgery. 2007;193(6):797–804.

25. Ali MR, Mowery Y, Kaplan B, DeMaria EJ. Training the novice in laparoscopy: more challenge is better. Surg Endosc. 2002;16(12):1732–36.

26. Kohls-Gatzoulis JA, Regehr G, Hutchison C. Teaching cognitive skills improve learning in surgical skills courses: a blinded, prospective, randomized study. Can J Surg 2004;47(4): 277–83.

27. Coleman J, Nduka CC, Darzi A. Virtual reality and laparoscopic surgery. British Journal of Surgery. 1994;81(12):1709–11.

28. Tak Gopal R, Singh AG, Ganpule AP, Sabnis RB, Desai MR. Office Laparoscopic Endotrainer or Commercially Available Laparoscopic Endotrainer. Podium presentation, WZUSICON 2016.

29. Gladwell M. Outliers: The story of success. Hachette UK; 2008, Nov 18.

30. Gawande A. Top athletes and singers have coaches. Should you. The New Yorker 2011 Oct 3:44–53.

2

Basics in Laparoscopic Urologic Instrumentation

Arvind P Ganpule, Abhishek Singh, Sudharsan Balaji, V Mohan Kumar

INSTRUMENTS USED FOR GAINING ACCESS

Veress Needle (Fig. 2.1)

This is the key instrument for gaining access using the closed technique for pneumoperitoneum insufflations. Veress needle can be classified as disposable and nondisposable.

The different parts of the Veress needle are: (a) Shaft, (b) tip and (c) hub.

- *Shaft:* The Veress needle is available in a size of length 80 mm, 100 mm and 120 mm. Longer 150 mm needle for obese patients is also available. Disposable needle is 14 gauge in diameter. Reusable needle is larger in diameter (3 mm). The shaft is metallic and radiopaque. It has got a conduit for passage of gas for insufflation.

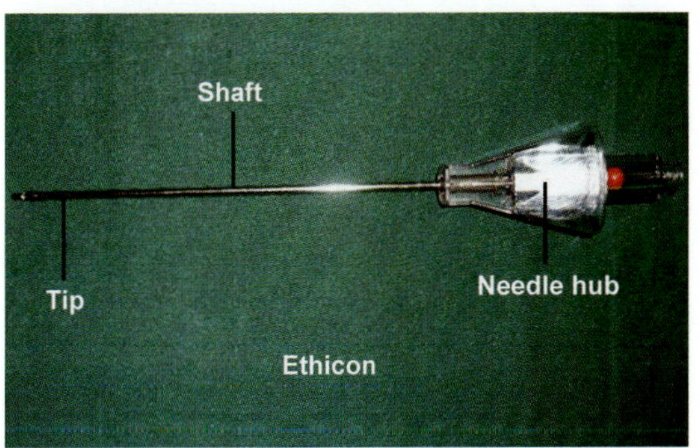

Fig. 2.1: Veress needle and its parts

- *Tip:* The tip of the Veress needle will show a vent for insufflation of the gas. The tip is always beveled. The beveled tip just a few centimeters beyond the blunt needle. The blunt needle springs forward once the tip of the bevel enters the abdomen.
- *Hub:* The hub of the needle shows a floating ball. The floating ball remains suspended when the needle is in a negative milieu. The ball also helps in performing the hanging drop test for ascertaining the accuracy of access. Ball (red or green) at the center of the hub floats when the tip of the needle is in the peritoneum. The hub has a Luer lock arrangement, which helps to attach syringe. The indicator suggests the position on the needle. Green color in the indicator suggests that the needle is in a negative milieu (peritoneum), red color indicates that the needle is in preperitoneal space or is in the mesenteric fat or the needle is blocked. This safety mechanism is seen in Ethicon™ needle.

The four steps which should be meticulously followed to ensure that the position of the Veress needle is proper are as follows:

1. *Aspiration:* The hub of the needle is aspirated to check for red (blood), yellow (bowel contents), green (bile). If in the peritoneal cavity, only air is aspirated.

2. *Hanging drop test:* A drop of saline is placed on the hub of the needle, and we see for a rapid drop of fluid column. Rapid drop of saline indicates a peritoneal placement of the needle tip.
3. *Low initial intra-abdominal pressure:* Initial pressure should be less than 5 mm Hg at a rate of 1 litre/min and should gradually go on increasing. In case the needle is perfectly placed, an initial negative pressure reading may be seen. If an initial pressure of 8 mm of Hg is seen, but it starts to go down immediately, this scenario is also acceptable as needle may be against some tissue initially.
4. *Uniform distension:* After achieving complete insufflation the abdomen should be uniformly distended and tense like a football. At this stage the abdominal pressure should be equal to set pressure.

Hasson's Cannula (Figs 2.2A and B)

The original Hasson cannula was a metal cannula. It consisted of a metal shaft with a rubber hub. This cannula is typically used when an open access is gained, in children and in hostile abdomen (multiple scars). The newer version of these cannulas is disposable. It consists of a cuff that remains outside abdomen and snugly fitting the port site. The part of the trocar which is supposed to remain inside the abdominal wall has an inflatable balloon. These two features help in maintaining the position of the cannula.

Ports

The ports are classified as follows:
- *Depending on the make (Fig. 2.3):* (a) Disposable, (b) nondisposable
- *Depending on the tip:* (a) Cutting tip, (b) non-cutting or dilating **(Figs 2.3, 2.4A and B)**
- *Depending on the size:* 2 mm, 5 mm, 10 mm, 12 mm, 15 mm, 20 mm
- *Depending on the type of valve:* (a) Flap valve, (b) trumpet valve **(Fig. 2.4C)**

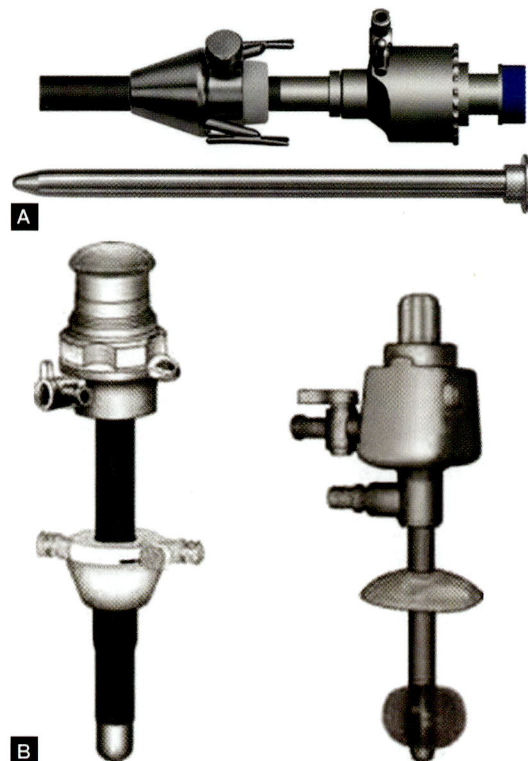

Fig. 2.2A and B: Hasson's cannula

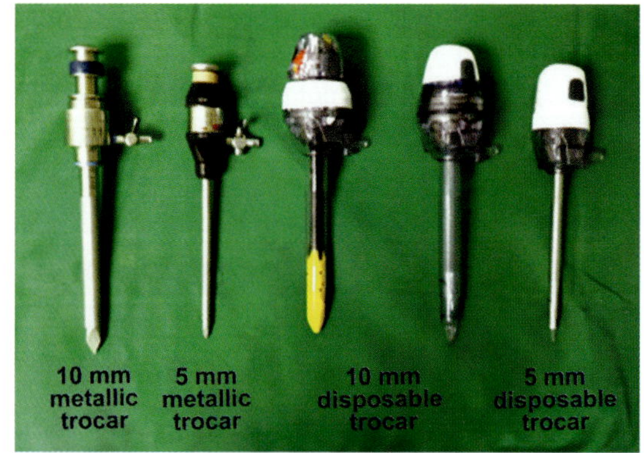

Fig. 2.3: Types of trocars

The different parts of the trocar are
- *Obturator:* The obturator can be blunt with a dilating tip **(Fig. 2.4B)**, cutting tip or blunt tip. The dilating tip trocars like the one by Ethicon™ (EndoPAT Xcel™

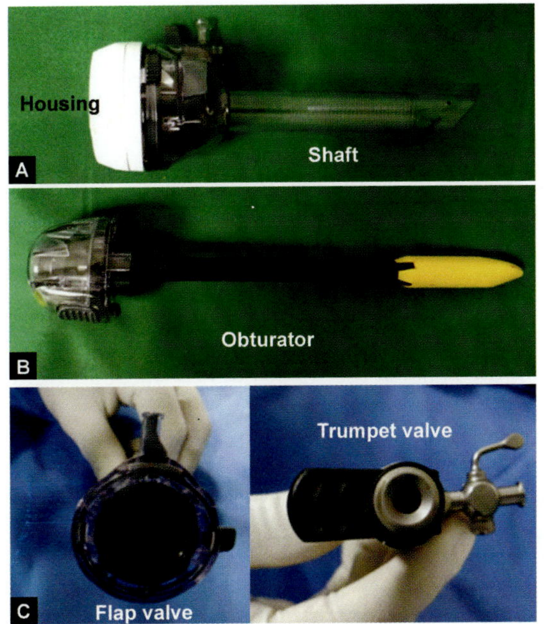

Fig. 2.4A to C: (A and B) Parts of a trocar; (C) Types of valve

B series) have a transparent shaft with a facet for telescope placement at the top and a lock by the side. This trocar can be used to gain entry in the abdomen under vision. The dilating tip dilates through the anterior abdominal wall muscles rather than cutting through it. The cutting tip trocars cut through the anterior abdominal wall to gain entry into the peritoneum, these can be either metallic or made of plastic. The cutting tip trocars have a blade (EndoPAT Xcel™ D series by Ethicon™), the blade is to be loaded with a push button. Once the trocar meets the resistance of the anterior abdominal wall, the blade cuts through the muscle and fascia of the abdominal wall, the moment of the blade crosses the abdominal wall and into the peritoneum, there is a loss of resistance and the blade retracts back making trocar a blunt end trocar. A blunt trocar is the one which is used to gain access in the open method and also used to get a re-entry into the abdomen once the port which was placed slips out during the procedure.

- *Housing and the cannula (**Fig. 2.4A**):* This is the part of the trocar that acts a conduit for the instruments. The housing features the valve (flap valves in disposable trocars and trumpet valves in non-disposable trocars). The trumpet valves will only allow the passage of instrument which is equal to size of the trocar used with the cannula, if a smaller size instrument is used it will cause leakage of gas. A multiseal flap valve is made of multiple rubber leaflets, which coapt around the passing instrument and hence, it allows passage of instrument which are equal to or smaller in size to the trocar, without leakage of gas. The gas vents in all trocars lies distal to the valves. This prevents smudging of the lens during introduction or removal of the telescope.
- *Special variants of trocars:*
  - *Trocars with pistol handles:* They have handle which can be used to place a trocar.
  - *Hybrid trocars:* They are trocars with 5 mm as well as 10 mm channels so that both size instruments can be placed through them.

Instruments used for retraction and dissection: Retracting and dissecting instruments are of the most commonly used instruments in laparoscopy. Some of the commonly used ones are:
- Maryland forceps
- Bowel grasping forceps—double jaw action type and single jaw action type
- Allis laparoscopic forceps
- Right angles laparoscopic forceps

These instruments can be disposable or reusable. The reusable ones are made of three parts, namely (a) handle, (b) outer sheath and (c) insert.

Handle: It is the part used for holding a laparoscopic instrument, it has finger grip. The handle may have a locking mechanism depending on the make of the instrument, the locking mechanism can be of ratchet type (KarlStorz™) or button type (Wolf™). The instruments like Maryland forceps have a pillar for attachment of a monopolar cautery cable. These instruments have circular knob which is used to rotate the shaft.

Outer shaft: It is an insulated hollow housing which holds the insert. The insulation should be checked regularly as breech in insulation can cause thermal injury to bowel.

Insert of the instrument: The purpose for which the instrument will be used depends on the insert. The insert can have a Maryland tip or a bowel grasping tip or an Allis tip. The insert get locked into the outer shaft which get attached to the handle **(Fig. 2.5)**.

Fan retractor: It is a retractor used to retract bowel or solid organs. It has 3–5 blades which open like a fan and aid in retracting the organs laparoscopically. Available as 5 mm or 10 mm instrument.

Needle Holders (Figs 2.6A and B)

Laparoscopic needle drivers are used for intracorporeal suturing. Needle driver has a beak, shaft and a handle. The needle holders are classified depending on the beak of the

needle holder as straight beak, parrot beak and self-riding. They have different grips, namely handle grip and a pistol grip.

Laparoscopic Scissors (Fig. 2.6C)

Like the retracting and dissecting instruments the non-disposable scissors also have three parts which are the outer sheath, handle and the insert.

The disposable scissors are one piece instrument. All the scissors can be classified on the basis of the tip as curved tip or straight tip, they can have short or long jaws. A special type of scissor which is articulating and rotating jaws is available, this feature allows the scissor to access relatively difficult angles and locations.

INSTRUMENTS USED FOR HEMOSTASIS

Clips: The variety of clips available:
- *Non-interlocking titanium clips:* They are available in a cartridge of six clips. They are cheap in comparison to other clips available. One clip costs approximately 60 INR (Indian national rupee). They are radiopaque. They require separate applicator for the application of the clips. As they are not absolutely secure in comparison to other clips they should be used for securing bleeders over the Gerota's fascia or small venous tributaries, particularly in donor nephrectomy. The

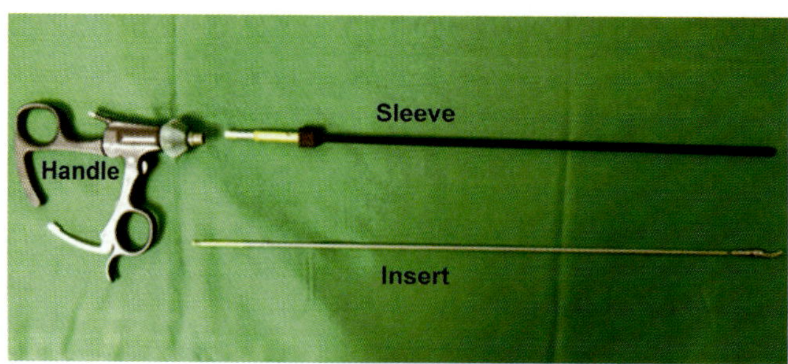

Fig. 2.5: Parts of laparoscopic instrument

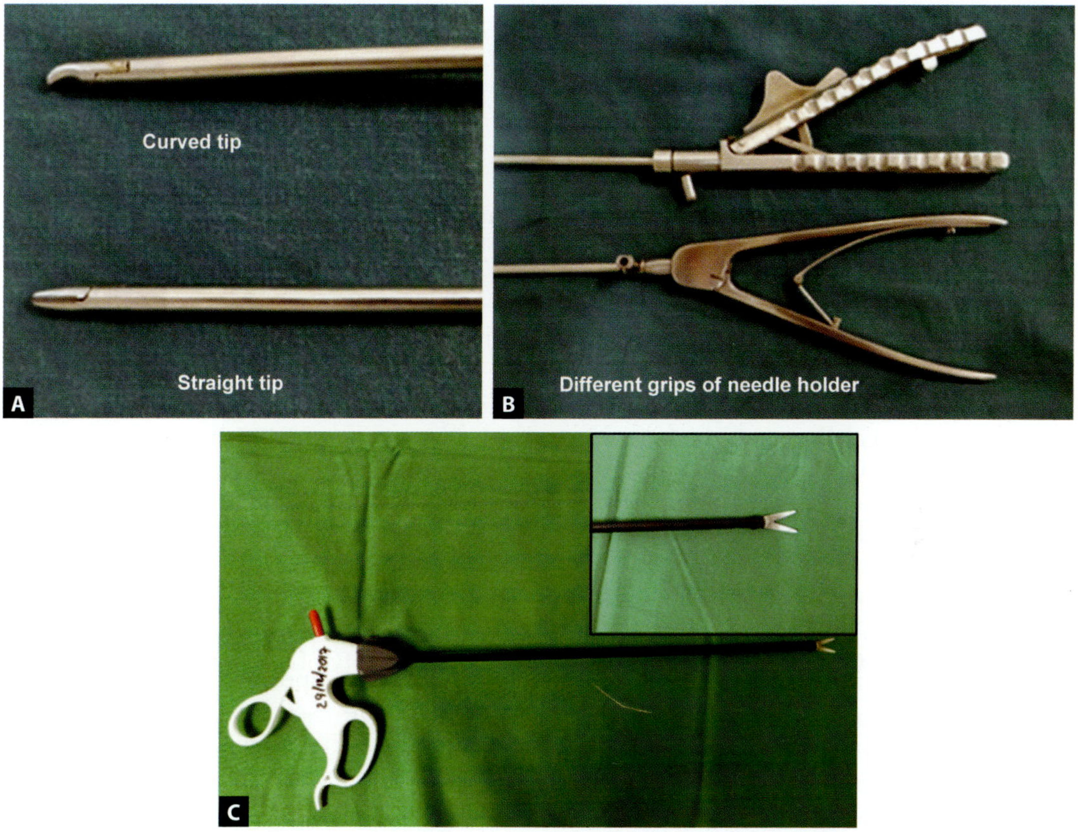

Figs 2.6A to C: (A and B) Needle holder tip and handle; (C) Laparoscopic scissors

advantage of these clips is that, they can be removed during bench surgery.

- *Interlocking clips* **(Fig. 2.7):** A number of variety of clips is available (allport, ligamax). The clips are extremely secure and can be used for securing the renal vein and the renal artery. The length of the clip is approximately 16 mm. They are available with preloaded clip appliers, each clip applier has 20 preloaded clips. Every time the handle is pressed one clip is deployed. These instruments are preloaded; multiple clips can be deployed, without taking the instrument out of abdominal cavity. The clips are radiopaque. The clips have to be twisted open with the help of two hemostats if they have to be unclipped.

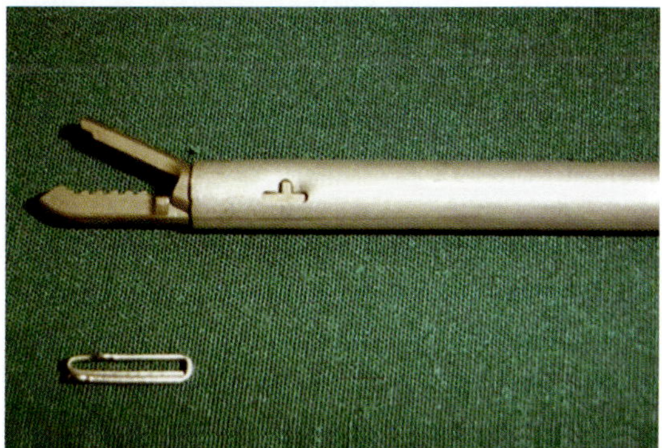

Fig. 2.7: Interlocking clip with applicator

A few of the clip applicators have an indicator, indicating the number of the clips left to be deployed.

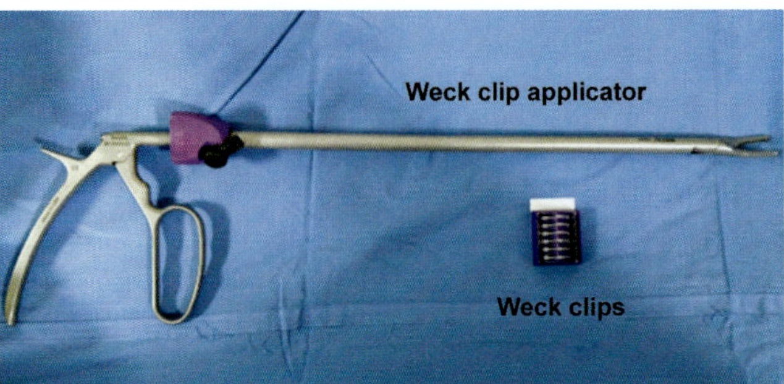

Fig. 2.8: Weck™ clip with applicator

- *Weck clips (Fig. 2.8):* The Hem-o-loc clips (Teleflex Medicals), popularly known as Weck™ clips, are available in three variants (Teleflex, NC, USA)—green (5 mm), purple (10 mm) and gold clip (15 mm). The clips are made of nonabsorbable polymer, extremely secure and are radiolucent. The clips are used for securing the renal vein, renal artery. The 5 mm clips can be used for securing the gonadal vessels. Golden clips are used to secure large renal veins, especially right renal vein. Following the US FDA warning (black box) the clips have been contraindicated for use in laparoscopic donor nephrectomy. The warning came following reports of deaths following the use of these clips in donors. A multicenter study by Ponsky et al included over 1000 patients with 486 donor nephrectomies did not find any of the clips that slipped.

The authors suggested the following steps to be followed while applying Weck™ clips:
1. The vessels to be secured should be circumferentially dissected.
2. The knob of the clip should be seen.
3. Two clips should always be applied on the patient side.
4. Always keep a cuff of 2 mm beyond the clip.
5. Once the clip is applied the surgeon should be able to feel the click and all the people in the theater should be able to hear the click.
   The Weck clips can be removed by custom made specific unclippers. In addition, an innovative way of unclipping Weck clip is to use ultasonic energy like harmonic and burn the clip at the level of knob or the 'V' of the clip. The clip immediately disengages.

STAPLERS

Staplers are devices used for tissue approximation **(Fig. 2.9)**. Different tissues have different properties and hence different types of cartriges are used for different tissues. In addition, an innovative way of unclipping weck clip is to use ultrasonic energy like harmonic and burn the clip at the level of knob or the 'V' of the clip. The clip immediately disengages.

Classification of Stapler
- Depending on the form: Linear, curved and circular staplers.
- Depending on whether it has a blade or not it can be called cutting or a non-cutting stapler.
- It can be classified as articulating or non-articulating staplers. The tip of the articulating stapler can be moved around to confirm to the shape of the tissue to be stappled.
- Stapler can be disposable or reusable.
  The staples of the stapler are made of different materials, titanium is one of the most commonly used materials, which is a stable metal and does not produce any immune reaction. Other materials which are used for

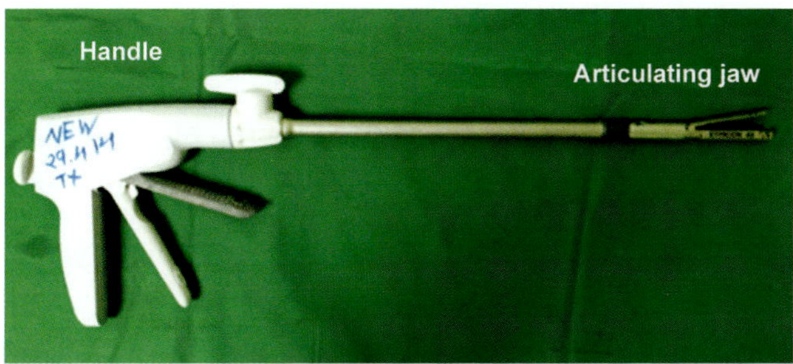

Fig. 2.9: Laparoscopic stapler

Sl. No.	Stapler (manufacturer)	Advantage
	Table 2.1: Some frequently used laparoscopic staplers	
1.	Echelon Flex™ GST (Ethicon)	Better grip on movement, least slippage
2.	The Echelon Flex™ Powered Endopath (Ethicon)	Battery power stapler, more stability, less tissue trauma
3.	Endopath® EMS (Ethicon)	Multifeed stapler for single use
4.	EndoGIA™ Tri-Staple™ Technology (Coviden)	Ergonomic design, can be used on wide range of tissue, precise articulation and one hand grasp

making staple include stainless steel and synthetic absorbable materials.

Cartridges are the cassettes containing the staples and are to be loaded onto the stapler gun. They are color-coded and depending upon the tissue to be stapled appropriate cartridge is used. The cartridges differ for different types of stapler. The height of the staples is determined by the tissue to be stapled, mesentery requires lesser height of the staples as compared to bowel. Color coding for various cartridges varies as per the height of the staples. For Ethicon™ staplers blue-colored cartridges are used for bowel and the white-colored ones are used for vascular pedicles.

Factors determining choice of the laparoscopic staplers **(Table 2.1)**:
- Whether it can access the target site
- Ability to articulate and rotate
- Ability to complete the staple line and cut
- Minimal movement of the gun during firing of the stapler
- Size of the gun will determine what size of the trocar should be used.

Currently there are two major players in the laparoscopic stapler market, Ethicon™ and Medtronics™ (Coviden earlier) and these companies occupy 70% of the market share of the sales.

HEMOSTATIC AGENTS

Hemostatic Agents are Either Available as Sheets or Solutions

Agents commonly used and available as sheets
- *Surgicel™ (Ethicon, USA):* It is oxidized cellulose polymer which is a unit of poly-anhydroglucuronic acid. It induces blood clot formation.
- *Surgicel SNoW™, Fibrillar™:* It is same as Surgicel™ but woven or knitted so that it has better tissue adherence.

Agents commonly used and available as solutions
- *Floseal™ matrix (Baxter):* It contains thrombin made from human plasma and gelatin granules. The gelatin granules swell up

and give a mechanical tamponade effect. The thrombin in Floseal interacts with normal coagulation mechanism and accelerates conversion of fibrinogen to fibrin, resulting in accelerated clot formation.

- *Surgiflo:* Hemostatic matrix (Ethicon) is absorbable porcine gelatin paste, it is put over the sutured surface of bleeding organ for hemostasis.
- *Evicel™ (Ethicon):* It is a human fibrin-based hemostatic agent, can be stored at room temperature for 24 hours. It is available as airless spray and is not dependent on patient's coagulation profile.

Rescue Stitch and Tray

To salvage bleeding in minimal access surgery a rescue stitch can be used. Bleeding in minimal access environment can be very challenging for the surgeon. Rescue stitch can save the day, when used judiciously.

Rescue stitch is not available commercially but, is made by taking 4 inches of polyglactin 0 or polypropylene 3–0 on a large needle, ideally CT1 needle is suitable as it can be seen in the pool of blood. A thread is knotted at the end of the suture and a Weck™ clip (Teleflex, NC, USA) is applied proximal to it. Once the bleeding vessel is identified, the suture is passed through both the edges of the vessel and then the Weck clip is sinched over the bleeding vessel, this will control more than 50% of the bleeding. Another throw is now passed through the vessel walls making it a figure of 8 stitch and then two ends of the thread are tied to make a secure knot. Rescue stitch is a part of the rescue tray which contains, a Maryland forceps, a needle driver, a Satinsky clamp, Surgicel™ (Ethicon, Somerville, USA) bolster and a cartridge of Weck clip. The Maryland forceps is used to hold the edges of the vessel, needle driver is kept in the tray with a rescue stitch held in the jaws and is used to pass the needle through the bleeding vessels. Satinsky clamp can be used to clamp vessels and Surgicel bolster is used to pack the bleeding area. The rescue stitch should be plasma sterilized and then stuck to the wall of the operating room in accessible position so that it can be readily available for use in emergency.

3

Basics in Port Placement and Abdominal Wall Entry

Sudharsan Balaji, Arvind P Ganpule, V Mohan Kumar

POINT OF ENTRY (Fig. 3.1)

Multiple authors have identified different points of initial entry into the abdomen like umbilicus and Palmer's point. We prefer to insufflate the abdomen at the point of first port placement. The surface marking is arrived with the marking of the anterior superior iliac spine of the ipsilateral side and lower border of umbilicus. The midpoint of the line joining these two points is the reference point. It is wise to measure the distance of this point from the subcostal line in the long axis of the patient. A minimum of 12–14 cm is the usual and adequate distance to provide the necessary space for instrument handling and to avoid clashing between instruments. Account should be made for the increase of this distance in the long axis after pneumoperitoneum by 2–3 cm. For example, if the distance of this reference point from the subcostal line is 15 cm, then the actual distance after insufflation will be around 18 cm and in which case, we prefer to place the first port about an inch (2.5 cm) above the reference point. This correction is mandatory as caudal placement may be detrimental for upper polar dissection. On the contrary, if the distance of the reference point from the

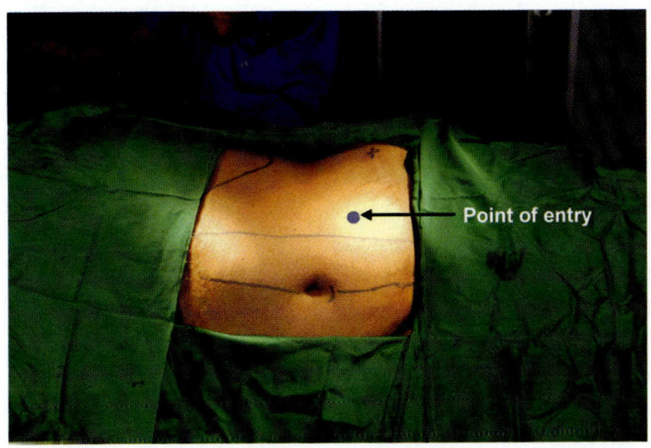

Fig. 3.1: Point of entry

subcostal line is only 12 cm, after insufflation it usually becomes 14 to 14.5 cm. In this case, we have to place the first port on the reference point as further cranial shifting may cause crowding of the ports externally with subsequent instrument clashing.

Another correction that is usually done is the lateral correction that is required in obese patients. Hence, in obese patients or those with falling abdominal pannus in the lateral position, the reference point is shifted up to a maximum of one inch (2.5 cm) laterally.

Entering the Abdomen at the Palmer Point

Dr Raoul Palmer, a gynecologist, described entry into the abdominal cavity through the left upper quadrant. He described the point of entry as Palmer's point. Palmer point is a point 3 cm below subcostal margin on the left side along the midclavicular line.

Though authors do not use this point of entry on a regular basis, it has been used by them in cases where access is failed from the left iliac fossa in left upper tract surgeries.

With these corrections on the longitudinal and mediolateral axes of the patient in specified circumstances, the corrected reference point is marked. We prefer creating pneumoperitoneum using Veress needle in all adult patients. The Veress needle is held like a dart and advanced into the abdomen. A typical three passes are observed—first at the fascia, second through the muscle and the last the most obvious, the peritoneum with a loud click as the inner sharp tip retracts inside. The position is confirmed with the marker on the hub, aspiration to check for blood/bowel contents followed by instillation of 3 cc of saline and confirming free flow under gravity. This is then followed by insufflation up to a preset pressure of 20 mm Hg.

We use a bladed 12 mm trocar for the first port at this reference point. Free flow of gas through the gas vent after removal of obturator confirms the entry into peritoneal cavity. The 30° camera should be kept ready and white balanced, before this port placement and an immediate check laparoscopy is done to see for proper insufflation, to check for underlying bowel, mesenteric, solid organ or vascular injury.

Port Placement for Laparoscopic Urological Surgeries

*Laparoscopic Nephrectomy **(Fig. 3.2)***

The next port is placed in the same line as the first port, one finger breath below the costal margin. Typically this is a 5-mm dilating port for the left side and a 12-mm port on the right side. Right hand port in case of a nephrectomy should be a 12-mm port, as it will allow passage of Weck clip applicator, which would be used to secure the renal hilum. Third port (camera port) is placed at the junction of upper one-third and lower two-thirds along the lateral border of rectus.

The liver retraction port should be at the level lower border of liver, in the midline or on the opposite side, it should pass through the falciform ligament. The position of the port can be pre-confirmed by using a syringe filled with saline and needle. The needle is inserted and saline injected to look for the trajectory of the port. If the above principles are followed, a proper liver retraction can be achieved. Similarly, a fourth port is placed at least four finger breaths lateral from the first port and two finger breaths cranial to the anterior superior iliac spine. This port is used to retract the ureterogonadal packet and place traction on the kidney. A needle-syringe with saline is injected from the outside to note the trajectory of these ports before placement.

*Laparoscopic Pyeloplasty **(Fig. 3.3)***

The port placements are similar for a pyeloplasty barring a few minor changes. For reconstructive surgery, all the ports are placed

4

Energy Sources in Laparoscopic Surgery

Abhishek Singh, Arvind P Ganpule

INTRODUCTION

Energy sources have become an integral part of surgery for cutting, coagulation, hemostasis and sealing during dissection and surgeries.

Electrosurgery: It is the use of radiofrequency alternating current during surgery to increase the cellular temperature to vaporize or coagulate the tissue.

Electrocautery uses direct current in which current is passed through a resistant metal wire electrode which generates heat. [1]

A regular electrosurgical generator uses current of 50/60 Hz and increases the frequency of current to 200,000 Hz. Such frequencies are radio frequencies, when current passes at such high frequency through the human body, no neuromuscular stimulation occurs, and patient does not get an electric shock.

Classification

It can be classified based on the type of electrosurgical unit (ESU) generator used:
- *Simple generator:* Monopolar/bipolar cautery
- *Advanced bipolar systems:*
  - Ligasure
  - Enseal
- Ultrasonic: Harmonic scalpel
- Integrated (ultrasound and advance bipolar) : Thunderbeat

Monopolar Generator[1]

These are the most commonly available electrosurgical units in all operating rooms **(Fig. 4.1)**.

Monopolar circuit traverses from generator—active electrode—patient—patient return electrode.

Various waveforms generated by electrosurgical generators **(Fig. 4.2)** are[1]:
- *Cut:* Waveform is constant, heat is generated rapidly leading to tissue vaporization or cutting.
- *Coagulation:* Waveform is interrupted, less heat is produced, and no tissue vaporization occurs instead coagulation occurs.
- *Blend current:* It is modification of duty cycle. It uses a lower cycle, so less heat is produced and decreased heat produces coagulation.

Electrosurgical Tissue Effects (Fig. 4.3)

Cutting

By using this mode, the probe acts like a hot knife, as the intense heat produced will vaporize the tissue. When the electrode is kept slightly away from the tissue, the maximum

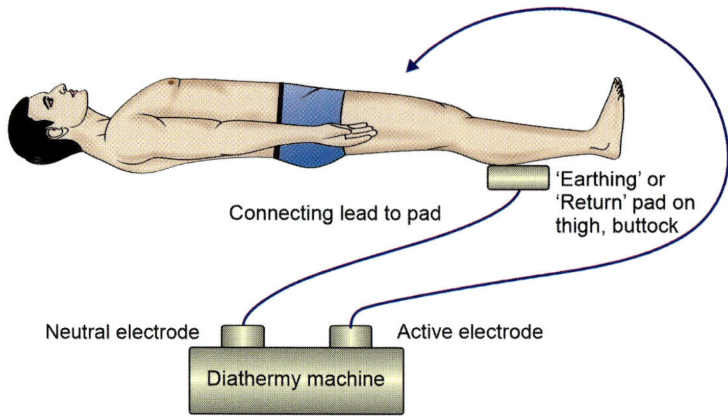

Fig. 4.1: Monopolar circuit

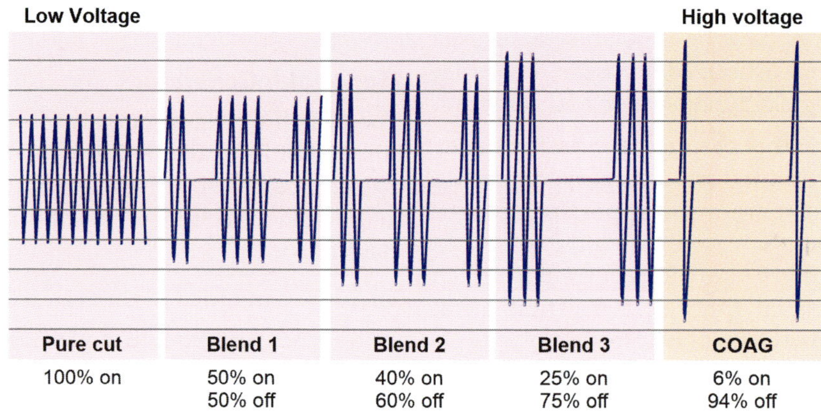

Fig. 4.2: Waveforms of cutting and coagulation

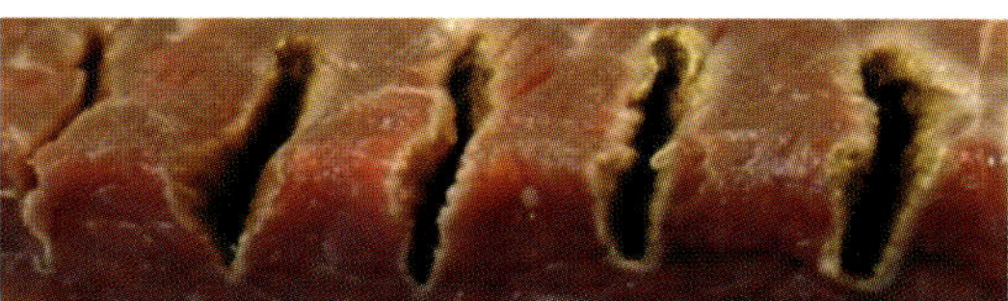

Fig. 4.3: The cutting current makes a deep incision and coagulation current has lateral spread

current concentration and cutting can be done.

Coagulation

In this mode, charring occurs involving a large area. In coagulation mode, the duty cycle (on time) is only 6%, this leads to heating up of tissue and coagulation rather than vaporization.

Patient pad placement: Patient plate should be in contact over a large muscular surface area. Bony areas should be avoided. Soft pads are better than metallic plates as they give uniform area of contact. The pads should be placed near the area of interest of surgery so that the pathway of current in the body is minimum.

Bipolar[1]

In this form of electrosurgery, active and the return electrode are the part of the bipolar

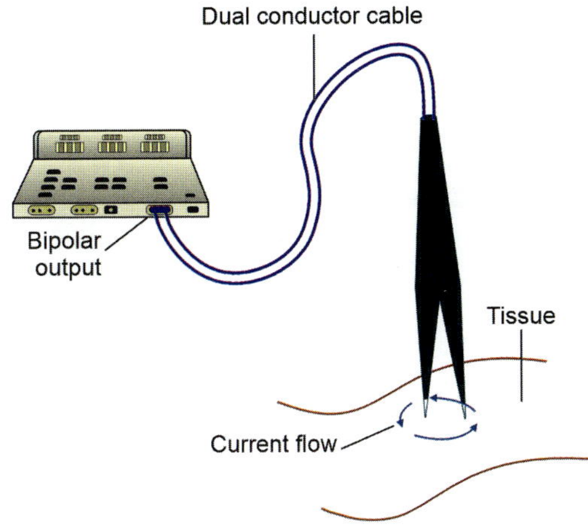

Fig. 4.4: Bipolar circuit

device and no patient plate is required. The current passes from one prong of bipolar device to the other through the tissue in between and circuit is completed **(Fig. 4.4)**.[2,3]

Advanced Bipolar Systems

- *Ligasure (Medtronic):* It is an advanced bipolar energy source which combines pressure and energy to create a seal. It consists of a specialized generator system that has vessel sealer capability also **(Fig. 4.5)**.[6] Ligasure is an advanced bipolar system that uses a combination of high current, lower voltage and pressure by the instruments to work as a hemostatic and a vessel sealer. It has a low mist generation, minimal charring, minimal sticking and less

thermal spread. It has a feedback mechanism, which gives a beep sound once the tissue is adequately sealed. Even vessels up to seven millimetres can be sealed using this device. The seals are created by melting the collagen and elastin in the vessel walls and forming it into a permanent seal. It does not rely on proximal thrombus for hemostasis. Sealed blood vessel can withstand up to three times higher blood pressure than normal.

Enseal™ (SurgRx, Inc. Palo Alto, CA) (Fig. 4.6)

The Enseal system uses an advanced bipolar technology to seal the tissue within the blades of the instrument. It uses a patented blade technology that has a strong uniform compression along the tissue sealing line. It includes conductive particles embedded in the jaws of the instrument, which is temperature sensitive. These particles control the current that goes into the contact tissues.[4,5] Once the tissue heats above a critical level, these nanoparticles interrupt the flow of current. This cycle is continued till the entire tissue segment is uniformly heated and fused. The vessel walls are fused through coagulation, compression and protein denaturation. It can seal vessels up to 7 mm with a seal strength of 7 times the systolic pressure.

Ultrasonic Generators

High power ultrasound waves can be used to produce surgical cutting, coagulation, and dissection of tissues **(Fig. 4.7)**.[7]

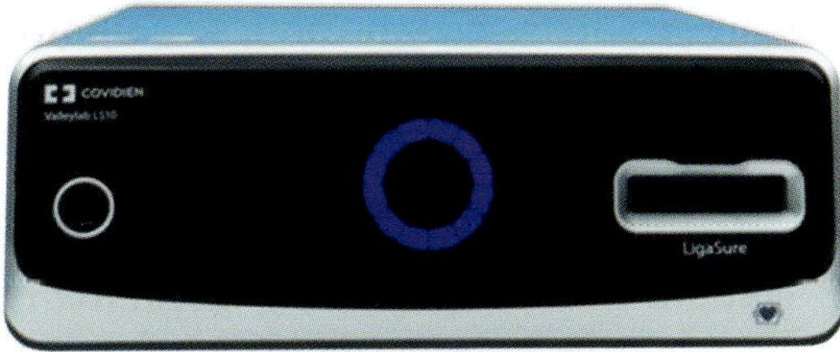

Fig. 4.5: Ligasure

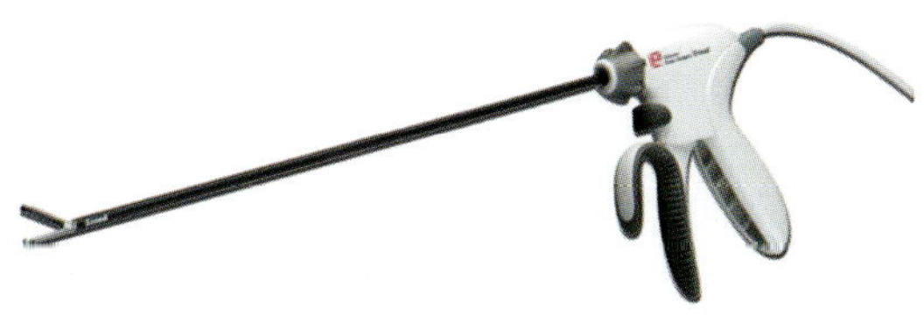

Fig. 4.6: Enseal

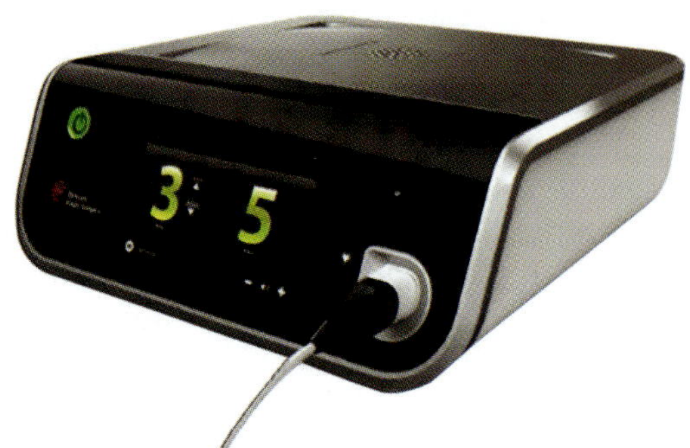

Fig. 4.7: Ultrasonic generator

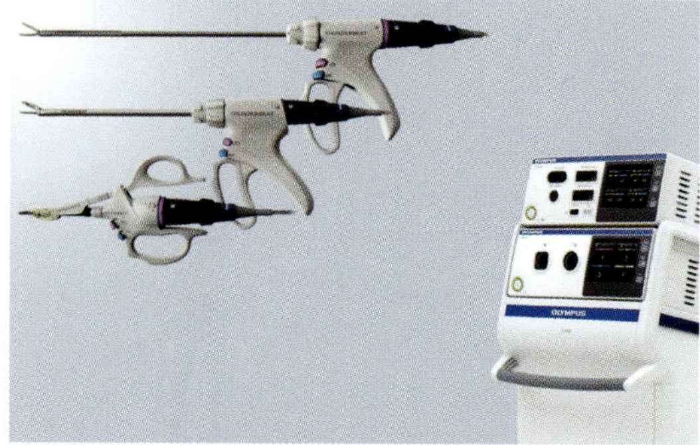

Fig. 4.8: Thunderbeat

These systems operate at high frequency of 55 kHz, which cleave loose tissues by frictional heating providing cut and coagulate at the same time.

The handpiece contains piezoelectric crystals which are present under pressure amid metal cylinders. On activation, piezoelectric ceramic disks in handpiece become excited and this electrical energy is transferred into mechanical energy. Mechanical energy is amplified at nodes and a maximum amplitude of 55,000 Hz is reached at blade tip. It causes compression of tissues, broken hydrogen bonds and cell protein denaturation. Ultrasonic surgery causes slower coagulation as compared to electrosurgery. However, excessive heating of ultrasonic dissectors is an issue which causes lateral thermal spread. So, one must be careful while using this instrument as a dissector.

Integrated Ultrasound and Advanced Bipolar Generators

Thunderbeat

The Thunderbeat™ (Olympus), was the first device to integrate the ultrasonic and advanced bipolar generator **(Fig. 4.8)**.

Ethicon has also come up with an integrated generator: Ethicon Endo-Surgery™. The sealing capabilities of this device are same as ultrasonic or advanced bipolar depending on the generator used.[8]

They have advantages of both the bipolar system and the ultrasonic system. Since both energies are used together, the heat generation of combined bipolar is lesser.

Safety Considerations

- *Direct application*: Direct application of an active electrode to an unintended area can cause direct tissue injury.
- *Direct coupling*: When the activate active electrode touches a nearby metallic instrument, the instrument gets energised and this energy may travel through another path to the patient plate causing injury. For example, a monopolar energy touches a laparoscopic telescope and if the telescope is with bowel, then telescope will cause thermal injury to the bowel **(Fig. 4.9)**.
- *Insulation failure*: If there is a break in the insulation, the energy through the instrument can cause tissue injury. For example, if a portion of monopolar instrument has an insulation break and this area comes in contact with bowel, it can lead to bowel injury **(Fig. 4.10)**.
- *Capacitive coupling*: It happens when the charge generated within an insulator separates two conductors. It completes circuit and cause surrounding organ injury. For example, hybrid cannula with suction and hook has metallic hook covered by an

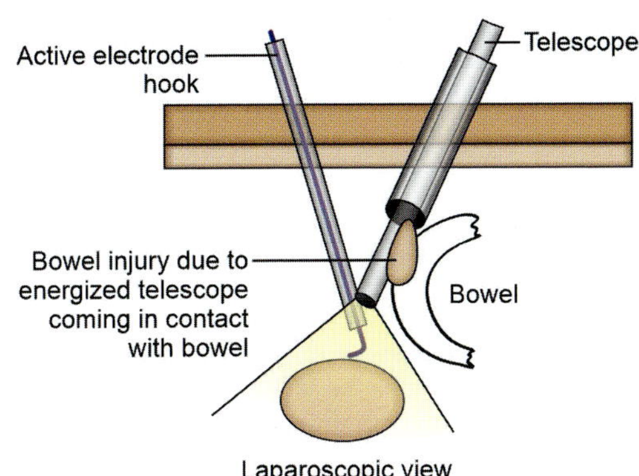

Fig. 4.9: Direct coupling of current

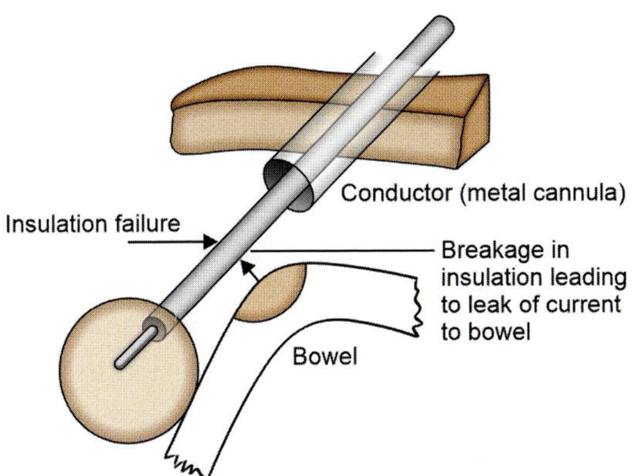

Fig. 4.10: Insulation failure

insulator which is fixed within a metallic suction cannula. The insulator can act as a capacitor and when it comes in contact with adjacent bowel, it may cause bowel injury **(Fig. 4.11)**.

REFERENCES

1. www.asit.org/assets/documents/Prinicpals_in_electrosurgery.pdf
2. Chen J, Jensen CR, Manwaring PK, Glasgow RE. Validation of a Laparoscopic Ferromagnetic Technology-based Vessel Sealing Device and Comparative Study to Ultrasonic and Bipolar Laparoscopic Devices. Surg Laparosc Endosc Percutan Tech. 2017;27(2):e12-e17. doi: 10.1097/SLE.0000000000000385. PMID: 28234706; PMCID: PMC5377999.
3. Hubner M, Demartines N, Muller S, Dindo D, Clavien PA, Hahnloser D. Prospective randomized study of monopolar scissors, bipolar vessel sealer and ultrasonic shears. Br J Surg. 2008 Sep;95(9):1098-104. doi: 10.1002/bjs.6321. PMID: 18690630.
4. http://www.ethicon.com/healthcare-professionals/products/advanced-energy/enseal/enseal-g2-tissue-sealers
5. Heniford BT, Matthews BD, Sing RF, Backus C, Pratt B, Greene FL. Initial results with an electrothermal bipolar vessel sealer. Surgical endoscopy. 2001;15:799-801.
6. Ping H, Xing NZ, Zhang JH, Niu YN, Zhang JZ, Wang JW. A single institution experience using the LigaSure vessel sealing system in laparoscopic nephrectomy. Chin Med J (Engl). 2011;124(8):1242-5. PMID: 21543004.
7. Tomita Y, Koike H, Takahashi K, Tamaki M, Morishita H. Use of the harmonic scalpel for nephron sparing surgery in renal cell carcinoma. J Urol. 1998 Jun;159(6):2063-4. doi: 10.1016/S0022-5347(01)63247-6. PMID: 9598518.
8. http://medical.olympusamerica.com/products/thunderbeat-1.

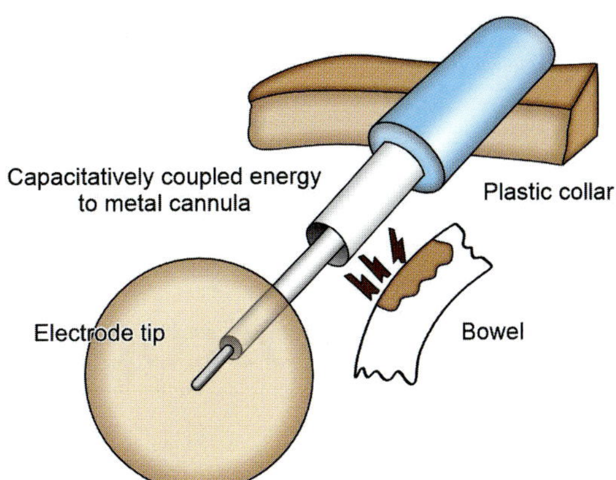

Fig. 4.11: Capacitative coupling

5

Tips and Tricks in Laparoscopic Adrenalectomy

Arvind P Ganpule, Sudharsan Balaji, V Mohan Kumar, Abhishek Singh

LEFT SIDE TRANSPERITONEAL ADRENALECTOMY

Port Positioning

The port position is dictated by the size of the adrenal lesion, the pathology and the laterality of the mass.

Port Placement

The principles of port placement are that the area of interest should be at the apex of the angle formed by the two working ports with the camera in center **(Figs 5.1A and B)**.

Pneumoperitoneum

The pneumoperitoneum is created either with the open technique or the Veress needle technique. The site of creation of the pneumoperitoneum depends on the approach utilized. If the open technique is employed, the umbilicus is the choice of access. If the Veress needle is used, it is inserted in the ipsilateral iliac fossa. Once the pneumoperitoneum is created, the ports should be inserted in such a way that the camera port lies in front of the adrenal. The ports are inserted as follows:

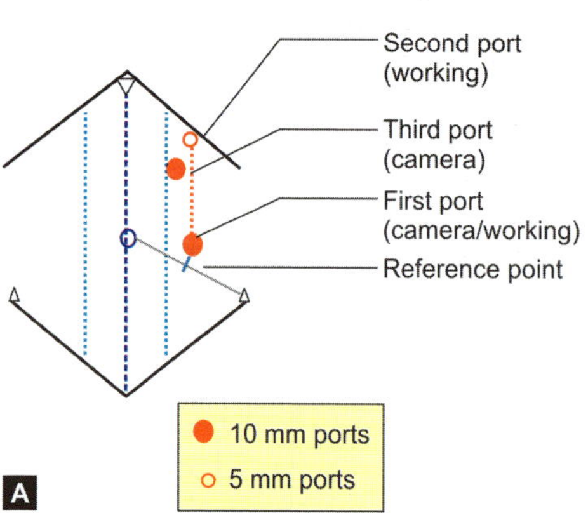

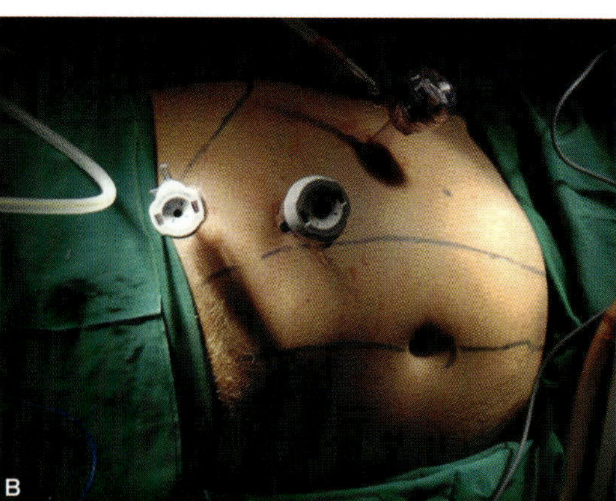

Figs 5.1A and B: Ports for laparoscopic left adrenalectomy

Three ports are inserted. The 10 mm camera port is at the lateral border of the umbilicus in front of the adrenal gland. The other two ports are placed on either side 5–7.5 cm away from the camera port. The right hand port should always be a 10-mm port and is placed one finger breath below the costal margin in the midclavicular line on the right side. The left hand port is 5–7.5 cm caudal and lateral to camera port on the right side. Principle of placing a liver retractor is same as nephrectomy in right. Proper positioning of liver retracting port is critical to exposure of adrenal gland. The port position for a left-sided adrenalectomy mirror is the right side. An additional 5 mm retraction port can be placed along the anterior axillary line at the level of lower pole of the kidney.

Steps

Bowel Mobilization

The line of Toldt is incised and the colon is mobilized inferiorly **(Fig. 5.2)**. The extent of the caudal mobilization is not as extensive as that in nephrectomy. The aim being to expose the renal vein. In contrast, the mobilization of the splenocolic and lienorenal ligaments should be extensive. On the left side, the spleen is extensively mobilized giving an appearance of a open book **(Fig. 5.3)**. This part of the dissection is vital in adrenalectomy on the left side. Unless the spleen is mobilized

extensively the renal vein and the adrenal vein dissection would not be optimal. If this step is not done aggressively, the spleen keeps on obstructing the vision of the surgeon. The splenorenal ligament is preferentially taken down with harmonic scalpel. The advantage of using this modality is that, it helps in securing the small vessels in the ligament. It is essential that, this step is done prior to identifying the renal vein, allowing full medial rotation of the spleen away from the surgical field.

Identification of the Renal Vein

The renal vein is identified as a bluish hue with subtle venous pulsations seen through the Gerota's fascia **(Fig. 5.4)**. If the identification of the renal vein is challenging, one can identify the gonadal vein and trace it till its confluence with the renal vein. The next

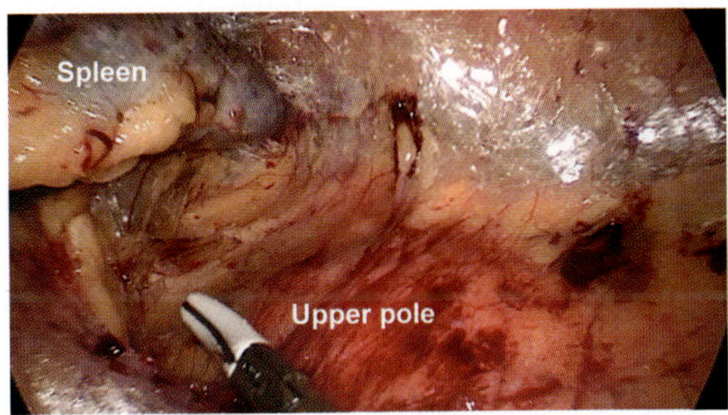

Fig. 5.3: Dissection of upper pole

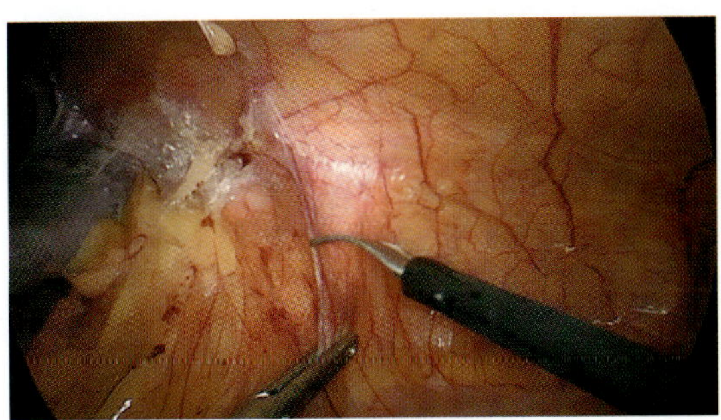

Fig. 5.2: Reflection of colon

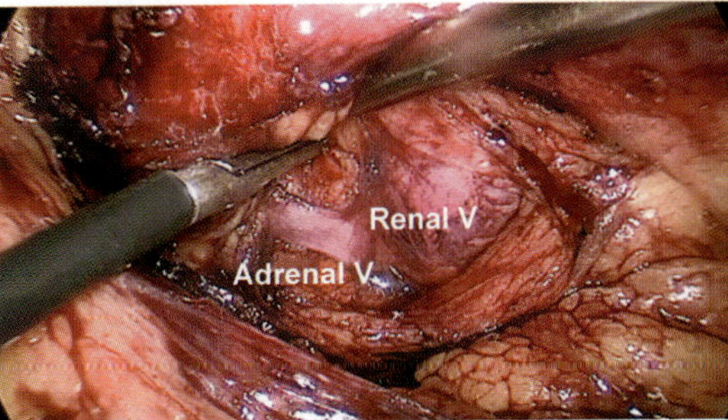

Fig. 5.4: Identification of renal vein and adrenal vein

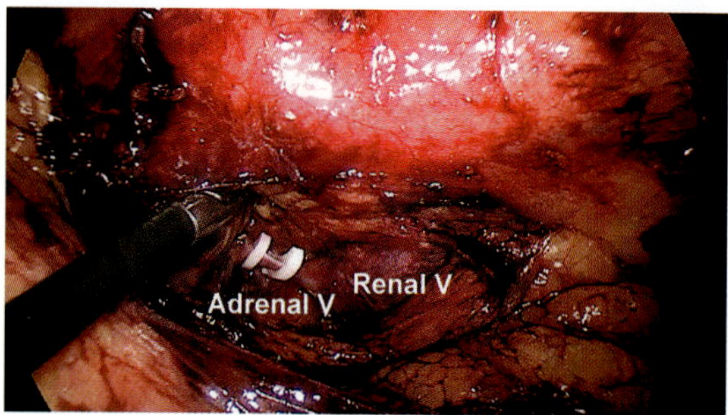

Fig. 5.5: Clipping of adrenal vein

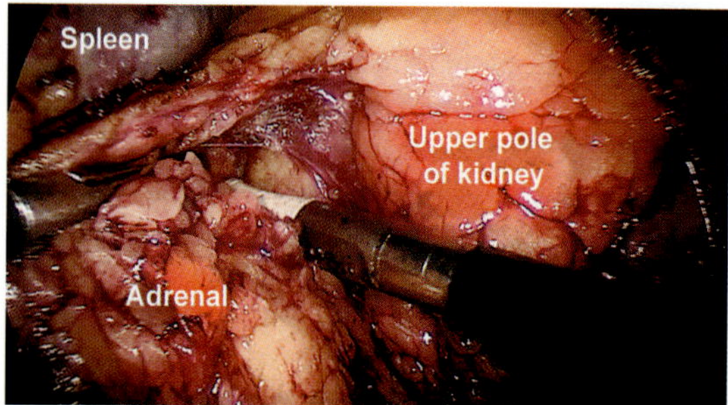

Fig. 5.6: Dissection between kidney and adrenal

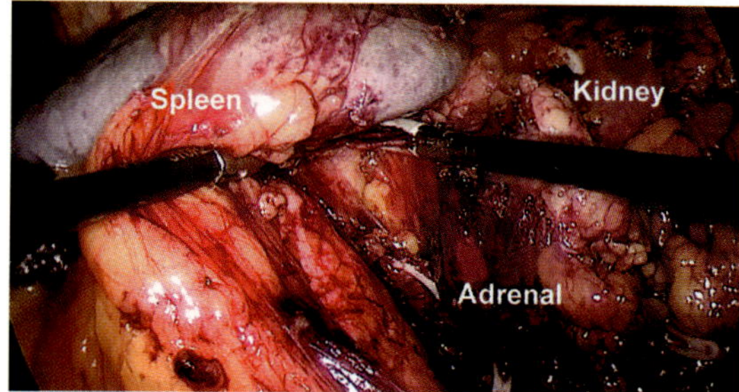

Fig. 5.7: Dissection between adrenal and spleen

step in the procedure is securing the adrenal vein **(Fig. 5.5)**. The dissection of the adrenal vein starts at its confluence with the renal vein. The dissection should be adequate to allow safe clipping and transection of adrenal vein. The dissection is deemed to be adequate if the adrenal vein is seen entering the adrenal gland or the lower border of the adrenal gland is clearly seen. The inferior phrenic vein is considered to be the landmark to assess the adequacy of the dissection. The adrenal vein is secured with the help of either interlocking clips or hemolok clips. It is essential to keep an adequate amount of cuff of adrenal vein at the renal vein end. In addition, a cuff should be left beyond the clips to ensure that the clips do not slip. The controversy exists as regards the need to secure the adrenal vein prior to dissection or it is necessary to dissect and secure it after the dissection of the tumour. The authors prefer to secure the adrenal vein prior to dissection of the SOL in pheochromocytoma and other functional tumors.

Dissection of the Plane between the Adrenal and the Upper Pole of the Kidney

The Gerota's fascia over the upper pole of the kidney is opened to expose the upper pole of the kidney and the adrenal gland. Special precaution to be exercised, include avoiding injury to a upper polar branch of the renal artery or an accessory renal artery. This information can be obtained from the review of preoperative CT images. The dissection should proceed between the adrenal gland and the upper pole of kidney till the posterior and lateral abdominal wall muscles are seen **(Figs 5.6 and 5.7)**. The gland is gradually separated from the upper pole of the kidney, throughout its length and breadth. It is important to avoid grasping the adrenal during the course of the dissection.

At this point adrenal gland is separated all around and advanced energy sources are used to secure hemostasis at the gland is supplied by multiple small arterial branches, and after separation, the adrenal gland is entrapped in the specimen retrieval bag (Nadiad bag).

Right Side Adrenalectomy

The port placement varies on the right side that a 5-mm port is required for retraction of the liver **(Fig. 5.8)**.

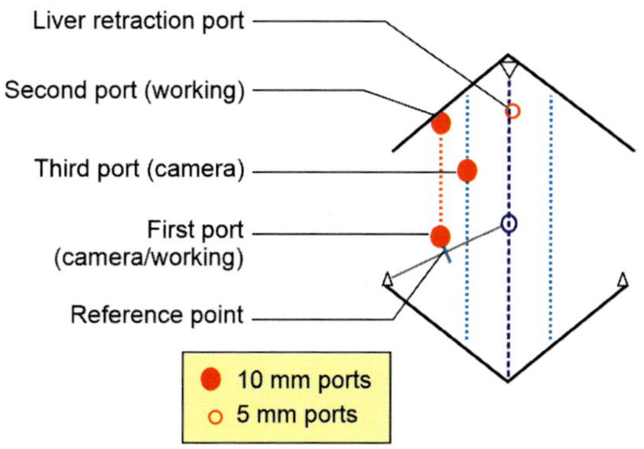

Fig. 5.8: Port placement for laparoscopic right adrenalectomy

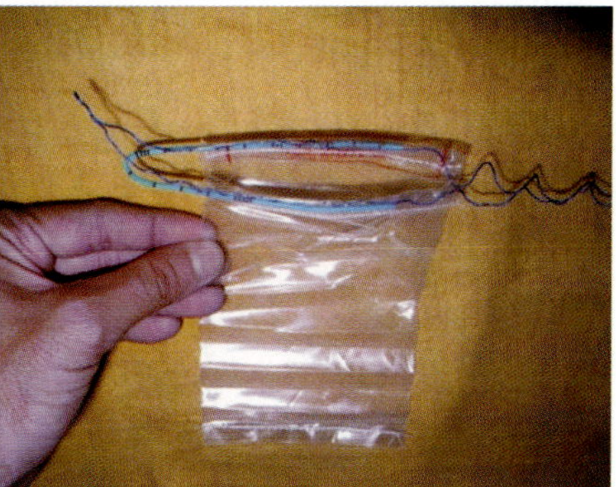

Fig. 5.9: Kocherization of duodenum and identification of IVC

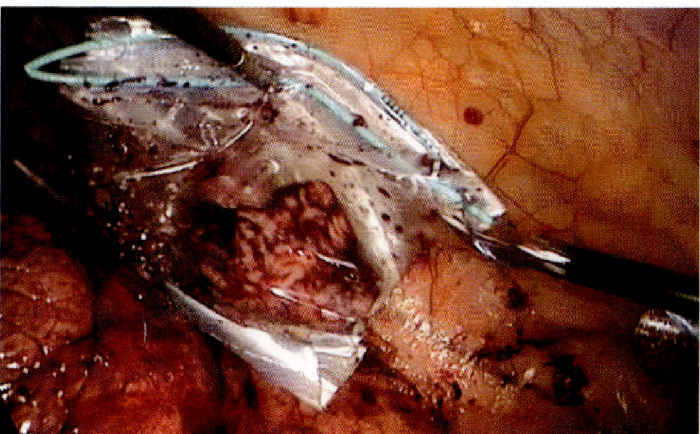

Fig. 5.10: Entrapment of specimen in Nadiad bag

The duodenum is kocherized and the inferior vena cava completely exposed **(Fig. 5.9)**.

On the right side, the renal vein is exposed. This acts as a landmark. Once the renal vein is exposed, it is traced till its junction with the inferior vena cava. The dissection proceeds along the upper border of the inferior vena cava. Once the IVC is identified, the plane in between the psoas muscle and the inferior vena cava (IVC) is found. This is essential as unless the adrenal gland is lifted, the adrenal vein does not tent up. The course of the adrenal vein on the left side is parallel to the IVC, tenting or lifting the adrenal makes the adrenal vein vertical. The adrenal vein as on the left side is secured with the help of hemolok clip.

Dissection in between the Kidney and the Adrenal

As on the left side all care should be taken to safeguard the accessory renal artery and the branches of the renal artery.

Specimen is entraped using Nadiad bag **(Fig. 5.10)**.

Issues with Management of Pheochromocytoma

Management of pheochromocytoma involves preoperative, intraoperative and postoperative periods.

Goals: The goals in management are to control hypertension, pheochromocytoma related symptoms and to avoid complications.

Preoperative Management

The preoperative management of pheochromocytoma patient starts 2 weeks before surgery. A thorough cardiac evaluation is a must in all the cases. The patient should be started on alpha blockers. Phenoxybenzamine is commonly prescribed. Prazocin is more commonly used. Phenoxybenzamine is started 7 to 14 days prior to surgery with a starting dose of 10 mg twice daily which can be titrated up to 1 mg/kg. Prazocin can be started at the dose of 2.5 mg daily. Selective alpha blockers such as terazocin or doxazocin can be used sometimes. The advantages of selective alpha blockers are the dose can be titrated, the tachycardia will be less and it can be taken on the day of surgery.

Beta blocker is started 2 days later as patient may develop reflex tachycardia and arrhythmia due to alpha blockers. Beta blockers should never be started before alpha blockers. Selective β_1 blockers such as atenolol, metoprolol preferred. If BP is not controlled, then metyrosine can be given followed by calcium channel blockers. The measures to be taken one to two days prior to surgery are as follows.

Increase in intravascular volume by adequate fluids (1–2 L of bolus on the night before surgery). Last dose of alpha blockers should be taken on the night before surgery and the morning dose should be omitted. Blood pressure and heart rate should be monitored.

Surgery can be done if the following criteria (Roizen) are met

- In hospital BP hold not be more than 160/90 for at least 24 hours before surgery.
- Orthostatic hypotension should be present but upright BP should not be less than 80/45.
- No more than one extrasystole/5 min
- No ST/T wave changes in ECG for one week.

Intraoperative Period

Adequate precautions should be taken including preparation, minimal tissue handling, deep plane anesthesia, use of shorter acting drugs, and fluids after vein clamping. Adequate vascular access in the form of central line and two large IV lines is a must. Drugs such as sodium nitroprusside, NTG and esmolol should be kept ready. The crisis can occur during induction, tumor manipulation and vein clamping.

Postoperative Period

Hypotension should be avoided with adequate fluids. Pressor agents should be avoided in the postoperative period. We should be aware of the possibility of rebound hypoglycemia due to insulin excess and manage accordingly.

6

Tips and Tricks in Laparoscopic Pyeloplasty

Arvind P Ganpule, V Mohan Kumar, Sudharsan Balaji, Abhishek Singh

INTRODUCTION

Pyeloplasty regardless of the approach, namely open, laparoscopic or robotic offers excellent results. The approach to be chosen depends on the age of the patient, the degree of hydronephrosis, extent of extrarenal pelvis and surgical expertise available. Regardless of the approach the success rates exceed 95% in expert hands.

Stenting

In all pediatric open pyeloplasty cases, our choice of stenting is an antegrade splint. The antegrade splint is placed after completion of the medial wall of the reconstruction. The splint is typically a 3 of 4 Fr ureteric catheter. The ureteric catheter along with a percutaneous nephrostomy in the form of a Foley catheter is placed. The postoperative protocol for removal of these tubes is to remove the ureteric splint after 5 days and clamp the percutaneous nephrostomy. This ensures that the reconstruction is patent. The patient is observed for a day for any increasing hydronephrosis or pain and thereafter the percutaneous nephrostomy is removed. We believe employing this approach for this subset of patients helps to avoid manipulating the urethra for stent insertion as well as extraction of stent and thus preventing the possible complications.

In all the adult pyeloplasties, authors perform a preoperative retrograde pyelogram. The advantage of doing this was fourfold; it helped us to decide in initial part of the learning curve if a laparoscopic approach was feasible, it also helped to place a single J ureteric catheter which in turn helped in keeping the pelvis distended and helped in dissection. A collapsed pelvis makes the dissection extremely difficult. Second, the ureteric catheter offers an opportunity to keep the guidewire and perform a spatulation. If in the step of spatulation, the insertion of blade of scissors is difficult, the ureteric catheter can be removed and the spatulation can be performed over the guidewire. The single J ureteric catheter is replaced with double J stent after completion of the procedure.

In pediatric laparoscopic and robotic pyeloplasty an antegrade stent is placed either with a miniport or with a 18 Fr angiocath. The position of the stent is ascertained with efflux of urine from the side holes of stent.

Preoperative Imaging Assessment

Ultrasonography

The sonography gives the following information, namely degree of hydronephrosis, cortical thickness, amount of extrarenal pelvis and the echogenicity of the kidney. In the laparoscopic approach, giant hydronephrotic kidney's need decompression with a preoperative PCN. This apart from making the procedure less challenging also helps in additional assessment of the renal function.

CT Angiography

CT angiography in pelviureteric junction obstruction (PUJO) helps in assessing the presence or absence of crossing vessels which would further help in dissection of the PUJ. Although clinically useful, the guidelines do not suggest this imaging modality as the standard of care for investigations.

A preoperative imaging helps in understanding the lie of the pelvicalyceal junction. For instance, if a transperitoneal pyeloplasty is to be attempted, then a PUJO which is situated posteriorly would be an extremely challenging situation. The easiest lie for performing a pyeloplasty would be anteriorly located pelvis which is extrarenal.

Positioning of the Patient (**Fig. 6.1**)

The patient is positioned at the edge of the table with the upper leg extended and the lower leg flexed. The pressure points are secured using pillows and cushioned. The patient is strapped with two straps, one over the thigh and the other over the chest. The patient is placed in a 45 tilt if the transmesocolic approach is employed.

Port Positioning

The preamble for proper port positioning is that the camera port should be in front of the PUJO. The exact location of the port position can be ascertained with either imaging or retrograde pyelogram. A preoperative pyelogram will help us to mark the position of the port on the skin. The rest of the ports should be placed in such a way that the working and the retracting port are equidistant from each other (equal azimuth angle). The choice of size of the ports varies depending on surgeons' experience and personal preference. The instrument retraction port can be 5 mm or 10 mm in size. The port positioning has been discussed in detail earlier.

Steps in Port Positioning

Step 1: Retrograde pyelogram and ascertain the exact position of the ureteropelvic junction.

Step 2: Veress needle insertion at the midpoint of the ASIS and the umbilicus.

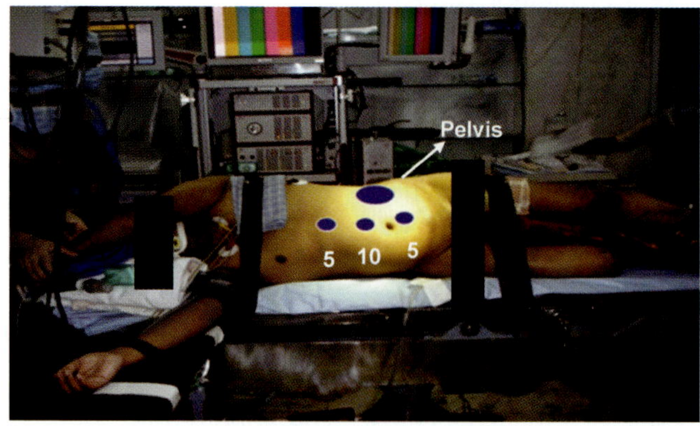

Fig. 6.1: Patient positioning and port placement for laparoscopic pyeloplasty

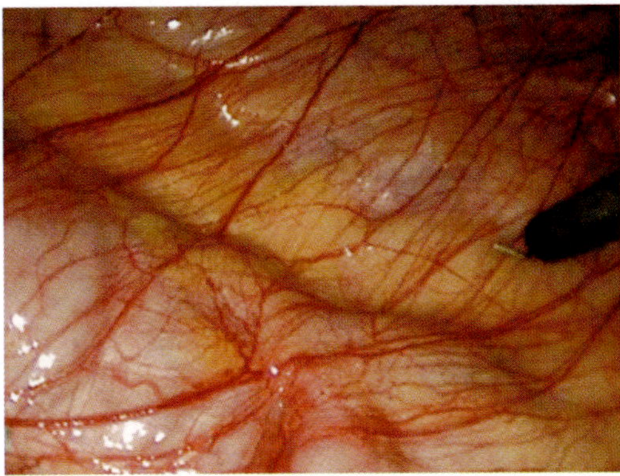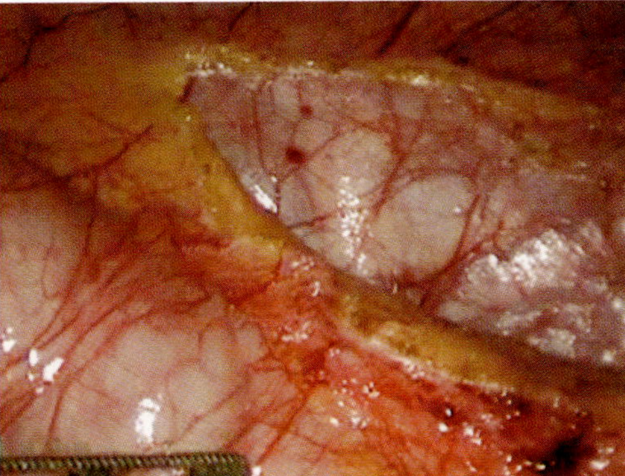

Fig. 6.2: Reflection of bowel

Step 3: Once the pneumoperitoneum is created the camera port is inserted in front of the renal pelvis.

Steps of Dissection

The steps of the dissection are as follows:

1. *Reflection of the bowel:* The reflection of the bowel need not be as extensive as in laparoscopic nephrectomy **(Fig. 6.2)**. The plane of the dissection should be initially outside the Gerota's fascia (extragerotal). The extent of dissection should extend from the iliac crossing up to the splenorenal ligament. It is not necessary to take down the splenorenal ligament. The dissection should delineate the PUJ adequately. The pelviureteric junction should be dissected either by starting the dissection at the ureterogonadal packet or proceeding from the renal pelvis. This helps in identifying the crossing vessels, if any. A preplaced ureteric catheter as described earlier is of benefit for this step as it keeps the pelvis distended and thus facilitating dissection.

2. *Transmesenteric approach:* The transmesocolic approach is employed if the mesenteric arcades are not thick, the arcades are easily visible and the mesenteric fat is not very dense **(Fig. 6.3)**. This approach is of particular benefit in pediatric patients as the

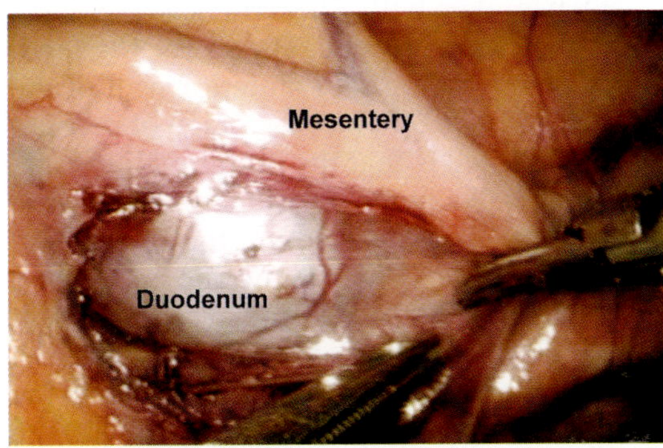

Fig. 6.3: Transmesenteric approach

mesenteric fat is not thick. This approach saves time of reflection of the bowel.

3. *Dissection of the crossing vessels:* The vessels should be circumferentially dissected. The dissection of the vessel can be aided by use of a vascular sling. The dissection of the vessel is considered to be complete if the PUJ is completely mobile behind the crossing vessel **(Fig. 6.4)**.

4. *The transabdominal hitch stitch:* The challenges in laparoscopic pyeloplasty include the need to avoid as many ports as possible. The more the number of ports and instruments inside the abdomen, the more will be the challenges involved. A transabdominal hitch stitch helps in offsetting this problem. This stitch should be taken on the anterior abdominal wall

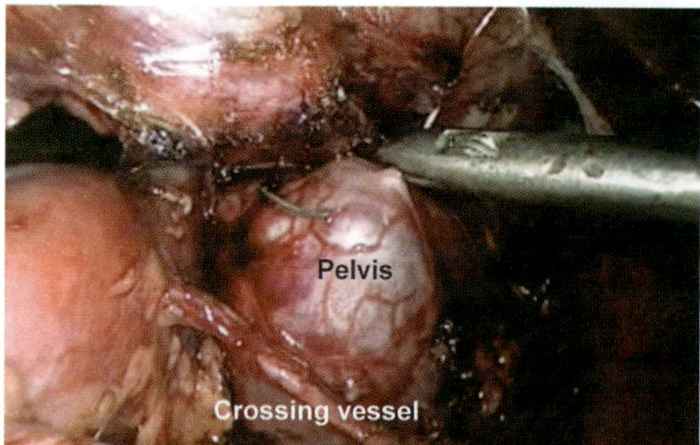

Fig. 6.4: Dissection of crossing vessel

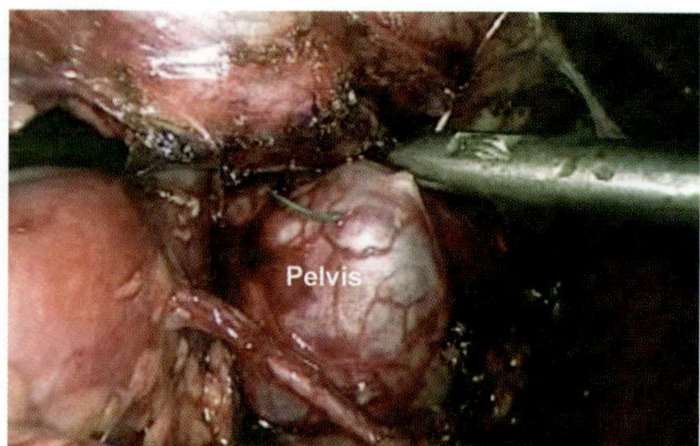

Fig. 6.5: Hitch stitch

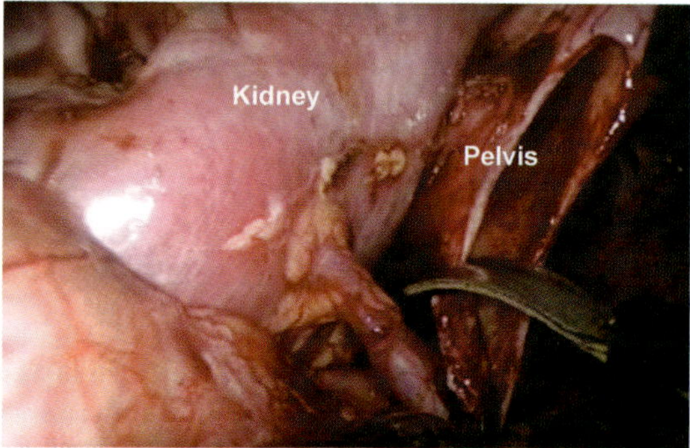

Fig. 6.6: Pyelotomy

opposite the pelviureteric junction. The stitch is taken with a straight needle either a silk or polypropylene. Thereafter, the stitch is passed through the anterior wall of the pelvis **(Fig. 6.5)**. The advantage of passing such a stitch is that the ureteropelvic junction is well aligned. In addition, during the critical step of spatulation the hitched up pelvis helps in aligning the dependent pelvis with the spatulated ureter. The position of the transabdominal stitch is important as the aim of this stitch is to lift the pelvis in the right direction. In addition, the advantage of a transabdominal hitch stitch is that it helps in identifying the most dependent part of the pyelotomy.

5. *Pyelotomy:* We prefer to perform the pyelotomy by starting the incision near the hitch stitch. Typically from an ergonomic perspective it is easier to perform the pyelotomy using the left hand for a left-sided procedure and using the right hand for a right-sided procedure. The caveat for this step is that the incision should not extend to the lower pole calyx. This, if done, runs the risk of developing a lower pole infundibular stenosis. The incision on the pelvis should be done till the dependent part of the incision is reached **(Fig. 6.6)**.

6. *Spatulation:* Optimal spatulation of the ureter is the key to success. The different surrogate markers to define appropriate spatulation are evidence of opening up of the strictured segment. Adequate spatulation is evident if longitudinal ureteral folds are seen. It is easier to spatulate the right ureter with the right hand of the surgeon while the left ureter is preferentially spatulated with the left hand **(Fig. 6.7)**.

7. *Suturing:* The important points to be considered are the length of the suture, the type of suture material and the needle used.

Length of suture material: The ideal length of suture would be between 10 and 14 cm. The length of the suture is decided on the length of the pyelotomy incision and the suture line. Too long a suture would make the suturing difficult.

Type of Suture Material

Vicryl: The suture material has a good memory. It has a good knot tying ability.

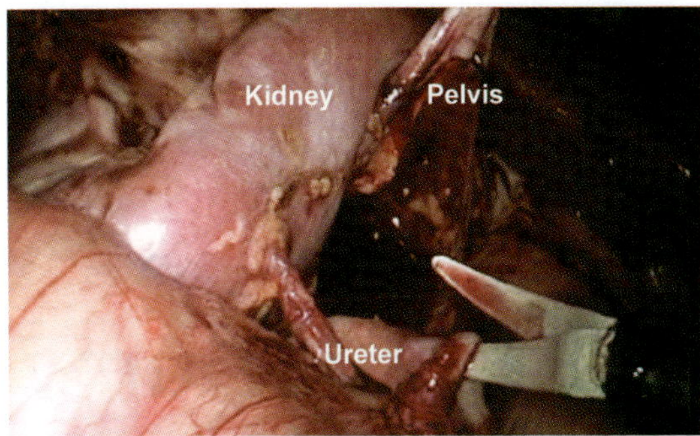

Fig. 6.7: Spatulation

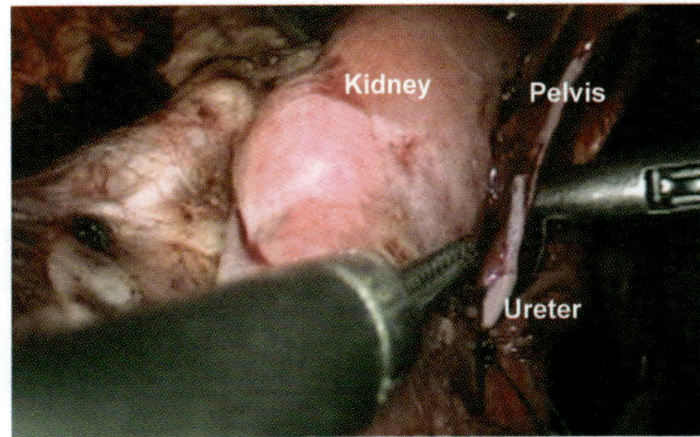

Fig. 6.9: Posterior wall closure

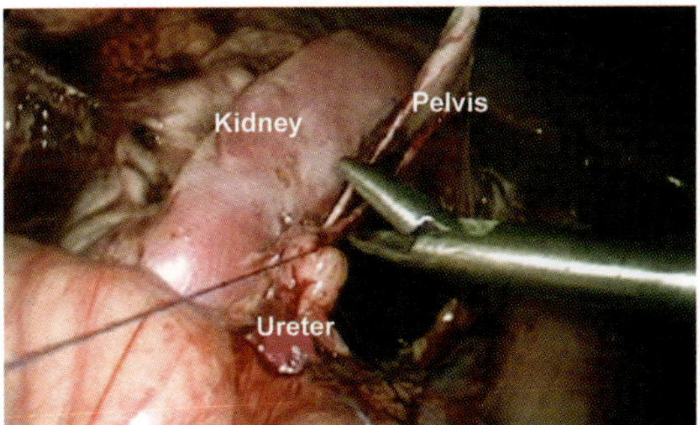

Fig. 6.8: Corner stitch

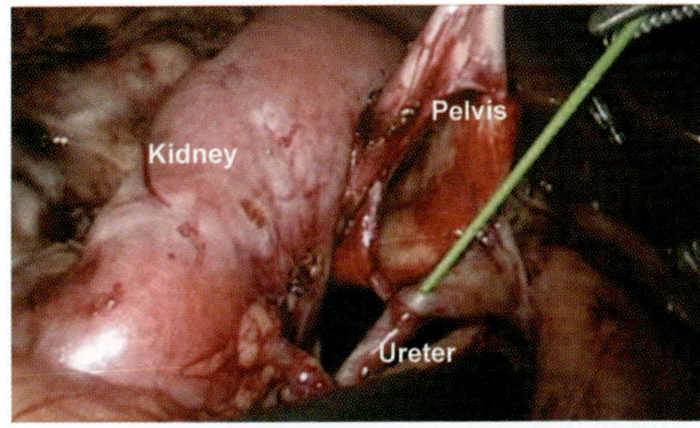

Fig. 6.10: Anterior wall closure with DJ stenting

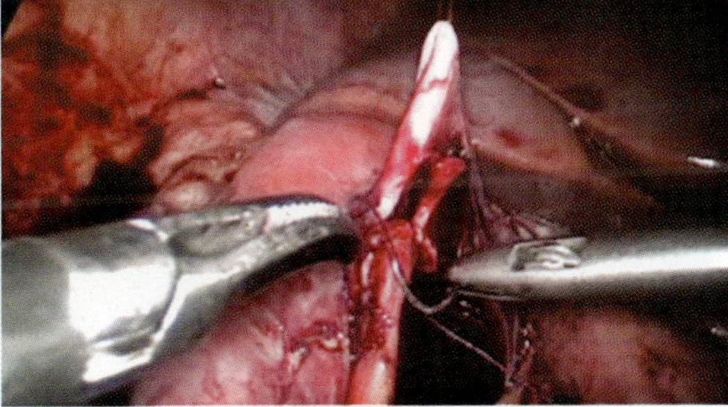

Fig. 6.11: Pyelotomy closure

Monocryl: It has good tissue holding property. However, this suture material does not have memory and hence the knot tends to loosen.

Bidirectional sutures: Typically used if the surgeon is not careful about as in robotic prostatectomy.

The angle stitch is critical and this should pass exactly through the "V" of the spatulation. The redundant pelvis should not be excised **(Fig. 6.8)** till the end as this acts as a handle for manipulating and adhering to the principles of no touch technique in pyeloplasty. Once the spatulated ureter is sutured to the dependent pelvis, the needle is brought below the neo UPJO so that the medial/posterior wall is sutured **(Fig. 6.9)**, and following this the anterior/lateral wall is sutured **(Fig. 6.10)**. A stent when deemed necessary can be passed through a miniport after the completion of the medial/posterior wall. On the contrary, the pigtail/ureteric catheter placed at the beginning can be changed to a DJ stent at the completion of the procedure under fluoroscopy. The pyelotomy is closed as a continuation of either the medial or lateral wall suture **(Fig. 6.11)**.

Postoperative drain is indicated if the pelvis friable, sutures are cutting through or if the surgeon that the anastomosis is not secure.

7

Tips and Tricks in Laparoscopic Radical Nephrectomy

Raghunath S Krishnappa, Nagaraja VH, Srivatsa N, KR Seetharam Bhat, Tejus C, Abhishek Singh, Arvind P Ganpule

There are currently five laparoscopic approaches to renal surgery: Transperitoneal, retroperitoneal, hand assisted, robotic, and laparoendoscopic single-site surgery (LESS) and natural orifice transluminal endoscopic surgery (NOTES). This chapter would focus on the transperitoneal and retroperitoneal approaches.

The choice of surgical technique should be based on patient-specific considerations (e.g. tumor location and size) and the technical expertise available. In most institutions, laparoscopic radical nephrectomy (LRN) has replaced open radical nephrectomy (ORN) in many patients, especially if the tumour size is less than 10 cm. Numerous studies have established the oncologic outcomes of LRN to be equivalent to that of ORN.

TRANSPERITONEAL APPROACH

Preparation, Positioning and Port Insertion

As described in the section of port positioning for renal surgery **(Fig. 7.1)**.

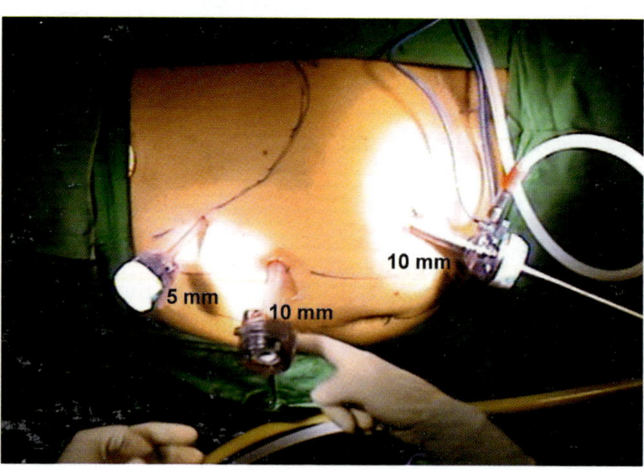

Fig. 7.1: Port placement for laparoscopic radical nephrectomy

Operative Technique

- Reflection of colon and dissection of upper pole of kidney **(Fig. 7.2)**

Left: The white line of Toldt is incised from the level of iliac vessels inferiorly, through the splenophrenic attachments. Splenocolic ligament should be incised to allow the spleen, colon and tail of pancreas to fall medially. The thin colorenal attachments are incised and the plane between the mesentery of the ascending/descending colon and anterior surface of Gerota's fascia is identified. Mesenteric fat has a brighter hue of yellow compared with the retroperitoneal or Gerota's fat, which allows for identification of the correct plane of dissection. Identifying these natural tissue planes are easier with proper traction-countertraction maneuvers. The main distinguishing feature between simple and radical nephrectomy is that the Gerota's fascia and fat are removed with the kidney in LRN as against the simple nephrectomy.

Right: Incise the white line of Toldt from base of cecum, extending cephalad and then through the triangular ligament of the liver. The 5 mm port in the epigastrium is used to pass a self-retaining forceps, which is passed beneath the liver edge and affixed to the upper edge of the incision in the line of Toldt. Medial traction on the colon reveals colorenal attachments that should be divided to complete the colon reflection. Avoid thermal injury to gallbladder and duodenum. A Kocher maneuver may be required to fully expose the medial portion of the kidney and the connective tissue overlying the renal hilum and inferior vena cava.

- Dissection of the lower pole of kidney and ureter **(Fig. 7.3)**

Left: At the lower pole of the kidney, the ureter and gonadal vein are identified. In the upper 1/3 of its course, the gonadal vein is medial to the ureter. A plane is created medial to the gonadal vein and ureter, and continued until the psoas muscle is encountered. Transection of the gonadal vein in male may result in transient testicular pain in the postoperative period. Left renal vein receives gonadal vein, adrenal vein and lumbar vein. Knowing where to look for the veins is vital for preventing vascular injury and minimizing blood loss. The most insidious of the three tributaries into the left renal vein is the lumbar vein which is posterior to the renal vein and can result in significant bleeding if injured. Ureter is

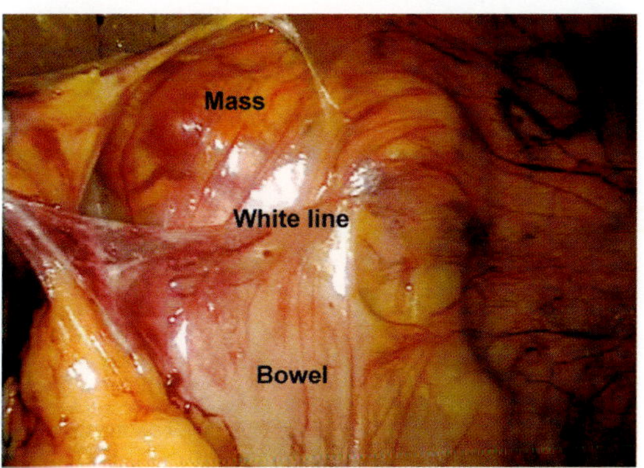

Fig. 7.2: Bowel reflection

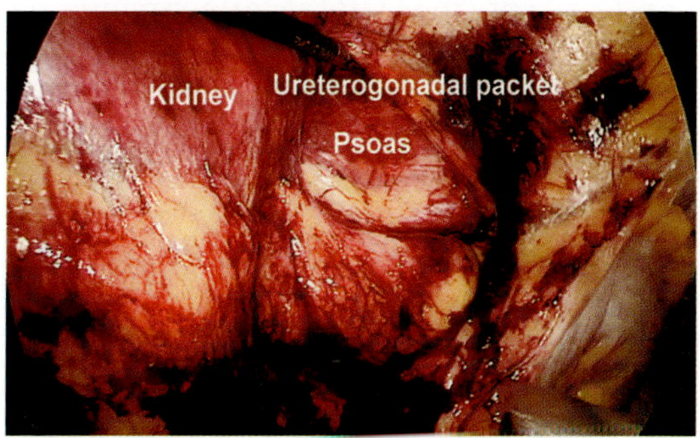

Fig. 7.3: Dissection of lower pole with lifting of ureterogonadal packet

identified just deep to the gonadal vessels ("water under the bridge"). The ureter is not divided at this time, because it can be used to help elevate the kidney. Care should be taken to stay above the psoas fascia to minimize postoperative thigh numbness.

Right: The gonadal vein enters the IVC near the lower pole of the kidney so it is usually preserved.

- *Renal hilar dissection:* There are generally three ways to address the renal hilum: Anterior (most commonly done), posterior, and inferior approach with a "renal lift" maneuver. The renal vein is usually clearly seen and is readily exposed by blunt dissection, but the renal artery is surrounded by a thick layer of lymphatic tissue that requires sharp dissection before it is clearly exposed. Safe dissection of the hilum requires medial retraction of the colon and bowel, and anterolateral retraction of the kidney **(Fig. 7.4)**.

  For an anterior approach, on the right side, the vena cava is dissected to expose the origin of the renal vein. The renal artery is usually located directly posterior or slightly inferior to the right renal vein.

  On the left side, the renal vein is found by following the left gonadal vein superiorly, to its insertion into the renal vein.

  The posterior approach requires the release of the lateral attachments of the kidney for complete medial rotation of the kidney. The renal artery pulsations will be first encountered. One must be aware that the artery crosses posterior to IVC on the right side **(Fig. 7.5)**.

- Ligation of renal blood vessels
  Three options: Endovascular gastrointestinal (GI) stapler, Weck Hem-o-lok clips and titanium clips **(Figs 7.6 and 7.7)**.

  First the artery is divided and then the vein. In 2006 and 2011, the manufacturer of Weck Hem-o-lok ligating clips (Teleflex Medical) and the Food and Drug Administration respectively issued alerts stating that Weck Hem-o-lok ligating clips are contraindicated for the ligation of the renal artery during laparoscopic donor nephrectomy owing to a few donor deaths

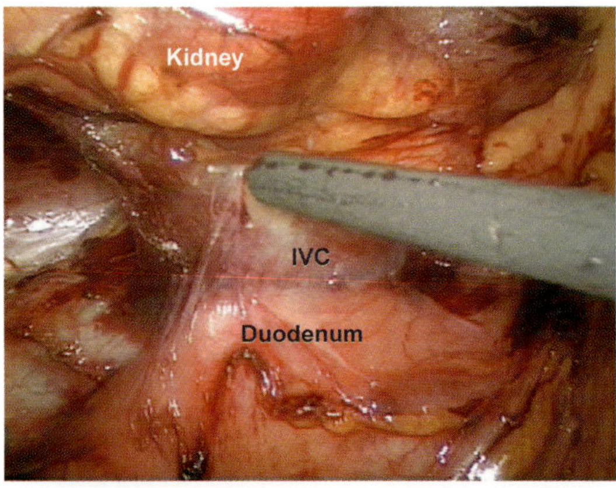

Fig. 7.5: Kocherization on right side

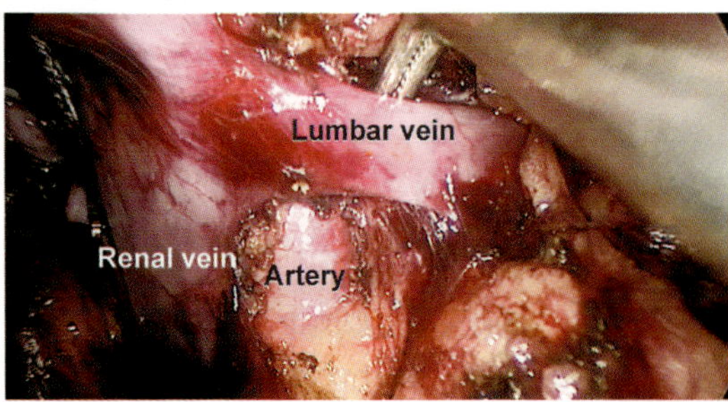

Fig. 7.4: Hilar dissection

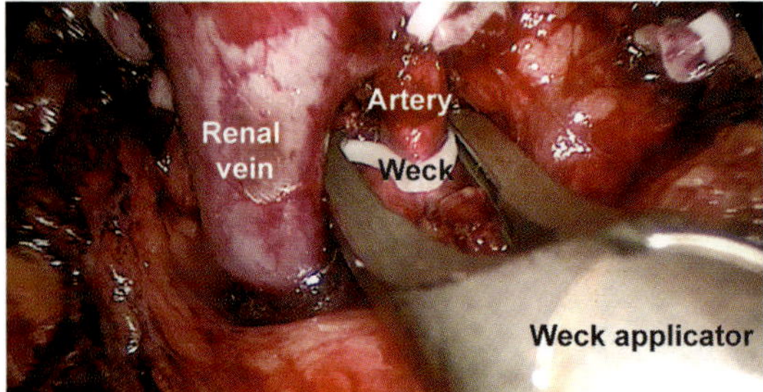

Fig. 7.6: Renal artery clipping

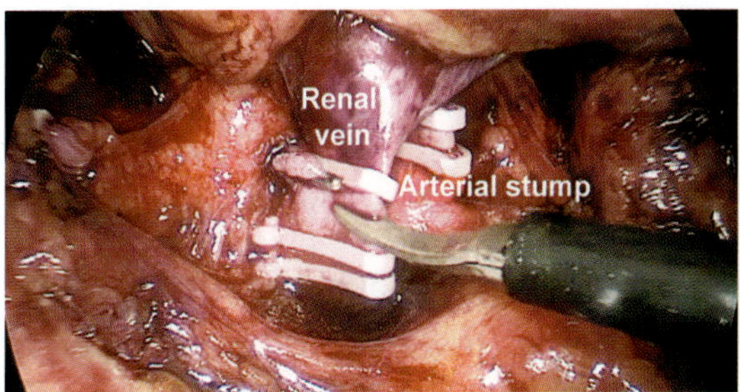

Fig. 7.7: Renal vein clipping

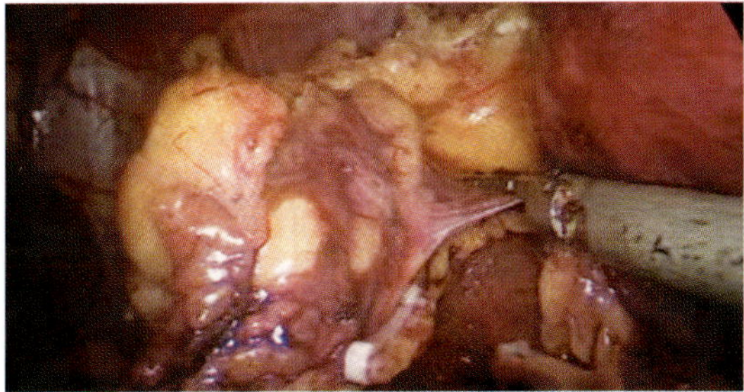

Fig. 7.8: Isolation of upper pole and adrenal gland

linked to failure of the clips in ligating the vessel. But Hem-o-lok clips are still being used safely in majority of the LRN cases in India.

- *Isolation of upper pole and adrenal gland:* The adrenal may be removed en bloc with the kidney when indicated **(Fig. 7.8)**. In adrenal sparing surgery, the Gerota's fascia is opened over the upper medial aspect of the kidney. The perinephric fat is then gently peeled off circumferentially above the upper pole of the kidney. It may be necessary to clip and transect the ureter at this point, to reflect kidney anteriorly for easy upper pole dissection.
- *Regional lymphadenectomy:* Suspected lymph nodes may be removed, and a full hilar or retroperitoneal dissection can be carried out if necessary based on preoperative factors.

    For left-sided renal masses, the lymphatic tissue on the anteromedial surface of the aorta from the level of the superior mesenteric artery cranially to the bifurcation of the aorta caudally is removed.

    For right-sided renal masses, when lymphadenectomy is considered, the paracaval, precaval, retrocaval, and inter-aortocaval nodes from the right crus of the diaphragm to the bifurcation of the IVC are sampled.

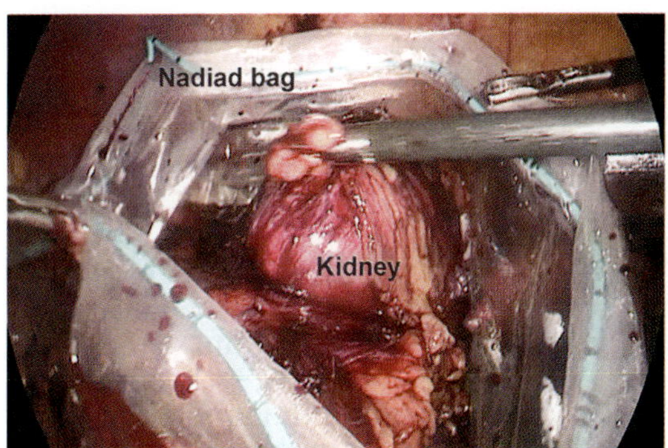

Fig. 7.9: Bagging of specimen

- *Organ retrieval:* The kidney can be removed intact through a separate incision or by morcellation in a sac **(Fig. 7.9)**. Histopathology report may be compromised if morcellated.
- *Port site closure:* As a rule, all midline ports greater than or equal to 10 mm, and all non-midline ports greater than 12 mm are closed. In more obese patients, Carter-Thomason device is used to approximate fascia under direct vision.

Scan QR Code for Video on
Laparoscopic Radical Nephrectomy

RETROPERITONEAL APPROACH

The patient is placed in the lateral flank position with a kidney bridge or flexing the table. The primary port is placed using a 1.5 cm incision below the 12th rib at mid-axillary line, deepened down to the thoracolumbar fascia. A retroperitoneal space is created using Gaur balloon (tying the finger of a glove over a K-90 catheter) and inflating it with saline up to 500–700 ml. Two secondary ports are inserted under laparoscopic vision. Second port (10 mm) at renal angle, at least 3 finger breadths distant from first port and third port (5 mm), 3 finger breadths anterior to first port, forming a straight line with the other ports.

After port insertion, standard surgical steps in sequence are followed: Ureter identification → hilar vessel dissection and division → kidney mobilization.

Transperitoneal Versus Retroperitoneal Laparoscopic Radical Nephrectomy (LRN)

Several retrospective and a few prospective studies have been performed comparing the transperitoneal and retroperitoneal approaches for LRN. The retroperitoneal approach seems to have the disadvantage of a limited working space and difficulty in orientation due to the absence of clear landmarks. However, it can provide a rapid and direct access to the renal hilum.

The transperitoneal approach, in contrast, has a large working space with easier orientation, but the access to the renal hilum requires mobilization and retraction on the bowel. Despite these technical differences, there appear to be no differences in terms of complications between these two approaches.

In practice, the choice of approach is influenced by tumor location, patient's body habitus, previous intra-abdominal surgery, and surgeon factors such as personal preference, technical skills and learning curve.

Important Surgical Caveats (Bail me out)

- If you are struggling, do not hesitate to place a 5 mm port to provide a better working angle.
- When dissecting the midportion of the kidney medially on right side, the first structure encountered will always be the duodenum, not the IVC. Temporarily lowering the pneumoperitoneum to 5 mm Hg will help it to fill out.
- The hook can be used to dissect on the anterior wall of IVC. When approaching the lower pole, beware of the insertion of the gonadal vein on the anterolateral surface of the IVC.
- *Bowel injuries:* Minimize use of monopolar energy. Use cold scissors/bipolar/ultrasonic energy instead.
- *Splenic injuries:* Minimize traction.
- *Diaphragmatic injuries:* Minimize use of cautery at the upper pole of the kidney.
- *Renal hilum injuries:* Avoid metallic clips. When stapler is used, pay attention not to include metallic clips in the staple line. Always inspect the cartridge of the stapler before use. When Hem-o-lok clips are used, follow the above instructions.
- *Local and port-site metastases:* Use endobag and avoid morcellation.
- *Chylous ascites and lymphoceles:* Clip large lymphatics that crossover the left renal vein.

8

Tips and Tricks in Laparoscopic Ureteric Reimplantation

Rohan Batra, Arvind P Ganpule

INTRODUCTION

Laparoscopic ureteric reimplantation is the procedure used to correct lower ureteric strictures or reflux. The most common causes of lower ureteric pathologies in adults are iatrogenic (endourological procedure or other pelvic surgeries), primary obstructive megaureter, reflux (VUR), inflammatory or malignancy. The treatment of lower ureteric pathology depends on the etiology of the disease. Cases which are not amenable to endoscopic treatment require a ureteric reimplant. Certain cases may require adjunct procedures like a psoas hitch or a boari flap. The laparoscopic technique offers numerous advantages over traditional open surgery, including reduced postoperative pain, shorter hospital stays, faster recovery, and improved outcomes. Here, we will explore the step-by-step approach to performing laparoscopic ureteric reimplantation, highlighting key considerations, potential challenges, and the benefits associated with this technique.

Evaluation and Patient Selection

Before undertaking laparoscopic ureteric reimplantation, a comprehensive preoperative evaluation is crucial. This evaluation includes a thorough medical history review, physical examination, laboratory tests, imaging studies (such as ultrasound, CT scan, DTPA scan) to assess renal function and identify any associated abnormalities. Patient selection is vital, and factors such as anatomical variations, body habitus, previous surgeries, and comorbidities must be considered.

Patient Preparation and Anaesthesia

This involves ensuring the patient is adequately informed about the surgery, risks, benefits, and expected outcomes. Bowel preparation is not necessary before this procedure. General anesthesia is required with a lithotomy position with Trendelenburg position.

A cystoscopy should be done before the procedure to see the ureteric orifice. We prefer to place a 5 Fr ureteric catheter before embarking upon the laparoscopy part of the procedure. After placing the ureteric catheter, a Foley's catheter is placed.

In some cases, the DJ stent is already placed in the ureter. In that case, the DJ stent can be replaced with a 5 Fr ureteric catheter. In case the ureteric catheter does not pass through the stricture part, the guidewire can be passed through while the ureteric catheter is kept up to the lower part of the stricture.

Trocar Placement and Instrumentation

The pneumoperitoneum is established through an umbilical incision. A 10 mm

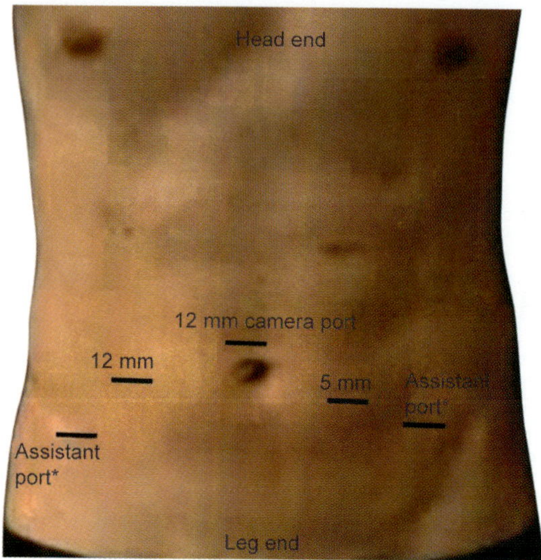

Fig. 8.1: Port position for the surgery

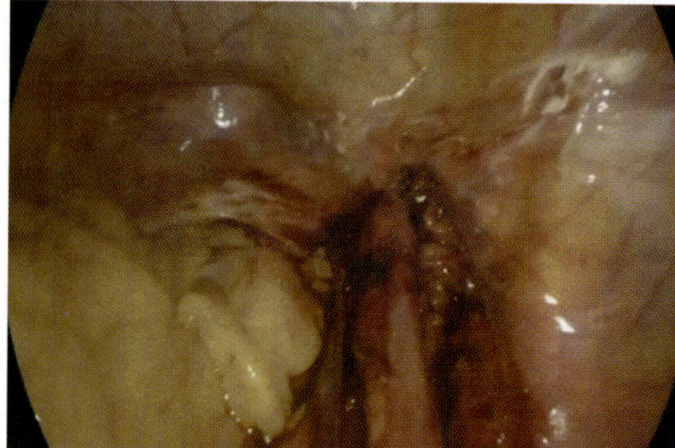

Fig. 8.2: Laparoscopic view of ureter and bladder after ureteric dissection

umbilical port is used for the laparoscope. After visualising the peritoneum for any adhesions and ruling out any injury, the patient is placed in a Trendelenburg position. This helps in visualization and bowel displacement. Additional 10 mm and 5-mm ports are placed 7–8 cm away from the midline. It is important to ensure proper trocar placement to optimize exposure and minimal instrument movement **(Fig. 8.1)**.

Exposure and Dissection

Once the trocars are in place, adequate exposure of the surgical field is important. This involves mobilizing and dissecting the lower ureters to the level of the ureterovesical junction. The ureter is identified beneath a layer of peritoneum just at the bifurcation of iliac vessels. Gentle tissue handling and meticulous dissection are crucial to avoid inadvertent injury to adjacent structures and preserve blood supply of the ureters. Careful attention should be made to the vascular supply, particularly in cases where previous surgeries or inflammatory processes may have caused anatomical distortions. Ureterolysis is

carried out in caudally to preserve the blood supply of the ureter. Gentle handling of the bladder helps in reducing postoperative bladder spasms.

Ureteral Mobilization and Reimplantation

After adequate exposure is achieved, the next step is ureteral mobilization and reimplantation **(Fig. 8.2)**. The ureter is carefully dissected from the surrounding tissues, maintaining its blood supply. This is followed by transection of the ureter at an appropriate distance from the bladder, creating a healthy segment for reimplantation. The position of the neo-hiatus should be such that it should correspond well with the anatomical course of the ureter. The distal ureter is then spatulated medially to create a wider opening for anastomosis, while ensuring that the ureteral blood supply is preserved. The rugosities of the ureteric mucosa will indicate that the spatulation has been adequate and ureter at spatulation area is healthy **(Fig. 8.3)**.

Then the bladder is filled and the bladder is dissected from the anterior abdominal wall between the obliterated umbilical ligament and umbilicus. The space of Retzius is entered and a proper place is decided for neocystotomy **(Fig. 8.4)**. At this juncture, the bladder is filled with around 150–200 ml

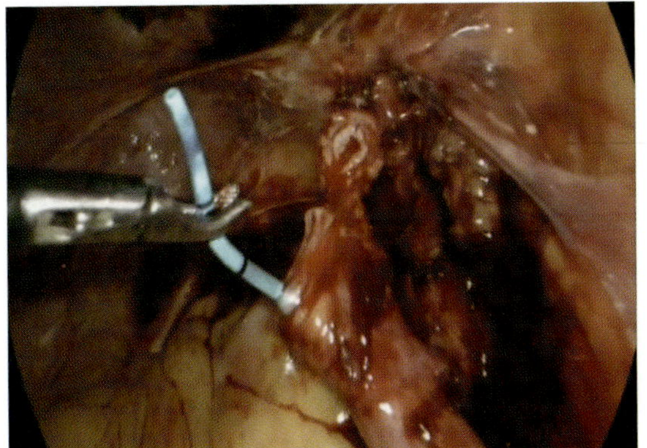

Fig. 8.3: Dissection of ureter, ureteric catheter is seen

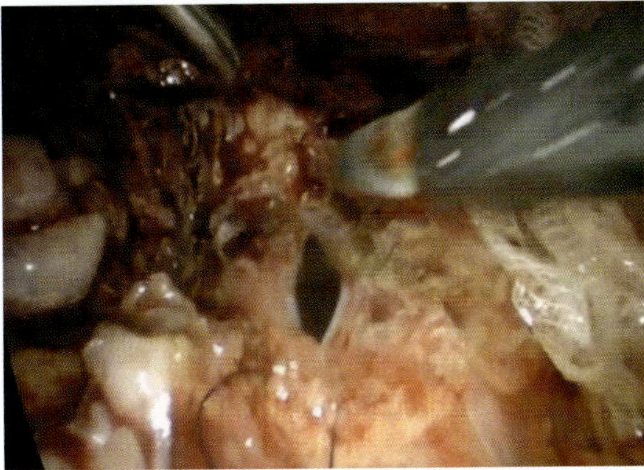

Fig. 8.5: Cystotomy incision

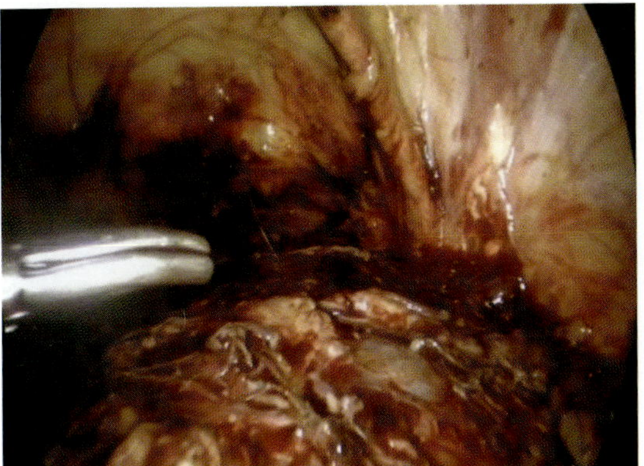

Fig. 8.4: Dissection of urinary bladder and marking of cystotomy site

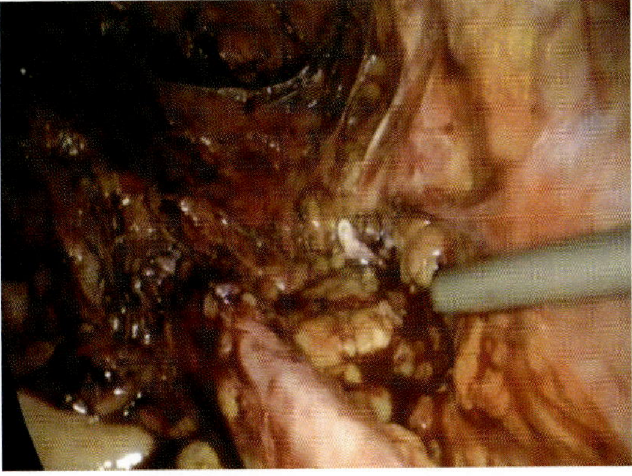

Fig. 8.6: Ureteric reimplant completed

saline. The bladder serosa and muscle fibers are divided with the help of hook cautery and blunt dissection until the bladder mucosa is visualized. If there is a megaureter, then tailoring of the excess ureter can be made and excess ureter can be cut **(Fig. 8.5)**. The corner stitch is taken with the help of 3–0 polyglactin sutures (vicryl or monocryl) with mucosa of bladder and whole thickness of ureter. After that, one wall of the anastomosis is closed with the help of continuous sutures. After that, DJ stent over guidewire is placed with the help of a miniport inserted infraumbilically in midline. After proper placement of the DJ stent, other wall of anastomosis is done in the same manner **(Fig. 8.6)**. The detrusor fibers can be closed with interrupted sutures. In some cases, if the anastomosis is in tension, then psoas hitch is done. The DJ stent is kept for 4–6 weeks and removed thereafter. If the lower end of the ureter does not reach the dome of the bladder, then Boari flap is made of approximately 5 cm base. The principle is that the anastomosis should be tension free. If any suspicion of impaired blood supply is there, the anastomosis site can be covered with an omental wrap.

The integrity of the anastomosis is tested by either performing a cystoscopy, filling of bladder with saline or injecting methylene blue dye into the bladder and assessing for leakage. However, it is not done routinely. An intraperitoneal drain can be kept for 2–3 days. The trocars are then removed, and the incisions are closed.

Postoperatively, patients are closely monitored for any signs of complications such as infection, bleeding, or urinary leakage. Pain management, early ambulation, and appropriate antibiotic prophylaxis are essential. Patients are typically discharged within 2–3 days. The catheter can be removed between 5 and 10 days and a 1-month follow-up appointment is scheduled to assess their progress and remove DJ stent.

CONCLUSION

Laparoscopic ureteric reimplantation is an effective and minimally invasive surgical technique for treating ureteral defects or reflux. With careful patient selection, meticulous surgical technique, and appropriate postoperative care, it offers several advantages over open surgery, including reduced pain, shorter hospital stays, faster recovery, and improved cosmetic outcomes.

9

Tips and Tricks in Laparoscopic Orchiopexy

Rohan Batra, Arvind P Ganpule

INTRODUCTION

Undescended testes, also known as cryptorchidism, is a common congenital condition characterized by the absence of one or both testes in the scrotal sac. If left untreated, it can lead to long-term complications such as infertility and an increased risk of testicular cancer. Laparoscopic orchiopexy is a minimally invasive surgical technique through which we can bring the intra-abdominal testis to the scrotum. Here, we will explore the step-by-step approach to perform laparoscopic orchiopexy, highlighting its benefits, potential challenges, and outcomes associated with this surgical technique.

Preoperative Evaluation and Patient Selection

A comprehensive preoperative evaluation is crucial before undertaking laparoscopic orchiopexy. This includes a detailed medical history review, physical examination, and imaging studies such as ultrasound. In many cases, USG cannot determine the position of testis, so magnetic resonance imaging (MRI) can be done to identify the position and location of the undescended testis. However, a diagnostic laparoscopy has to be explained to the patient and parents. Patient selection is essential, as factors such as age, testicular

position, and associated anomalies can influence the surgical approach and success rate. Also, any syndromic associations, endocrine disorders have to be determined before any surgical procedure. The ideal definitive management of an undescended testis should take place between 6 and 12 months of age. However, many a times, patients present very late in their teens. At that point, a detailed discussion should be done regarding the success of procedure with respect to fertility issues.

Patient Preparation and Anaesthesia

The patient and their parents or guardians should be well-informed about the procedure, its risks, benefits, and expected outcomes. Bowel preparation is not required. Patient requires a general anaesthesia with either a modified lithotomy position or a frog-leg position.

Always do a proper examination under anaesthesia again. 18% of the non-palpable testis become palpable under general anaesthesia.

Trocar Placement and Instrumentation

Once the patient is properly anesthetized and positioned, trocars are inserted for laparoscopic access. The pneumo-peritoneum is usually created using an open access in small

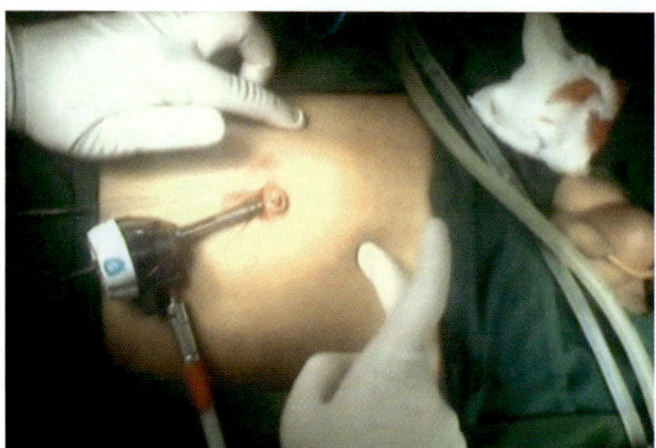

Fig. 9.1: Port placement for left laparoscopic orchiopexy

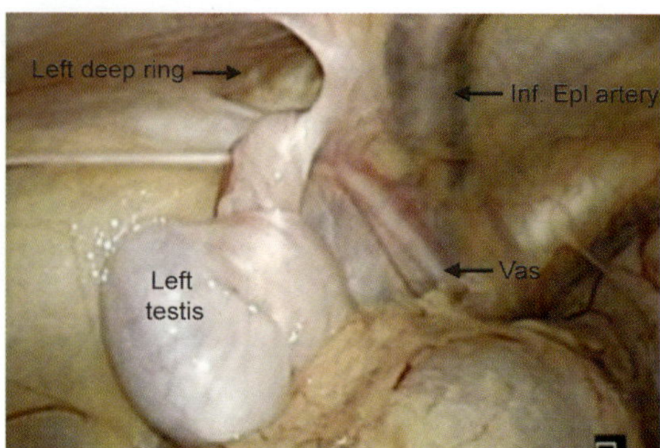

Fig. 9.2: Laparoscopic view of left UDT with deep ring, vas and inferior epigastric artery

children at the umbilicus. A 5-mm umbilical port is usually used for the laparoscope. Additional 5-mm ports are placed strategically for instrumentation considering the rules of triangulation. The working trocars are placed 6–8 cm away from the camera port with triangulation done towards the ipsilateral deep inguinal ring. Proper trocar placement is crucial for optimal visualization and instrument maneuverability **(Fig. 9.1)**.

Exploration and Identification of the Undescended Testis

The laparoscope is introduced, and the abdomen is insufflated to create a pneumoperitoneum. Then, the undescended testis is located and relations with iliac vessels is determined. This can be done by systematically examining the inguinal region, the inguinal canal, iliac vessels and vas. Careful identification of the testicular blood vessels and the vas deferens is necessary to ensure their preservation during the procedure. The anatomy of an undescended testis is of utmost importance. Care should be taken to identify if there is a long looping vas, as it is the most important structure that should not be damaged.

The variations that can be encountered during the laparoscopy are patent processes vaginalis, peeping testis (with external pressure on the inguinal canal, the peeping testicle can be visualized) and vanishing testis (blind ending vessels) **(Fig. 9.2)**.

Mobilization of Testis and Examining Vessel Length

Once the undescended testis is identified, it is mobilized. This is achieved by gently dissecting the testis from its surrounding lateral attachments first while preserving its blood supply. Sometimes, the lateral dissection has to be proceeded higher up. After dissecting the lateral attachments, median attachments up to the medial umbilical ligaments are released. After dissecting lateral and medial attachments, the gubernaculum is dissected. The gubernaculum can be clipped or taken down with advanced energy. It helps in holding the testis. To assess the adequate length of the testis, it should reach up to the opposite deep inguinal ring. If it reaches the opposite deep inguinal ring, then it is ready to be taken down into the scrotum. The testis is then brought into the inguinal canal or scrotum **(Fig. 9.3)**.

There are various ways in which the testis can be brought down through a scrotal incision.

- Open incision and dilatation through an artery forceps

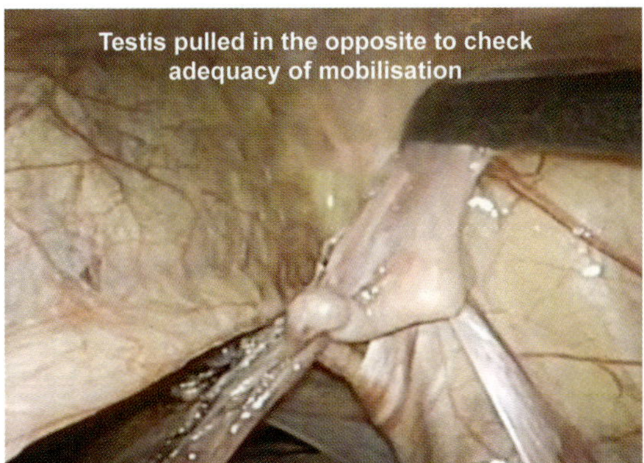

Fig. 9.3: Traction on testis to check the adequacy of mobilisation of testis

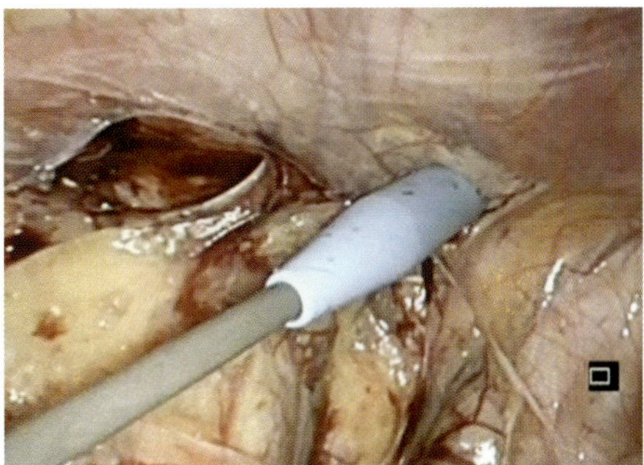

Fig. 9.4: Dilatation of tract with amplatz

- Using a laparoscopic port
- Using Amplatz sheath and dilators **(Fig. 9.4)**

One potential disadvantage of using an open incision and dilatation through an artery forceps is that there is sudden loss of pneumoperitoneum and can lead to difficult manoeuvre during bringing down of testis. A 10 mm laparoscopic port helps in circumventing that disadvantage. Alternatively, we use serial dilatation and Amplatz dilators to create a tunnel. This helps in serial dilatation of tissues which is atraumatic. Also, we can know the exact position of the dilators over guidewire which has to be lateral to the median umbilical ligament. After dilating up to 30 Fr Amplatz, the testis is easily delivered down up to the scrotum.

Closure and Postoperative Care

After successful mobilization, fixation of the testis is done in the subdartos pouch. Care must be taken whether there is any torsion or twist to the cord or not. After placing the testis in the scrotum, a check laparoscopy should also be done to check any tension on the cord, and to ensure full haemostasis. Meticulous closure of the port sites and wound is performed through subcuticular absorbable sutures. Postoperative care includes pain management, observation for any signs of complications, and proper wound care. The patient is usually discharged within two days and scheduled for a monthly follow-up visit to monitor healing and testicular position.

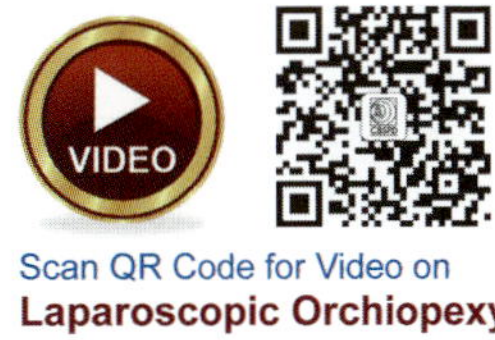

Scan QR Code for Video on
Laparoscopic Orchiopexy

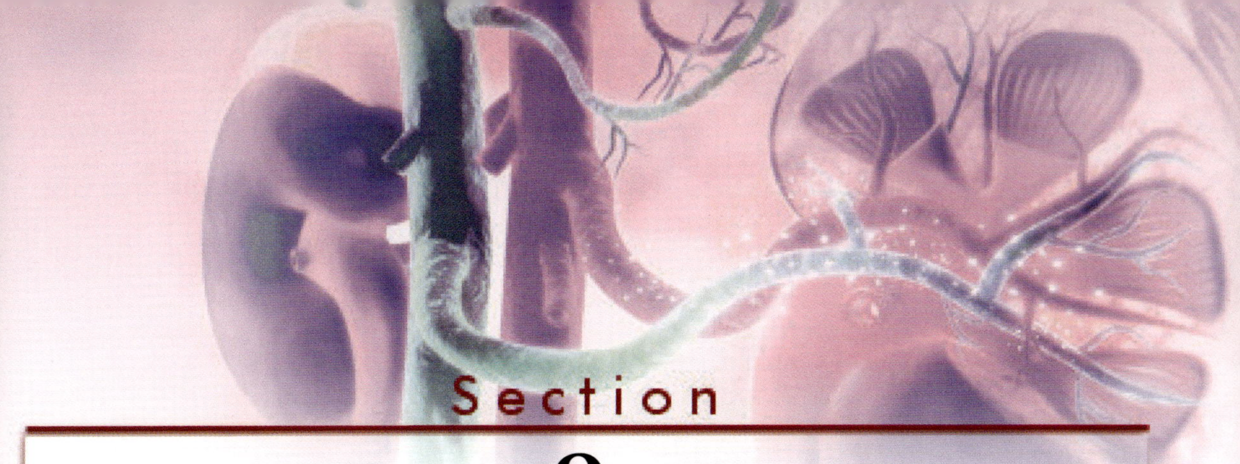

Section

Section

2

Tips and Tricks in Endourology

CHAPTERS

10

Puncture of the Renal Pelvicalyceal System for Percutaneous Renal Surgery

Rajesh Kukreja

HOW SHOULD AN IDEAL PUNCTURE BE?

An ideal puncture should fulfil all of the following criteria **(Fig. 10.1)**:

- The path should be a straight line from the skin passing through the cup of the calyx and the infundibulum to the pelvis.
- It should traverse the minimum renal parenchyma.
- It should give access to the maximum stone burden and the ureteropelvic junction when necessary.
- There should have nil or minimal angulation or torque on the renal parenchyma and the infundibulum.
- Access should be from the cup or fornix of the posterior calyx. Such a puncture would traverse or traumatize the least. Puncture through the infundibulum of a calyx is associated with a significant risk of significant bleeding from interlobar vessels.
- Puncture through the infundibulum of the upper, middle and lower poles was associated with vascular injury in 67.6%, 38.4% and 68.2% of kidneys, respectively. Puncture through the fornix proved to be much safer and it was associated with a venous injury rate of less than 8% and no arterial lesions. Direct puncture into the renal pelvis injured large retropelvic vessels in a third of cases and is also associated with potential prolonged urinary leakage and easy tube dislodgment.[1,2]

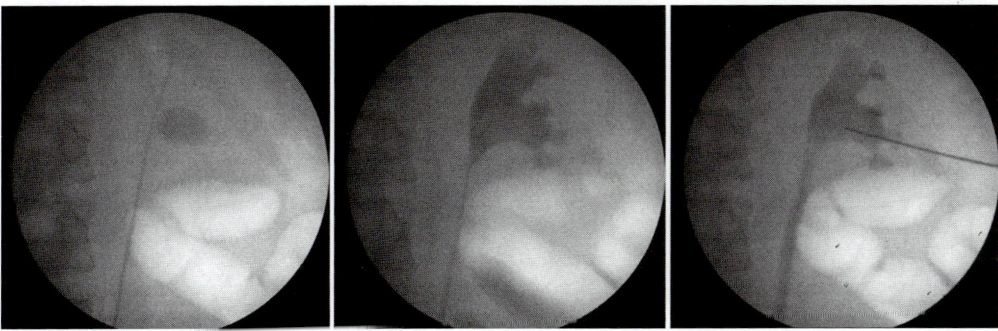

Fig. 10.1: An ideal puncture: The shortest distance from the skin to the cup of calyx in line with the infundibulum and renal pelvis and providing access to the maximum stone burden

The Ideal Initial Puncture Needle

The axial force of a needle during insertion in soft tissue is the summation of different forces distributed along the needle shaft such as stiffness force, frictional force and cutting force. Needle deflection and tissue deformation are major problems for accurate needle insertion.

- A diamond tip needle and not a bevel-tip needle should be used for the initial puncture. A diamond tip needle has symmetrical tip which exerts equal force in all directions on the tissue. Hence, the tissue is cut in the moving direction of the needle tip. A bevel-tip needle exerts forces asymmetrically, so cutting of the tissue occurs at an offset angle depending on the bevel angle, needle flexibility and tissue properties[3] **(Fig. 10.2)**.
- The size of the needle used for puncture is a matter of debate. The options are a 21-gauge needle (which allows a 0.018 inch guidewire) or an 18 gauge needle (which allows a 0.035 inch guidewire). The 18 gauge needle is stiffer but more traumatic. The 21 gauge needle is less traumatic but less stiff and hence cannot maintain the trajectory adequately. Also, the 0.018 inch guidewire that passes through

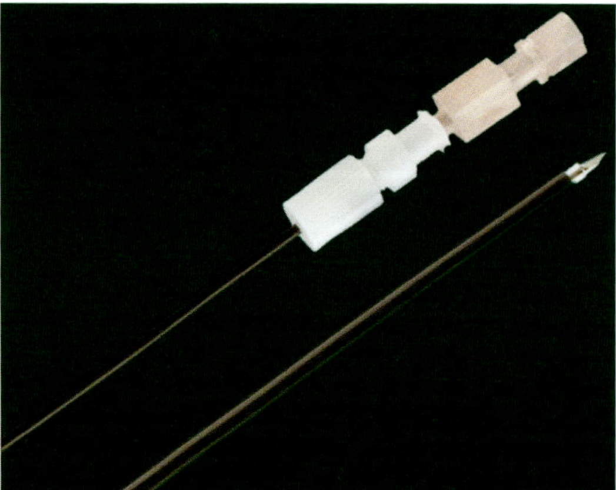

Fig. 10.2: Echotip diamond tip 18G needle (Cook Medical): The Echotip helps visualization during ultrasound-guided puncture

the 21 gauge needle must be exchanged for a standard 0.035 inch guidewire for subsequent tract dilatation. This requires an extra step, which adds to the complexity of the procedure and increases the risk of loss of access. Weighing the pros and cons of both, it would be rational to use the 21 gauge needle when the surgeon is less experienced or if minimizing trauma is the need of the moment. The 18 gauge needle should be used by an experienced surgeon who is confident of attaining access with minimum attempts.[4]

- The safest initial 0.035 inch guidewire to use for upper urinary tract percutaneous access is a PTFE-coated J-wire. The "J" tip makes the guidewire unlikely to perforate out of the collecting system. This guidewire may not easily pass down the ureter, however. A floppy-tip PTFE-coated guidewire or a hydrophilic guidewire with a straight or angled tip passes down the ureter much easily.

Choosing the Correct Entry Calyx

- The calyx of entry should be selected based on the distribution of the stone to be treated. It should give access to the maximum stone burden and the ureteropelvic junction when necessary. The remaining stones if any can be addressed with a second (and rarely a third or more) access or with flexible instrumentation through the initial access site.
- An upper pole calyx is generally the most versatile site to enter the upper urinary tract collecting system. The renal pelvis, lower pole calyces, and ureter usually can be entered with a rigid nephroscope from a well-placed upper pole access. The upper pole access is relatively made simpler due to comparatively dense adhesions of the Gerota's fascia leading to reduced mobility of the upper pole, in addition, anatomically the distance from the skin to the calyx is shorter as compared to the lower pole. Access to the middle calyces

will usually require a separate access or use of flexible instrumentation.

- Middle calyceal entry offers adequate access to the pelvis, ureteropelvic junction and upper ureter.
- Puncture of the lower pole may be slightly more difficult as the freely mobile lower pole moves away from the needle and dilators. Also, the lower pole tracts tend to be longer and more oblique, making stone removal from upper calyces with rigid instruments may be more difficult than the converse. Due to the posterior tilt of the upper pole of the kidney, the lower pole does not offer assured access to the upper pole.

Upper Calyceal Access: Subcostal or Supracostal

The upper portions of both the kidneys are located anterior to the posterior portion of the 11th and 12th ribs. A review of 90 normal supine intravenous urograms during full expiration noted that 85% of upper renal calyces are located above the 12th rib.[5] In the prone position, further cephalad movement of the kidney occurs in 80% of patients.[6]

Subcostal access is the safest route to the kidney because pleural injuries are rare with entry below the 12th rib. Nonetheless, if entry directly above the 12th rib (11th intercostal space) provides the best access to the optimal calyx, then the benefit generally exceeds the risk.

Entry above the 11th rib, however, has a greater potential for pleural and even lung injury, so when the best access calls for a direct puncture above the 11th rib, additional maneuvers could be considered to displace the kidney inferiorly. These include cephalad tilt of a subcostal access sheath placed into a lower calyx and attaining access during full inspiration. Smith et al[7] described the renal displacement technique wherein initial placement of a sheath or dilator is performed via a lower or midcalyx in order to allow for torque of the kidney downward. This can be held by an assistant while upper calyx puncture is performed via a subcostal route. This technique, however, mandates an unnecessary second tract. Another alternative is to angle the upper calyceal access tract cephalad from a subcostal skin entry site. This approach provides limited access to the rest of the kidney and traverses more of the renal parenchyma obliquely with increased chances of bleeding.[8] All of these alternatives can result in severe angulation and torque on the renal infundibula with damage to the infundibular vessels.

Stening and Bourne have discussed in depth the anatomic considerations in the supracostal approach for renal surgery.[9] The lower limit of the parietal pleura crosses the 12th rib obliquely at its midpoint such that the lateral half of the rib is uncovered by the pleura. In the midscapular line, the visceral pleura is in relation to the 10th rib, while the parietal pleura is at the level of the 12th rib **(Fig. 10.3)**. The parietal and visceral pleura

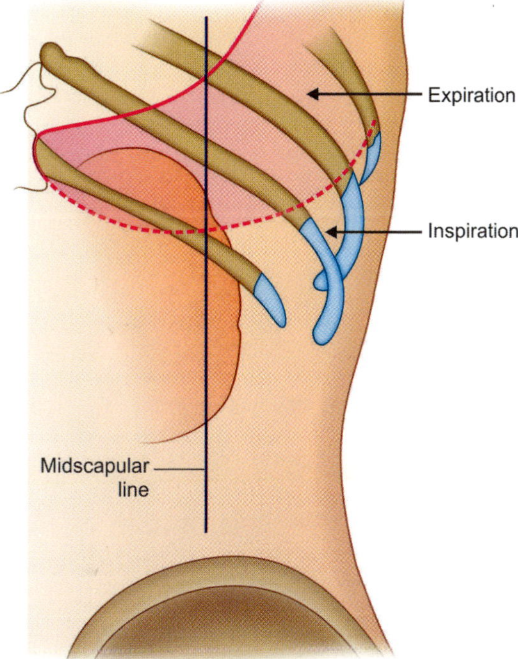

Fig. 10.3: Parietal pleura during phases of respiration: Diagrammatic representation (Stening and Bourne)

ascend cranially and laterally on the ribs, and further rise in deep expiration. Thus, a puncture made lateral to the midscapular line, below the 10th rib, in deep expiration would almost always prevent damage to the visceral pleura **(Fig. 10.4A)**.

Based on the study by Stening and Bourne, important guidelines to reduce thoracic complications would be:
- All intercostal punctures should be done while the lung is deflated during expiration to decrease the risk of pulmonary injury.
- Supracostal access should be performed lateral to the midscapular line to minimize injury to the pleura[9–11] and in line with the calyx of entry, infundibulum and pelvis **(Fig. 10.4B)**.

- The needle should be advanced along the upper margin of the rib during the expiratory phase. Needle passage along the inferior margin of the rib risks injury to the intercostal neurovascular bundle, which can result in significant bleeding.
- The supracostal skin puncture should be done over the lateral portion of the rib, and the puncture should be made during steady, quiet breathing or breath holding in expiration. However, once the needle has passed the diaphragm, the calyceal entry can be made during full inspiration when the kidney descends caudally.[12]
- Access above the 10th rib is associated with a high incidence of pleural violation and lung injury and should be avoided unless absolutely necessary. Thoracoscopic

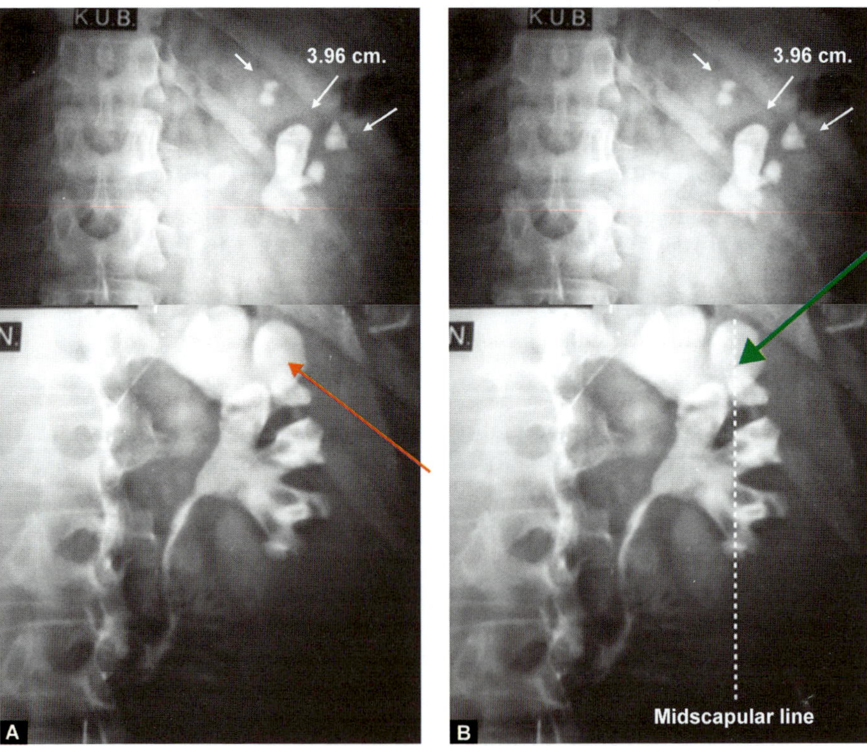

Figs 10.4A and B: Upper calyceal puncture. (A) Incorrect angulated subcostal puncture; (B) Correct supracostal puncture with entry from lateral to the midscapular line

guided access superior to the 10th rib can be performed to reduce the risk of lung injury.[13]

A multicenter retrospective study of patients undergoing percutaneous nephrolithotomy via upper pole access showed that patients with an intercostal approach experienced greater stone-free rates, fewer complications, and reduced operating times compared to patients with a subcostal approach.[14]

Risk of Visceral Injury

In the absence of splenomegaly or hepatomegaly injury to the liver and spleen is extremely rare when the access puncture site is below the 12th rib. However, supracostal access can be associated with an increased risk of injury to the liver and spleen, particularly if puncture is performed during the inspiratory phase of respiration rather than the expiratory phase or the puncture is above the 11th rib.[15,16] To decrease the risk of liver or spleen injury, the skin puncture site should be located as far medial as possible.

Placement of Ureteric Catheter

A retrograde ureteric catheter delineates the ureteral anatomy, as well as the exact stone location, degree of hydronephrosis, and the image of the selected calyx in order to plan the approach to the collecting system.

Advantages of a retrograde ureteric catheter:
- Opacification of pelvicalyceal system.
- Prevents fragment migration down the ureter.
- Retrograde saline flushing during puncture, tract dilatation, and flushing out of fragments.
- Retrograde guidewires can be passed up, if required.
- Injection of methylene blue for identification of the pelvic-ureteric junction (PUJ) or opening of calyceal diverticulum in difficult cases.

The rigid cystoscope is used to place a 0.038 inch Teflon-coated guidewire into the upper collecting system. When a tortuous area blocks the progress of the guidewire, a wire with a hydrophilic coating must be used. This wire is composed of an alloy core, a polyurethane jacket, and a thin hydrophilic polymer as the outer most layer. When in contact with fluid, the polymer binds water to create a lubricious coating with greatly diminished friction, avoiding excessive edema and creation of a false passage.[17] When the guidewire is in position, the 6F catheter is advanced over it to the renal pelvis, and the endoscope is removed. A 16 F Foley catheter is inserted and attached to a drainage bag at the same time. Both the catheters are tied with 2–0 silk to secure them in place. It is helpful to connect an empty syringe to the Luer lock adapter at the end of the ureteral catheter to prevent urine leakage.

Fluoroscopic Guided Access

There are two primary methods used to gain fluoroscopy-guided percutaneous renal access: The "bull's eye" technique and triangulation technique. Both the techniques need a target, most commonly generated by opacification of the collecting system with iodinated contrast that is administered retrograde via a ureteral catheter. A calyceal entry point is selected to avoid the larger vascular structures that are found at the level of the infundibulum.

Identifying the Posterior Calyx on Fluoroscopy

- Preoperative assessment with CT urogram or an IVU helps in identifying the posterior calyces.
- With the patient in prone position, diluted contrast when instilled will fill the dependent anterior calyces first. Thus, the posterior calyces will be filled later and would appear less dense. Injection of 5 to 10 ml of air via the ureteric catheter also

helps to identify the posterior calyces as air will preferentially enter these calyces when the patient is prone.

- The movement of the C-arm can help to identify the posterior calyx. In the prone position, the posterior calyces move in the opposite direction to the image intensifier on the C-arm. If the C-arm is rotated toward the surgeon, then the posterior calyces move away and shorten. Vice versa, if the C-arm is rotated away from the surgeon, then the posterior calyces appear elongated. Thus, by moving the C-arm, away from the surgeon one can identify the laterally placed calyces as posterior and by moving the C-arm toward the surgeon the posterior calyces appear more medially placed and appear end on.

Techniques[4,17–20]

Bull's eye technique: With the C-arm in the 30° position, an 18 G diamond tip access needle is positioned, so that the targeted calyx, needle tip, and needle hub are in line with the image intensifier, giving a bull's eye effect on the monitor. In effect, the surgeon looking down the needle into the targeted calyx. The needle is advanced to 1–2 cm increments using a hemostat to minimize radiation exposure to the surgeon. Continuous fluoroscopic monitoring is performed to ensure that the needle maintains its proper trajectory. Needle depth is ascertained by rotating the C-arm to a vertical orientation. If the needle is aligned with the calyx in this view, the urologist should be able to aspirate urine from the collecting system, confirming proper positioning.

The triangulation technique is based on simple geometric principles and is guided by biplanar fluoroscopy; one plane is antero-posterior (0°) to the line of puncture and the other is oblique (30°) **(Figs 10.5A and B)**. The C-arm can be tilted oblique in any of the four directions:

- Toward or away from the surgeon at right angles to the operating table or
- Toward head end (cephalic) or foot end (caudal) of the patient parallel to the operating table.
- The anteroposterior view may be consi-dered to be in a plane parallel to the

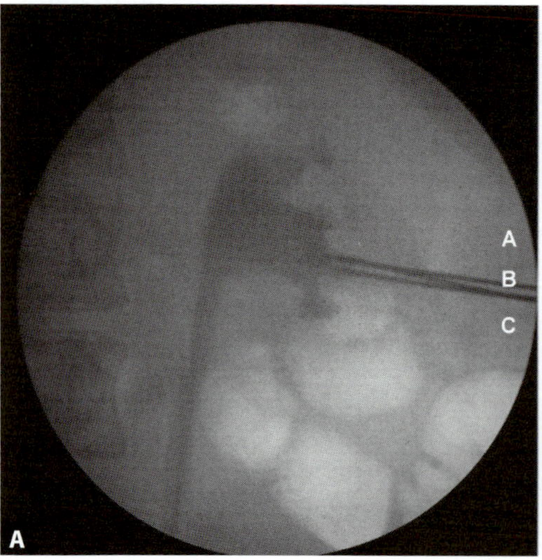

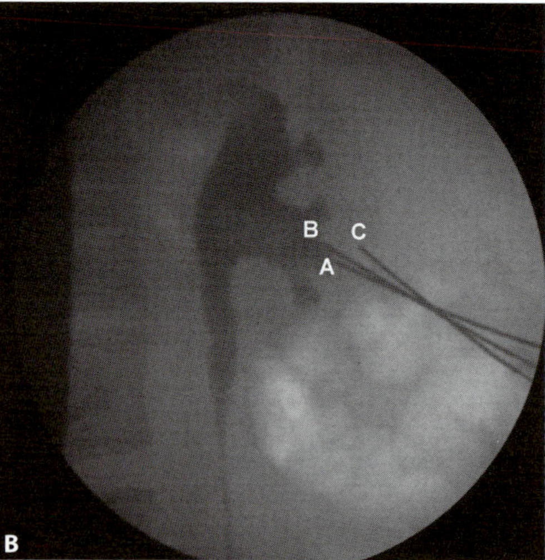

Figs 10.5A and B: (A) C-arm in 0°. All the 3 needles A, B, and C appear to be in the calyx. (C-arm in 30°); (B) Needle A is in the same calyx, needle B is posterior or superficial to the calyx (medial or towards the spine) and needle C is anterior or deep to the calyx (lateral or away from the spine)

axis of puncture and is used to monitor mediolateral (left–right) adjustments.

- The oblique view gives information regarding depth to the site of puncture and is used to monitor needle adjustments in the superficial/deep (posterior/anterior) orientation.
- When making adjustments in the mediolateral axis, care should be taken not to inadvertently move the needle in the cephalad caudad (superficial-deep) axis, and vice versa.
- It may be helpful for the surgeon to rest their arm on the patient during the access part of the procedure, as this minimizes unintended drifting of the needle away from the targeted axis and also provides additional needle stabilization. Once the needle is aligned with the targeted calyx in both the mediolateral and cephalocaudal (superficial-deep) orientations, it is advanced with continuous fluoroscopy.
- The needle should be advanced in the oblique view, which will allow for the assessment of the depth of the needle's penetration.
- It is helpful for the anesthesiologist to hold the patient's respirations while the needle is being advanced, to avoid having to "hit a moving target", as well as to minimize the risk of an inadvertent transthoracic puncture.
- After advancing the needle several centimeters in the oblique view, the anteroposterior view should be examined to confirm that the mediolateral trajectory of the needle is still properly aligned to the target. If necessary, the needle trajectory can be readjusted to maintain proper targeting.
- It is imperative that to minimize trauma to the renal parenchyma, the adjustment of the needle plane should be done when the needle is outside the renal capsule and not when the needle is in the parenchyma.

Manipulating the needle after entering the renal parenchyma may displace and lacerate the kidney and alter the position of the targeted calyx. Again, it is critical not to alter the access needle's orientation in one plane while making adjustments in the other plane, particularly when advancing the needle.

- A slight jiggle of the needle causing indentation of the desired calyx is a further sign that the trajectory of the needle is correct.

Comparing the Two Techniques

- With the "eye-of-the-needle" technique, the proper cephalocaudal (superficial-deep) and mediolateral axes of the needle are verified and maintained on a single fluoroscopic view, and the confirmatory view is necessary only to assure the depth of the needle tip. For the "triangulation" technique, one fluoroscopic view is used to assess the mediolateral axis and another is used to assess the depth or cephalocaudal (superficial-deep) axis.[18]
- In the triangulation technique, the puncture is along the stone axis, i.e. in alignment with the infundibulum. This decreases the need for excessive torque on the renal parenchyma by the rigid instruments, which may cause renal trauma and bleeding. Tepeler et al[21] did a comparison of the bull's eye and the triangulation technique and found no difference between the two as regards operation time, fluoroscopy screening time, duration of hospitalization and blood transfusion rate. They found a slightly greater drop in hematocrit and complication rate in the group undergoing access by the bull's eye technique as compared to the triangulation technique. However, the difference was not statistically different.
- The advantage of the triangulation technique over the "eye-of-the-needle" technique is that the needle cannot be passed

too deeply because the depth of advancement is monitored continuously. Also, the triangulation technique alone fulfils the five criteria of a successful puncture.

- The disadvantage of the triangulation technique is that maintaining both the mediolateral and cephalocaudal (superficial-deep) planes are difficult because both are not being monitored at the same time as in the "eye-of-the-needle" technique. Multiple attempts with excessive use of fluoroscopy may occur especially with a beginner. Usually, during the learning curve the problem comes in the assessment of superficial-deep planes with the C-arm in the oblique position. Whether the needle is superficial-deep to the calyx, has to be ascertained by the surgeon and adjustments made accordingly. The easiest way to determine this would be to place another needle on the skin surface over the target calyx or correlate with the spine. If the calyx is between the two needles or between the spine and the puncture needle, then the puncture needle is deep and should be adjusted superficially. If the target calyx is below the two needles or below the puncture needle and the spine, then the puncture needle is superficial and should be adjusted toward the depth.

Hybrid Technique[19]

- The three most important things needed to achieve a successful percutaneous renal puncture are the site of skin entry, the angle of entry and the depth at which the puncture is achieved.
- Determining the correct point of skin puncture is important in the triangulation technique because a skin puncture that is too medial or lateral to the desired optimum point of entry would result in a tract of variable length and angle of entry in the calyx. This would interfere with

proper access and would cause excessive torque on the parenchyma during maneuvering of the rigid nephroscope in the pelvicalyceal system. To avoid injury to the colon, the puncture should be medial to the posterior axillary line but not too medial as it would traverse the paraspinal muscle causing increased postoperative pain and would probably be directly on the renal pelvis without traversing the renal parenchyma. The puncture that is too close to the rib may injure the intercostal nerve and vessels and hence is to be avoided.

- Sharma described the technique of determining the site of skin puncture, which amalgamates the advantages of both the bull's eye and triangulation technique and hence is called the hybrid technique. With the C-arm at 0°, the site of skin corresponding to the target calyx is marked as point A. The C-arm is then rotated 30° towards the surgeon. The point on the skin corresponding to the target calyx and forming a bull's eye with the needle is marked as point B. In the bull's eye technique we take a puncture at the point B. However, in the triangulation technique, the puncture is along the stone axis in alignment with the infundibulum. If we take the target calyx as the center of a sphere, then we have an imaginary circle on the skin where the point A is the center of the circle. The distance from point A to B will be the radius of the circle. The radius remains the same irrespective of the direction in which it is measured from the center of the circle. Thus, when we take a line along the stone axis where we intend to take a puncture—the site of skin puncture is marked using this principle. This means that the point B1 is marked on the skin such that the distance from point A to B1 is equal to the distance between A to B, i.e. the radius of a circle with the target calyx being its center. B1 is the site of entry on the skin.

- The angle of puncture: In the bull's eye technique, the angle at which the needle is seen as a dot is the angle at which the puncture is made. The hybrid technique utilizes this principle. With the needle at point B and the C-arm rotated 30° towards the surgeon and the needle forming the bull's eye; the angle that the needle makes with the skin surface is measured using a protractor. One needs to take care that the protractor is held parallel to the operating table. Using the principle of sphere and circle, if we are hitting the calyx by using the triangulation technique from the point B1—the angle of puncture would be the same with probably variations of 1–2 due to the not so perfectly flat contours of the body surface.

- The third component of the hybrid technique is to determine the depth of puncture. What we have till now is an imaginary triangle where we know: (1) One side—the distance between point A to B which is marked on the skin; (2) One angle, which is 90° with the C-arm at 0°; and (3) Another angle, which is measured using the protractor at the point B. With this information, by using the universal triangle solver application from Google play store we can determine the depth. In this application, if we put the two angles and one side, then by the law of sines, it calculates the other two sides and the angle. For example, if the distance AB is 4 cm and the angle calculated by the protractor is 65° and with the other angle always being 90° by universal triangle solver—the depth will be 9.5 cm.

Confirmation of an Ideal Posterior Calyceal Puncture

- If air has been instilled during opacification of the pelvicalyceal system, sudden release of air followed by a free flow of clear saline instilled through the ureteric catheter.

- When the glidewire is passed maintaining the angle of the needle, it enters the pelvis easily. No manipulation is needed. On the contrary, if the anterior calyx has been punctured, then the glidewire will be coiled in the calyx, will not enter the pelvis easily or will do so only after much manipulation.

- If at the point of withdrawing the trocar of the needle spontaneous output of urine has not been observed, it is advisable gently to try to introduce a hydrophilic guidewire, observing the advancement of the guidewire under fluoroscopy. Typically, it moves into the cavity of the calyx and progresses towards the renal pelvis.

- If no urine exits from the 18G needle and even a hydrophilic guidewire cannot be negotiated into the pelvicalyceal system, the needle is unlikely to be correctly placed. It is not advisable to inject contrast through the needle, since contrast can extravasate, creating a lake of radio-opaque material and making subsequent visualization of the pelvicalyceal system difficult.

- *Complex situations:* In situations where the volume of the stone occupies the entire volume of the calyx selected to be punctured, the needle is advanced until there is the tactile sensation of the needle tip touching the hard surface of the stone. In this situation the tip of the trocar of the needle is in contact with the stone but the cannula of the needle is at a distance of 1–2 mm from the surface of the stone. It is advisable to move the cannula on the trocar towards the stone until contact with the surface of the stone is felt. Then the trocar needle is removed and the hydrophilic guidewire is gently inserted into the narrow space between the urothelium of the calyx and the surface of the stone.

Sometimes this allows the advancement of the guidewire to the renal pelvis, but in other situations it is only possible to locate the guidewire in the punctured calyx.

Multiple Tracts

In the treatment of complex renal lithiasis with branches in multiple calyces, it is sometimes necessary to make multiple punctures through different calyces. Proper assessment of the pelvicalyceal system and planning of the tracts is a must. Multiple punctures when deemed probable should all be made initially. If the planned multiple punctures are made at the beginning of surgery, the injection of contrast through the initially placed ureteral catheter facilitates visualization of all calyces and the most suitable for punctures can be chosen in accordance with the silhouette of the stone. The injection of contrast distends the upper urinary tract and this facilitates insertion of the needles into the calyces. In contrast, if secondary punctures are made after debulking of the stone through the initial primary tract, the calyceal distension of the cavities may be hampered by the leaking of contrast and saline that is injected from the ureteral catheter through the Amplatz sheath.

If calculi are located in calyces that are in parallel or adjacent calyx, "Y" punctures are preferable.[18] After the calyx of initial puncture is cleared of stone the working sheath is retracted outside of the renal capsule and angled towards the second targeted calyx. The second puncture is made through the working sheath. One of the attractions of the Y puncture is that the second puncture is created through the same skin incision as the first puncture, minimizing the cosmetic effects of PNL. We do not advocate this technique as the second tract would become oblique with higher risk of bleeding and vascular injury.

It is better to have two separate skin entry points and reduce the amount of parenchyma traversed.

ULTRASOUND-GUIDED ACCESS

Percutaneous renal access can be achieved either with ultrasound or fluoroscopy guidance. The method of choice depends on training and personal preference. The side effects of extensive radiation during therapeutic procedures are well-known, which is the main drawback of fluoroscopy.

Ultrasound has several strengths as an interventional tool.[22]

- It is readily available, relatively inexpensive, and portable.
- It has no radiation hazards.
- It provides guidance for access in multiple, transverse, longitudinal, and oblique planes.
- It offers real time monitoring of the needle tip, which guides proper placement of the needle and avoidance of important viscera.
- An added advantage is that it can be used in conjunction with Doppler to avoid important vascular structures lying along the needle path.
- Percutaneous ultrasound-guided access is the simplest and most direct technique to drain a hydronephrotic collecting system in difficult clinical conditions as in placing a temporary urinary diversion due to an obstructing stone with infection, pyonephrosis or renal failure. It has also been used successfully to relieve upper tract obstruction secondary to malignancy. Ultrasound-guided nephrostomy puncture is preferred for patients in whom retrograde ureteral access is unsuccessful. It is also a method of choice in pregnancy when there is a need for deobstruction.

In a few comparative studies,[23–27] ultrasound-guided access has been associated with reduced radiation exposure time, reduced number of attempts to puncture and reduced blood loss as compared to fluoroscopy-guided access. Urologists trained in percutaneous access may be able to provide improved stone-free rates during percutaneous nephrolithotomy (PCNL) while minimizing access related complications.

Instrumentation

Convex probes produce rectangular scans and are most commonly used for gaining percutaneous renal access. Sector probes can be useful when performing nephrostomies in the pediatric age group. The ideal transducer for renal access is a convex transducer of 3.5 MHz, focused at 7–9 cm. If children or thin patients are to be scanned, then a 5 MHz smaller transducer with a focus at 5–7 cm is required. Alternatively, a sector probe can be used in this situation. The monitor used for intervention should ideally be equipped with an electronic dotted line which shows the needle path.

The rigidity of the 18G needle compared to the 21G needle is advantageous for accurately directing the needle tip as it is advanced through the fascial planes. The 18G needle tip is also readily identifiable with real-time ultrasonography guidance. Although routine needles can be used for this purpose, the echo tip needle (Cook Medical Inc., Bloomington, IN, USA) is helpful in achieving ultrasound-guided access; the needle tip is scored and this increases the reflectivity and visualization on ultrasound. Clear visibility of the needle is "key" to the success of ultrasound-guided needle access **(Figs 10.6A and B)**. The most common reason for non-visualization of the needle tip is nonalignment of the needle tip and transducer. This can be achieved by proper alignment using a puncture guide.

Technique (Figs 10.6A and B)

Ultrasound scanning commences posteriorly and proceeds until the posterior axillary line. If scanned in this way, the first calyx to be seen will be the posterior calyx. The site of needle entry is marked and the puncture performed with an 18G echo tip (Cook Medical Incorporated) needle. The key point at this crucial step is that there should be minimal respiratory and ultrasound probe movement. In order to ensure an accurate puncture, the needle tip should be seen along the electronic dotted line throughout its course. The position of the needle in the desired calyx is confirmed with return of clear fluid.

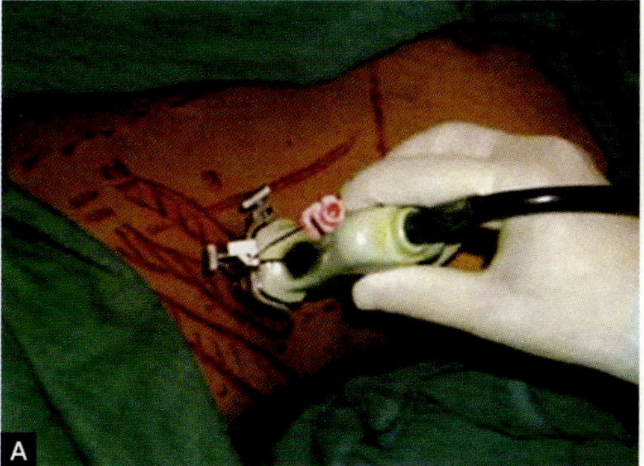
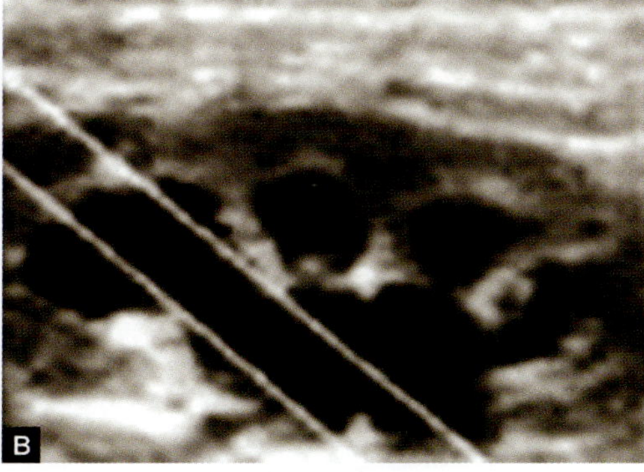

Figs 10.6A and B: (A) The puncture guide helps in directing the needle in the desired plane and depth; (B) The ultrasound probe should be aligned in such a way that the tract provides the shortest access from the skin through the cup of the calyx, infundibulum, and finally into the pelvis

Ultrasound-guided access satisfies all the attributes of a perfect renal access, i.e. shortest possible tract traversing the skin, cortex of the kidney, and cup of the desired calyx of puncture in a straight line and in alignment with the infundibulum and renal pelvis.

Ultrasound Punctures in Ectopic Kidneys and Transplanted Kidneys

A supine oblique position with a bolster under the ipsilateral hemipelvis is used. A mechanical bowel preparation with a low enema is used in all the cases. This helps in identification of gas in the sigmoid colon, which helps identify the bowel and prevents possible injury. Pressure on the ultrasound probe helps to displace the intervening bowel loops between the puncture line and targeted calyx. Similarly, contralateral pressure applied by the assistant helps displace the kidney close to the abdominal wall. All these maneuvers improve the chances of achieving a straight, short, and direct tract to the desired calyx. PCNL is feasible in transplanted kidneys with the help of ultrasound-guided access and this decreases the amount of radiation and intravenous contrast required. With the patient in a left-sided oblique position with a bolster under the ipsilateral hip, the bowel is displaced and a puncture into the superior calyx provides easy access to the ureteropelvic junction and stone in the pelvis.

The addition of Doppler to ultrasound imaging (which facilitates visualization of blood vessels) may be associated with less blood loss and/or lower transfusion rate than ultrasound alone.[28]

BLIND ACCESS

The upper urinary tract collecting system can also be accessed "blindly," without any imaging guidance.[29] The only situation in which this should be considered is when sonography is not available and there is complete ureteral obstruction (precluding retrograde instillation of contrast material or opacification of the collecting system with intravenous contrast). The lumbar notch, also known as the superior lumbar triangle or Grynfeltt lumbar triangle, has been reported as a reliable landmark for blind percutaneous renal access. The lumbar notch is an area of muscular insufficiency through which hernias can occur. It is located posteriorly below the 12th rib. The superior border is the 12th rib and the latissimus dorsi muscle, the lateral border is the transversus abdominis and external oblique muscles, the medial border is the quadratus lumborum and sacrospinalis muscles, and the inferior border is the internal oblique muscle. Insert a needle 3 to 4 cm deep into the notch at a 30° cephalad angle to enter the collecting system. Another blind approach to the collecting system is to inserta needle directly perpendicular to the body surface 1 to 1.5 cm lateral to the L1 vertebral body, which will lead directly to the renal pelvis if anatomy is normal. If fluoroscopy is available, then air and contrast material can be injected through a blindly placed needle to assess fluoroscopically its position and to guide another needle properly through a posterior calyx. In the only randomized clinical trial comparing "blind" access to image-guided access, entry into the collecting system was successful in 50% and 90% of cases, respectively.[30] Use of the technique is not recommended in most settings.

REFERENCES

1. Sampaio FJB. Surgical Anatomy of the Kidney in the Prone, Oblique, and Supine Positions. Smith's Textbook of Endourology, Third Edition:63–94.
2. Sampaio FJB, Mandarim-de-Lacerda CA. 3-Dimensional and radiological pelviocaliceal anatomy for endourology. J Urol 1988;140:1352–55.
3. Abolhassani N, Patel R, Moallem M. Needle insertion into soft tissue: a survey. Med Eng Phys 2007;29:413–31.

4. Wolf JS. Percutaneous approaches to the upper urinary tract collecting system. Campbell-Walsh Urology. 10th ed. Philadelphia, PA: Saunders Elsevier; 2011.

5. Payne, S.R., Webb, W.R. Percutaneous Renal Surgery, 2nd edn. Edinburgh: Churchill Livingstone, 1988, pp. 5–6.

6. Preminger, G.M., Schulez, S., Clayman, R.V., et al. Cephaladrenal movement during percutaneous nephrostolithotomy. J Urol. 1986;137:623–25.

7. Karlin, G.S., Smith, A.D. Approaches to the superior calyx: Renal displacement technique and review of options. J Urol 1989;142:774–77.

8. Ahmed R. El-Nahas, Ahmed A. Shokeir, et al. Post-percutaneous Nephrolithotomy Extensive Hemorrhage: A Study of Risk Factors. J Urol 2007;177:576.

9. Stening SG, Bourne S. Supracostal percutaneous nephrolithotomy for upper pole calyceal calculi. J Endourol. 1998;12;359–62.

10. Yates J and Munver R. Diagnosis and Management of Thoracic Complications of Percutaneous Renal Surgery. Smith's Textbook of Endourology, third edition.

11. Maheshwari PN, Mane DA, Pathak AB. Management of pleural injury after percutaneous renal surgery. J Endourol. 2009;23:1769–72.

12. El-Nahas AR, Shokeir AA, El-Kenawy MR, et al. Safety and efficacy of supracostal percutaneous nephrolithotomy in pediatric patients. J Urol. 2008;180:676–680.

13. Finelli A, Honey RJDA. Thoracoscopy-assisted high intercostal percutaneous renal access. J Endourol. 2001;15:581–85.

14. Lang E, Thomas R, Davis R, et al. Risks, advantages, and complications of intercostal vs subcostal approach for percutaneous nephrolithotripsy. Urology. 2009;74:751–55.

15. Hopper KD, Yakes WF. The posterior intercostal approach for percutaneous renal procedures: risk of puncturing the lung, spleen, and liver as determined by CT. AJR Am J Roentgenol. 1990;154:115.

16. Robert M, Maubon A, Roux JO, Rouanet JP, Navratil H. Direct percutaneous approach to the upper pole of the kidney: MRI anatomy with assessment of the visceral risk. J Endourol. 1999;13:17.

17. Bernardo NO. Percutaneous Renal Access Under Fluoroscopic Control. Smith's Textbook of Endourology. 3rd ed.

18. Miller NL, Matlaga BR, Lingeman JE. Techniques for fluoroscopic percutaneous renal access. J Urol. 2007;178:15–23.

19. Sharma G, Sharma A. Determining site of skin puncture for percutaneous renal access using fluoroscopy-guided triangulation technique. J Endourol. 2009;23:193–95.

20. Steinberg PL, Semins MJ, Wason SE, Matlaga BR, Pais VM. Fluoroscopy-guided percutaneous renal access. J Endourol. 2009;23:1627–31.

21. Tepeler A, Armagan A, Akman T, Polat EC, Ersöz C, Topakta R, Erdem MR, Onol SY. Impact of percutaneous renal access technique on outcomes of percutaneous nephrolithotomy. J Endourol. 2012;26:828–33.

22. Desai MR, Ganpule AP. Percutaneous Renal Access Under Ultrasound Control. Smith's Textbook of Endourology. 3rd ed.

23. Basiri A, Ziaee AM, Kianian HR, et al. Ultrasonographic versus fluoroscopic access for percutaneous nephrolithotomy:A randomized clinical trial. J Endourol. 2008;22:281–84.

24. Zegel HG, Pollack HM, Banner MC, et al. Percutaneous nephrostomy: Comparison of sonographic and fluoroscopic guidance. AJR Am J Roentgenol. 1981;137:925–27.

25. Kukreja R, Desai M, Patel S, et al. Factors affecting blood loss during percutaneous nephrolithotomy: prospective study. J Endourol. 2004;18:715–22.

26. Agarwal M, Agrawal MS, Jaiswal A, et al. Safety and efficacy of ultrasonography as an adjunct to fluoroscopy for renal access in percutaneous nephrolithotomy (PCNL). BJU Int. 2011;108:1346–49.

27. Watterson JD, Soon S, Jana K. Access related complications during percutaneous nephrolithotomy: urology versus radiology at a single academic institution. J Urol. 2006;176:142–45.

28. Tzeng BC, Wang CJ, Huang SW, et al. Doppler ultrasound-guided percutaneous nephrolithotomy: a prospective randomized study. Urology 2011;78:535–39.

29. Chien GW, Bellman GC. Blind percutaneous renal access. J Urol. 2002;16:93–96.

30. Basiri A, Mehrabi S, et al. Blind Puncture in comparison with fluoroscopic guidance in PCNL: a randomized controlled trial. Uro J. 2007;4:79–83.

11
Tract Dilatation in Percutaneous Renal Surgery

Rajesh Kukreja

Tract dilation is an essential step in the performance of percutaneous renal surgery. With proper tract dilation, an appropriate size working sheath can then be placed, facilitating the insertion of the endoscopes, working instruments, and nephrostomy tube. Dilatation is always performed over a guidewire.

Placing a Secured Guidewire

Establishing a secure wire is the key to successful tract dilatation and PCNL.
- Free flow of saline or urine from the 18 gauge needle confirms a correct puncture.
- A 0.038 or 0.035 inch hydrophilic nitinol core glidewire is then passed through the needle and into the collecting system. The nitinol core glidewire is preferred because it is quite maneuverable and resists kinking **(Fig. 11.1A)**. If a 21-gauge puncture needle that accepts a 0.018-inch wire has been used, transition dilators are necessary to upsize to a larger working wire.[1,2]
- Under fluoroscopic guidance an attempt is made to advance the glidewire down the ureter. If the wire does not pass easily into the ureter, it can be coiled in the renal pelvis.
- Maneuvers to negotiate the wire into the ureter include:
  - An 8 Fr fascial dilator is passed into the calyx, followed by a 5 Fr Cobra tipped angiographic catheter. The angiographic catheter helps direct the glidewire towards the ureteropelvic junction (UPJ), facilitating placement of the wire down the ureter.
  - With help of a stiff dilator like an Alken rod, the kidney can be tented cephalad. This helps in straightening any kink at the ureter or UPJ and negotiating the glidewire across. This maneuver is especially helpful in lower calyceal punctures at acute angle to the ureter.
- After the glidewire is positioned in the ureter it may be exchanged for a stiffer, polytetrafluoroethylene coated working wire, such as a Zebra or Amplatz super-stiff wire **(Fig. 11.1B)**. The lubricious nature of the glidewire makes it prone to displacement.
- An 8/10 Fr coaxial dilator or the dilatation cannula (Karl Storz) **(Fig. 11.2)** is used to place a second safety wire, usually a 0.035-inch wire. For beginners, it is imperative to have a safety wire in place before proceeding with percutaneous tract dilation.

Methods of Tract Dilatation

Several methods of tract dilatation are available, including metal telescoping dilators, semirigid Amplatz dilators and balloon dilators.

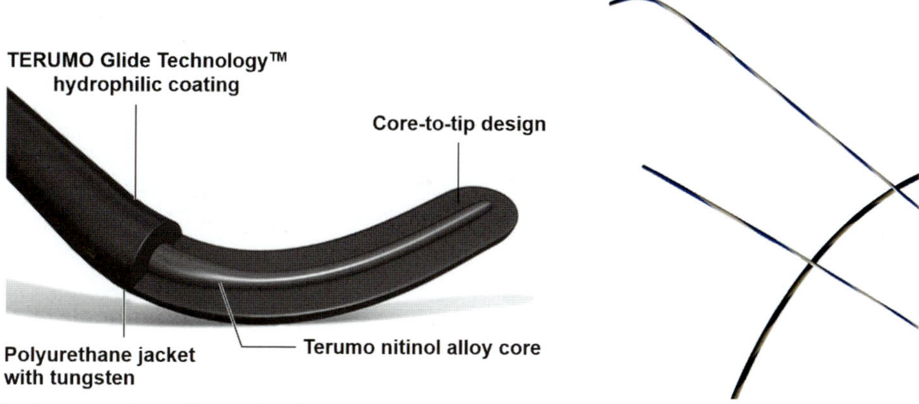

(A) Nitinol core hydrophilic guidewire

- *Core:* Nitinol core for flexibility and shape memory
- *Coating:* Polyurethane coating for smooth soft surface has tungsten added for radio-opacity
- *Hydrophilic material (M polymer):* Causes water to stick on surface making it smooth and slippery.
- *Diameter (Inch):* 0.018, 0.025, 0.035 and 0.038
- *Lengths:* 80, 150, 180 and 260 cm
- *3 cm floppy tip:* Straight/angle/J tip

(B) Zebra wire

- Kink resistant nitinol core with flexible PTFE jacket for torque ability
- Blue and white striped pattern for better endoscopic visualization and handling
- *Platinum distal tip:* Visible under fluoroscopy
- Lubricious uro-glide coating on distal 60 cm to reduce friction and make it kink resistant like a glidewire
- Advantages of both guidewire and glidewire and disadvantage of none

Figs 11.1A and B: Guidewires. (A) Nitinol core hydrophilic guidewire; (B) Zebra wire

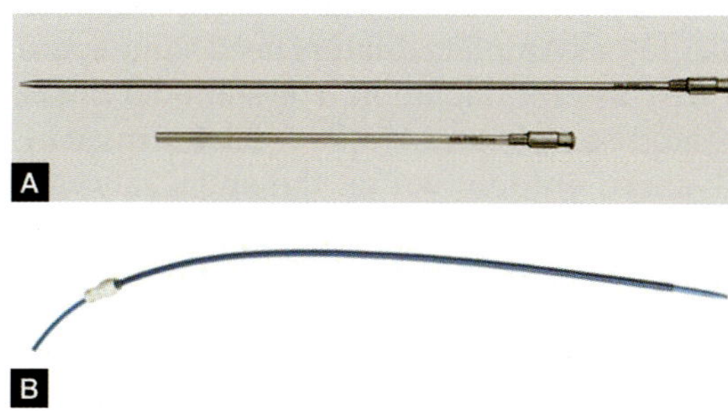

Figs 11.2A and B: Placement of safety guidewire. (A) 3 mm dilatation cannula (set of inner and outer cannula) (Karl Storz); (B) 8 Fr (70 cm long) Stylet with 10 Fr (30 cm long) introducer sheath; PTFE; kink resistant (Boston Scientific)

Alken's Dilators

These are rigid telescoping metal stainless steel dilators that are introduced over a central guide rod.[3] Progressively enlarging and telescoping coaxial stainless steel dilators starting from 9 Fr with successive increments of 3 Fr help to dilate the tract from the 7 Fr hollow guide rod up to 30 Fr **(Fig. 11.3)**. The guide rod (7 Fr) has a round bulbous end (9 Fr) that prevents the sequential dilators from overshooting.[4] The advantages of the Alken's dilator system are that it is reusable, hence inexpensive and importantly is able to dilate even when there is dense perinephric scarring. The ability of these dilators to dilate right till their ends is useful in difficult situations like a complete staghorn with minimal space between the calyceal wall and the edge of stone.

The disadvantage is that the same characteristics that make the Alken's dilator so effective are also the reasons why the rigid metal dilators can do considerable damage. They have an increased potential for iatrogenic injury, due to difficulty with controlling the pressure during dilation. Moreover, the

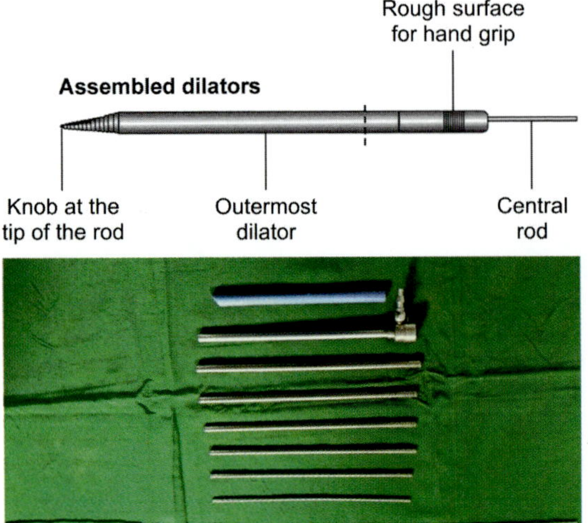

Fig. 11.3: Alken telescoping coaxial stainless steel dilators

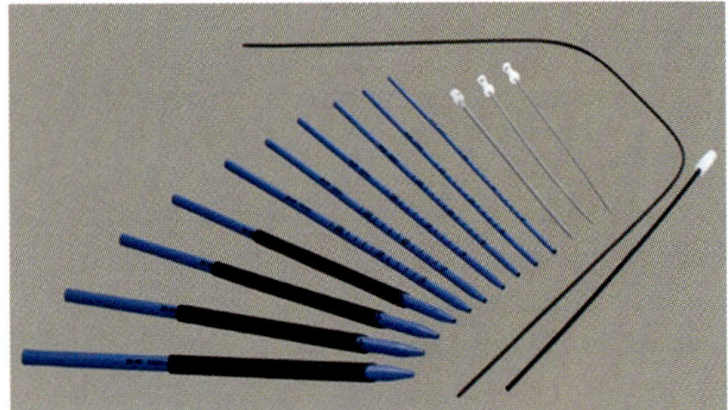

Fig. 11.4: Amplatz dilator set

necessity for manual stabilization of the central rod during the dilation increases the risk of perforating the renal pelvis.

Amplatz Dilators

These are semi-rigid tapered-tip polyurethane cylindrical dilators, of progressively increasing circumference, ranging from 8 to 30 F that are passed over an 8 Fr angiographic catheter that fits over a 0.035-inch guidewire **(Fig. 11.4)**.[5] They can also be passed over the Alken's guide rod. The dilators are passed one after the other, not coaxially like the rigid metal dilators but progressively, by advancing one dilator, removing it, advancing the next larger dilator, and so on until the final tract diameter is achieved. Finally, the working sheath is passed over the final dilator and then the dilator and 8 Fr catheter are removed, leaving the working wire and sheath in place. The dilators are made in increments of 2 Fr, but if the tissue being dilated is soft, then not every dilator needs to be used.

The advantages of Amplatz dilators are that trauma experienced by the collecting system is theoretically less than the trauma experienced by the collecting system using rigid metal dilators, but the disadvantage is that bleeding can happen each time a dilator is withdrawn. As these are disposable dilators, they are more expensive than the Alken's dilators.

There have been many comparative studies between the two dilator systems but experienced urologists have found no difference between the two systems in terms of safety. Alken's dilators may be preferred in patients who have a tight fitting staghorn calculus, as Amplatz dilators need some space in the calyx for dilatation. The shoulder or the tapered end of each Amplatz dilator must be advanced entirely within the entry calyx. In calyces that have no space, the dilatation may remain short due to tapered end of the dilator.

Balloon Dilators

The balloon dilator set consists of an expandable balloon, a working Amplatz sheath that is back-loaded before the inflated balloon is placed over the wire, and syringe inflator.[1] The balloon comes in inflated balloon diameters of 6, 8 and 10 mm with length of 15 cm and transparent or PTFE sheaths **(Fig. 11.5)** (Ultraxx, Cook Medical). Pressures of up to 20 atmospheres can be easily achieved with this system, although in general, much lower pressures are usually sufficient for tract creation. Balloon inflation is performed

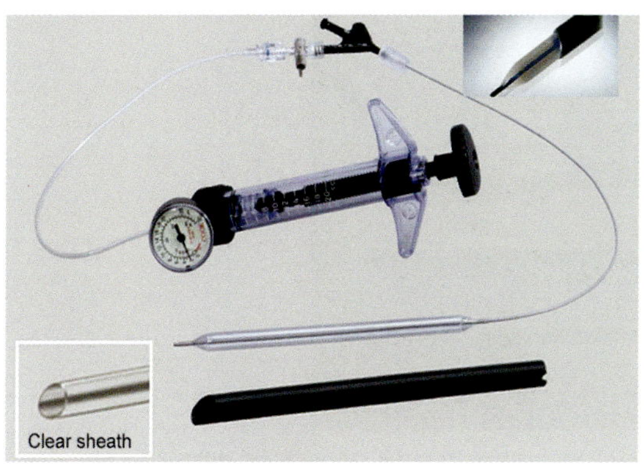

Fig. 11.5: Balloon dilator set

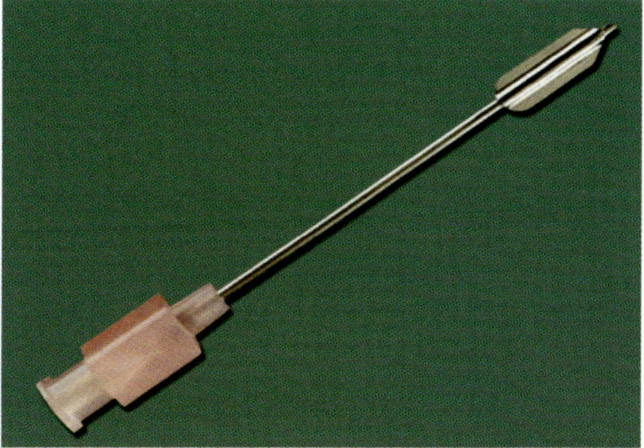

Fig. 11.6: Cook fascia incising needle

using radiographic contrast instilled within the injector syringe. The balloon should be inflated until no "waisting" or focal narrowing is evident. The pressure required to dilate the tract is generally under 15 cm H_2O. The balloon dilator should be manually stabilized during this procedure in order to avoid inadvertent displacement. Balloon inflation allows for full expansion of the balloon, which is followed by insertion of a working sheath over the balloon, in a rotational manner.

Balloon dilators have been reported to cause significantly less bleeding than sequential dilators because the radial force used to spread the renal parenchyma is less traumatic than the shearing or cutting action of sequential Amplatz dilators or metal telescoping dilators. The main disadvantage of the balloon dilator system is the cost. Sequential Amplatz or metal dilators may be useful in the setting of extensive perirenal fibrosis from previous renal surgery. However, an X-Force™ N30 nephrostomy balloon dilation catheter (Bard Urological, Covington, Georgia) can achieve 30 atmospheres. This may prove advantageous in the presence of flank scarring.[2] Alternatively, a 4.5 mm fascial incising needle **(Fig. 11.6)** (Cook Urological, Spencer, Indiana) can be placed over the working wire to facilitate balloon dilation.

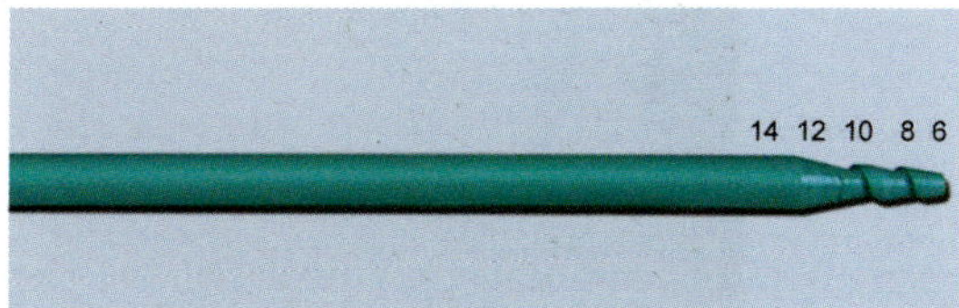

Fig. 11.7: Single step screw dilator

Single Step Dilatation

In an effort to make tract making rapid, easy, and blood less, multiple single step techniques have been described.

- The simplest is using the largest Amplatz dilators without the initial smaller dilators.
- *Screw dilators:* These have a screw-shaped tapered conical tip **(Fig. 11.7)**. They are available in 3 sizes—size 6 to 12 Fr, 6 to 14 Fr and 6 to 16 Fr (6 implies the size of tip and 12 implies the size of the shaft).
- The miniaturised PCNL sets have their own single step dilators **(Fig. 11.8)**.

Two new dilatation systems described have been a radially expanding single step dilator system[6] and the 5-PANG system **(Fig. 11.9)**.[7] In both the systems there is no need to remove the needle and hence mitigates the problem of tract loss. Also the dilatation would be faster.

There have been many comparative studies between the dilator systems but no

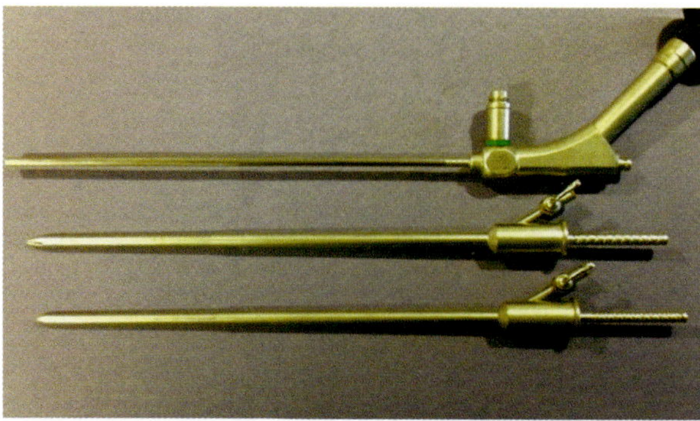

Fig. 11.8: Nagele modular MIP system (Storz): Each Mini perc sheath has its own single step dilator to be passed over the wire directly with the sheath back-loaded over its dilator

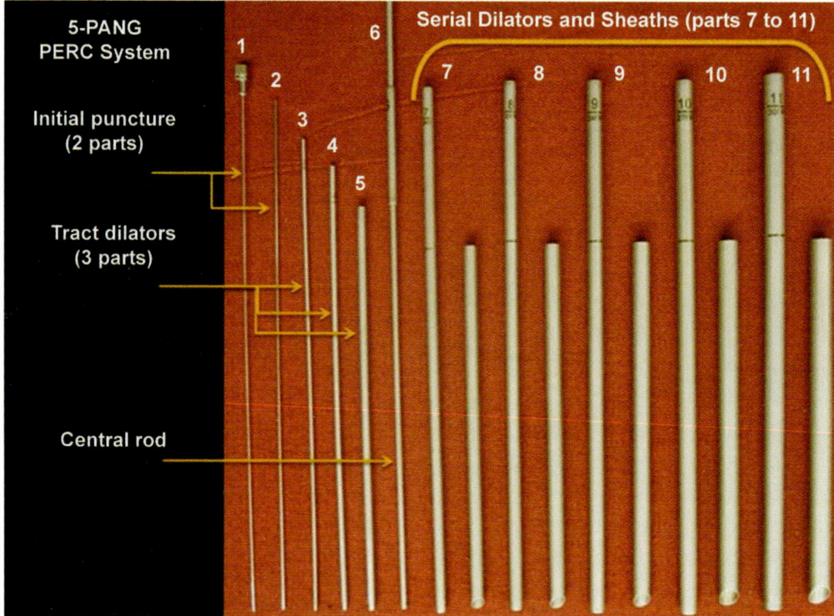

Fig. 11.9: 5-PANG system: Set of telescoping dilators with advantage of not removing the puncture needle, hence avoiding chances of kinking the wire

significant difference has been found between all the systems in terms of safety.[8–13]

Principles of Tract Dilatation

Whatever may be the mode of tract dilatation, certain principles need to be strictly adhered to.[8,14]

- The success of tract dilatation is dependent on maintaining the angle, depth, and the direction of the dilatation.

- Every step of dilatation should be monitored on fluoroscopy.

- The lumbodorsal fascia should be incised with a sharp blade knife passed along the needle under fluoroscopic guidance as a lumbotome or the 18 G Cook fascia incising needle **(Fig. 11.6)** passed over the wire. The fascia should be incised in two planes at right angles to each other. The fascia is the site of greatest resistance to the dilatation. This maneuver is especially helpful in case with retroperitoneal scarring and fibrosis due to previous surgeries. Care should be taken to avoid lacerating the nearby subcostal or intercostal neurovascular bundle on the inferior rib margin.

- The tract should be dilated only till the minor calyx. If overdilatation happens, it can traumatize the infundibulum, renal pelvis or ureteropelvic junction. Trauma to the anterior wall of the PCS can cause significant bleeding that may be difficult to control. It is always better to underdilate than to overdilate and cause trauma.

- Each dilator should be passed in the same phase of respiration as was during the puncture.

- Dilatation should always be rotating movements at the wrist joint (alternating supination and pronation) with minimal forward thrust. Attempt should be to dilate till the calyx and not till the calculus.

- The collecting system should be kept distended during dilatation by constant saline flushing through the retrograde ureteric catheter by the OR assistant. Free exit of the flushed saline from the dilators confirms entry of the dilator into the pelvicalyceal system **(Fig. 11.10)**.

- *Guidewire friction test:* Ridhorkar et al. demonstrated that free to and fro movements of the guidwire after every step of sequential dilatation indicates well-aligned dilatation without kinking of the guidewire.[15] Lack of free flow of saline through the dilators or presence of a kinked guidewire as confirmed by the guidewire friction test indicate improper dilatation due to wrong direction or angle of dilatation.

- Difficult conditions like retroperitoneal scarring or obesity are risk factors for guidewire kinking and loss of plane of dilatation.

Complications of Renal Tract Dilatation

- *Hemorrhage:* Acute hemorrhage can originate from either of these four sources: Intercostal vessels, renal parenchymal vasculature, branches of the renal vein and renal artery adjacent to the pelvicalyceal system. The reported incidence of serious arterial injuries ranges from 0.9 to 3% after percutaneous procedures.[1,10,12] The most clinically significant bleeding related to percutaneous tract dilation is due to over-advancement of the dilating instrument, resulting in splitting of the infundibulum. This occurrence can be avoided by understanding the anatomy of the entry calyx and infundibulum with retrograde contrast injection. Regardless of the dilating system used, the intention should

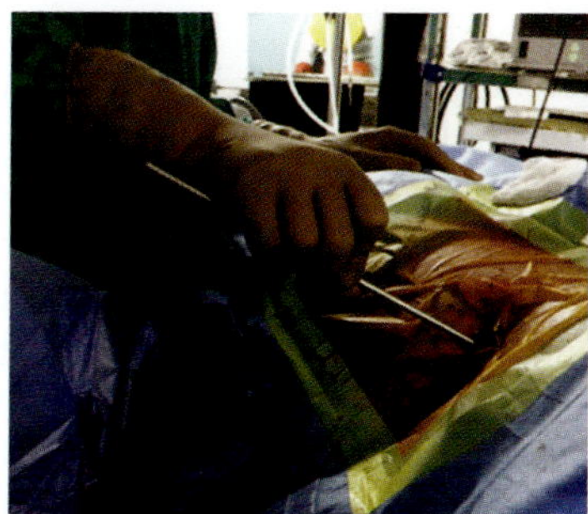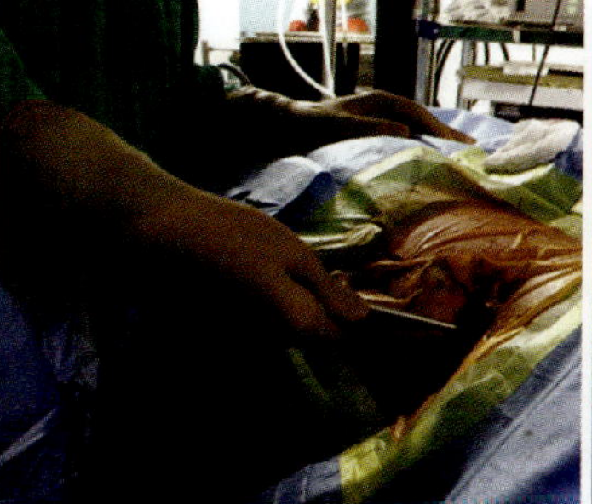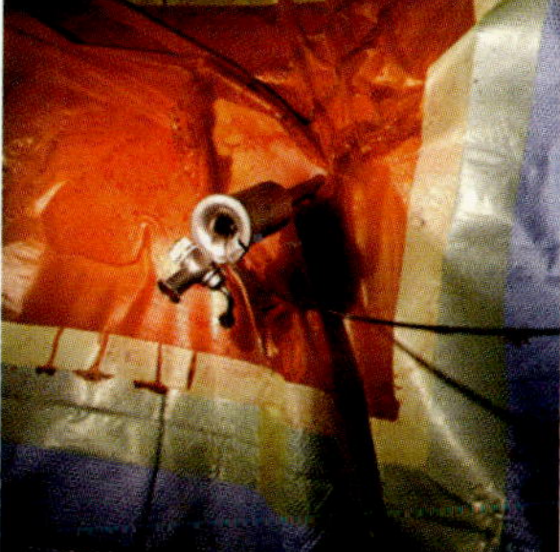

Fig. 11.10: Dilatation: Alternate pronation and supination movements of the forearm without any forward thrusting movements. Clear flow of saline from the sheath indicates well placed and nontraumatic dilatation

then be to place the widest part of the dilator into the entry calyx, but not into the infundibulum.

- *Renal pelvis perforation:* The most common cause of renal pelvis perforation is the aggressive use of serial dilators. The perforation is usually medial, following an over-advancement of the dilator. Renal pelvis perforation can also occur due to initial transgression of the puncture needle and in appropriate guidewire positioning. Initial advancement of the guidewire down the ureter and into the bladder facilitates dilation and greatly reduces the risk of this complication. The perforation is usually recognized intraoperatively by visualization of perinephric or renal sinus fat and contrast extravasation on fluoroscopy. Once recognized, it may require quick termination of the procedure and placement of a ureteral stent and a nephrostomy tube.

TROUBLESHOOTING DURING DILATATION

Underdilated Tract

- Identification
  - There is no free flow of saline from the exterior end of Amplatz sheath. Instead, hemorrhagic efflux is seen.
  - On passing the nephroscope, we see fat with the distal end of Amplatz sheath outside the pelvicalyceal system.
- *Cause:* This usually occurs early during the learning curve. Use of Amplatz dilators is associated with this as the terminal taper end of the dilator enters the calyx but the Amplatz sheath introduced over, it does not enter the calyx and remains outside the collecting system. This may cause brisk bleeding as there is a portion of parenchyma that has been partially dilated, which does not have the tamponade effects of the Amplatz sheath.

- Prevention
  - The collecting system should be kept distended during dilatation by constant saline flushing through the retrograde ureteric catheter by the OR assistant. Free exit of the flushed saline from the dilators and the Amplatz sheath confirms entry of the dilator into the pelvicalyceal system.
  - When using the Amplatz dilators, you need to pass the dilator well into the system so that the dilator beyond the terminal tapered segment has entered the calyx.
- Solution
  - Load the guide rod and Amplatz dilator corresponding to the sheath size over the guidewire. Pass the guide rod over the wire into the calyx and the dilator over the rod. Entry into the system is identified by free flow of flushed saline. Now reposition the sheath over the dilator.
  - If the wire has slipped out of the system, you may flush dilute betadine or methylene blue from the ureteric catheter and identify the opening in the renal parenchyma under nephroscopic vision. Pass the wire through the identified rent from where you can see betadine or methylene blue coming out. The wire should enter the pelvicalyceal system. Re-dilate now over the wire.
  - If this too fails, a new puncture may be required. This may be difficult as the contrast may extravasate or the calyx may not fill due to leakage of contrast. Choosing an access through another calyx or sonography-guided puncture may help.
  - In a rare situation, it may be needed to stage the procedure. The puncture site seals in 48–72 hours and a repeat procedure can be done after that time.

Overdilatation

- Identification
  - On passing the nephroscope, we see fat with the distal end of Amplatz sheath outside the pelvicalyceal system.
- *Cause:* Overdilatation is a state when the dilators have traversed the opposite wall of the PCS and the Amplatz sheath is now placed anterior to the kidney. Forceful dilatation is the usual reason for this problem.
- *Prevention:* Dilatation should always be by rotating movements at the wrist joint (alternating supination and pronation) with minimal forward thrust. Attempt should be to dilate till the calyx and not till the calculus.
- *Solution (Flowchart 11.1)*
  - The Amplatz sheath needs to be withdrawn back to get it in the PCS. The perforated pelvic wall will not have any tamponade effect and may bleed. Also, the irrigation fluid would leak through the hole and may cause significant fluid overload. Even the stone or stone fragments can migrate outside the PCS through the hole in the anterior wall.
  - The further plan after this would depend on the size of perforation, size of the stone and the amount of bleeding.
  - If the size of the perforation and the stone both are small, than one can get back properly in the system and quickly finish the procedure without causing much extravasation.
  - However, if there is a large perforation or a large stone or significant bleeding, then it is prudent to insert a nephrostomy tube, abandon the procedure. Always keep a large bore nephrostomy tube during such situations. The second procedure can be staged after 2 or 3 days, as the perforation usually heals during this period.

Kinking of Guidewire

- *Cause:* This usually occurs due to forceful dilatation in the wrong direction. This is like to occur when the tract is not in a straight line. Retrorenal fibrosis, obesity and an oblique or acutely angulated tract are risk factors. Once the guide rod is in place, this problem cannot occur.
- Prevention
  - The wire usually kinks at the level of the thoracolumbar fascia. Hence, the fascia needs to be incised well before starting the dilatation.
  - Dilatation should always be rotating movements at the wrist joint (alternating supination and pronation) with minimal forward thrust.

Flowchart 11.1: Algorithm for management of overdilated tract and pelvic wall perforation

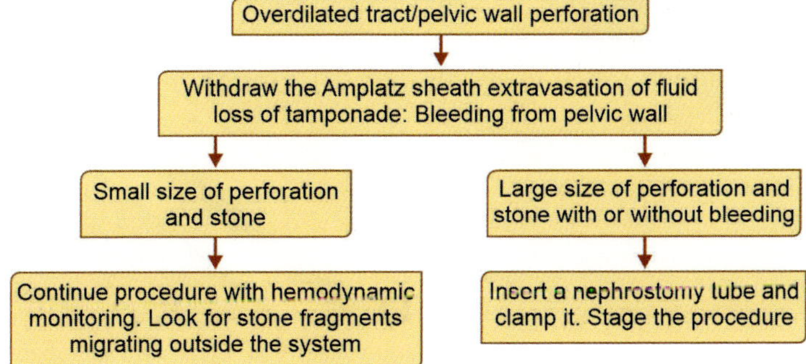

- If there is doubt regarding the correct direction, then moving the glidewire (friction test) gives a good indication. If the wire moves freely, then it indicates that the direction and trajectory is correct. Vice versa, if the glidewire does not move freely, then the direction and trajectory needs to be adjusted.
- Each dilator should be passed in the same phase of respiration was during the puncture.
- Use of the 5 part PANG needle system largely avoids this problem.[7]
- Solution
  - If a kink has occurred, then the initial dilator should be advanced close to the kink and the kinked portion of guidewire pulled inside the dilator. The correct direction should then be ascertained and further dilation should be done. Once the initial dilator (6 or 8 Fr) is inside the kidney, replace the wire with a new one.
  - At times a re-puncture is needed.
  - If a safety wire has been inserted, then it can be used for dilatation.

AMPLATZ SHEATH

No matter the type of dilator used, rigid or balloon, or the technique of track dilation, one-step or multi-stepped, an Amplatz sheath is always used for a standard PCNL. These are available in sizes ranging from 12 to 34 Fr with length ranging from 16 to 30 cm (Cook Medical). Opaque or clear sheath with radiopaque stripes are available **(Fig. 11.11)**.

Benefits of an Amplatz Sheath

- Amplatz sheath maintains the tract during procedure.
- It causes tamponade of the tract and reduces bleeding. The beveled end of the Amplatz sheath can be used to tamponade a part of renal parenchyma that is actively bleeding.
- It protects the renal parenchyma from injury by the instruments used in renal procedures.
- The use of Amplatz sheath maintains a low-pressure system and reduces fluid intravasation. Maintaining a low-pressure system would be important in patients with infected calculi as the risk of sepsis would reduce.

Care should be taken to avoid over- or under-advancement of the sheath on the dilators because this may cause bleeding and trauma to the renal parenchyma or collecting system.

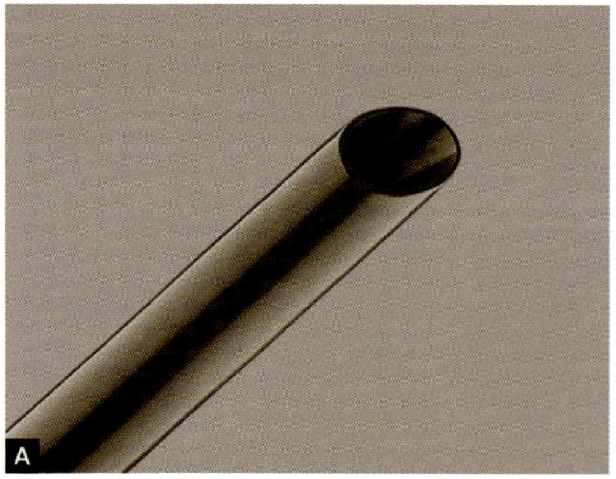
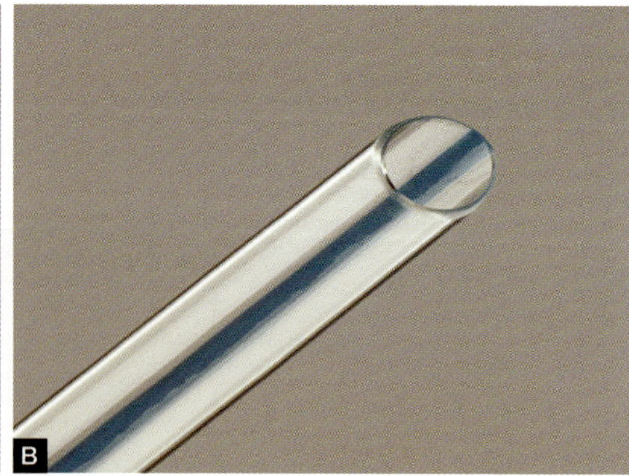

Figs 11.11A and B: Amplatz sheath. (A) Opaque sheath; (B) Clear with radiopaque stripe

REFERENCES

1. Petar Erdeljan, Hassan Razvi. Dilation of the Nephrostomy Tract. Smith's Textbook of Endourology. 3rd edn.
2. Miller NL, Matlaga BR, Lingeman JE. Techniques for fluoroscopic percutaneous renal access. J Urol. 2007;178:15–23.
3. Alken P. The telescope dilators. World J Urol. 1985;3:7–10.
4. Knoll T, Michael MS, Alken P. Surgical Atlas. Percutaneous nephrolithotomy: the Mennheim technique. BJU Int. 2007;99:213–31.
5. Rusnak B, Castañeda-Zúñiga W, Kotula F, et al. An improved dilator system for percutaneous nephrostomies. Radiology. 1982;144:174.
6. Goharderakhshan RZ, Schwartz BF, Rudnick DM, Irby PB, Stoller ML. Radially expanding single-step nephrostomy tract dilator. Urology 2001;58:693–96.
7. Patil AV. A novel 5-part Percutaneous Access Needle with Glidewire technique (5-PANG) for percutaneous nephrolithotomy: our initial experience. Urology. 2010;75.
8. Sharma GR, Maheshwari PN, Sharma AG, Maheshwari RP, Heda RS, Maheshwari SP. Fluoroscopy-guided percutaneous renal access in prone position. World J Clin Cases. 2015;3(3):245–64.
9. Davidoff R, Bellman GC. Influence of technique of percutaneous tract creation on incidence of renal hemorrhage. J Urol. 1997;157:1229–31.
10. Safak M, Gogus C, Soygur T. Nephrostomy tract dilation using a balloon dilator in percutaneous renal surgery:experience with 95 cases and comparison with the fascial dilator system. Urol Int. 2003;71:382–84.
11. Al-Kandari AM, Jabbour M, Anderson A, et al. Comparative study of degree of renal trauma between Amplatz sequential fascial dilation and balloon dilation during percutaneous renal surgery in an animal model. Urology. 2007;69:586–89.
12. Gonen M, Istanbulluoglu OM, Cicek T, et al. Balloon dilatation versus Amplatz dilatation for nephrostomy tract dilatation. J Endourol. 2008;22:901–04.
13. Dehong C, Liangren L, Huawei L, Qiang W. A comparison among four tract dilation methods of percutaneous nephrolithotomy:A systematic review and meta-analysis. Urolithiasis. 2013;41:523–30.
14. Wolf JS. Percutaneous approaches to the upper urinary tract collecting system. Campbell-Walsh Urology. 10th edn. Philadelphia,PA: Saunders Elsevier, 2011.
15. Ridhorkar VR, Desai RM, Sabnis RB, et al. Guidewire friction test: an aid to PCNL tract dilatation. Indian J Urol. 1998;14:74–76.

12

Tips and Tricks

Akshay Nathani, Abhishek Singh, Nitesh Kumar

INTRODUCTION

PCNL (percutaneous nephrolithotomy) is considered to be a standard of care and is traditionally being carried out in prone position since years.[1,2] Recent EUA Guidelines 2023 suggest both prone and supine positions are safe and efficacious, both have their own pros and cons.[3] Improvements in ergonomics and decrease in tract size of PCNL have led for better outcomes of patients with reduction in morbidity. Recent 2023 EUA (European Association of Urology) guidelines have mentioned prone and supine position both being equally safe with supine position having added advantages for ergonomics.

Fernström and Johansson are credited with description of first prone PCNL.[4] Prone position was accepted by urologists worldwide because the imaging modality available for preoperative planning was conventional X-ray intravenous urography for surgical planning.

In 1987, Valdivia, et al is credited with description of first supine PCNL[5] **(Fig. 12.1)**.

Recent imaging modalities available for preoperative planning of PCNL are

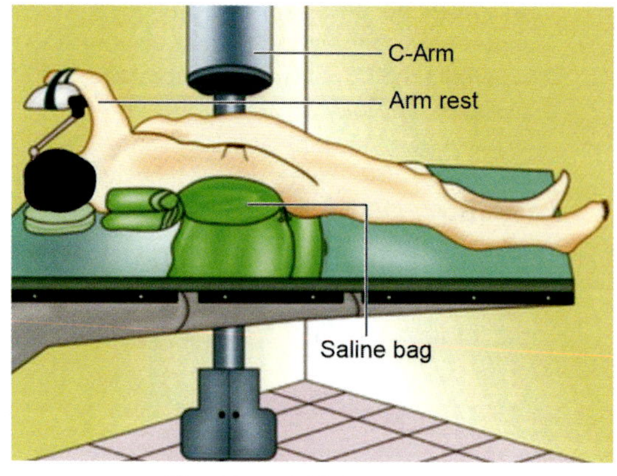

Fig. 12.1: Valdivia position

ultrasound, cross-sectional CT intravenous urography (IVU) which not only provides information regarding intrarenal but also perirenal anatomy, i.e. relationship of kidney with bowel, liver and spleen.

Over three decades, interest in supine PCNL has begun to rise significantly. CROES (Clinical Research Office of the Endourological Society) conducted a global study on supine vs prone position of PCNL in 2011 found that there was an increased interest in supine PCNL.[6]

Why Supine PCNL??

Disadvantages of prone PCNL led to make up of supine PCNL

- Difficulties from anaesthesia point—especially in obese, kyphotic, scoliotic and debilitated patients, difficult retrograde access if needed, patient discomfort, need of manpower for change of position from lithotomy to prone, lastly increased radiation hazards to operating surgeon as C-arm is in more vicinity.

Indications of Supine PCNL

- Calculi requiring simultaneous PCNL and RIRS
- Patient with metabolic syndrome
- Conditions precluding prone positioning such as skeletal anomalies

Pre-operative preparation: Clinical history, examination and investigations, i.e. laboratory hemogram, renal function test, coagulation profile and imaging in the form of X-ray KUB (kidney ureter bladder), CT IVU (intravenous urography) if renal parameters are normal or else plain CT KUB for pre-operative planning for stone size, location, stone burden Hounsfield unit. As per EUA guidelines, if urine culture suggests infection, then it should be treated and covered with appropriate antibiotics in perioperative period, if urine culture is sterile second generation cephalosporin is to be given at the time of surgery.[3]

Operative technique will be divided into following steps:

1. Operating room set up and armamentarium.
2. Patient positioning and ergonomics.
3. Armamentarium required.
4. Achieving access to target calyx.
5. Dilatation of tract.
6. Nephroscopy and intracorporeal lithotripters.

Operating Room Set up

Adequately spaced as to accommodate two sets of instruments, i.e one nephroscopy and one flexible ureteroscopy along with video trolly and light source should be kept handy in operating room as required. Supine approach does not mean ECIRS (endoscopic combined intrarenal surgery), but if needed it should be carried out at ease so the patient should be positioned in Galdakao modified Valdivia position. In this position one operating surgeon is spaced between the legs and another at patients flank side. Patient is positioned supine with slight rotation towards the opposite side to which will be operated, ipsilateral arm is placed over patient's chest, adequate high to ensure it does not interfere with C-arm during triangulation and enables proper flank exposure.

Patient Positioning and Ergonomics

Under general anesthesia the patient is moved to the edge of the table, the ipsilateral leg (PCNL side) remains straight on half of the table and the contralateral leg on the stirrup, this helps to avoid clashing of stirrup holder to instruments calyx pushing onto patient's body. Contralateral arm remains straight and the operating side arm is placed over the patient's chest high to avoid obscuring the angle of C-arm of mobile fluoroscopy.

Why the evolution of supine position from original Valdivia to Galdakao modification to Giusti's modification occurred??

Valdivia described the use of a saline bag to maintain and place the patient in position.[5]

The position is as described in the schematic **Fig. 12.2**.

Then *modification by **Galdakao*** which is most commonly used position was done for simultaneous access from retrograde manner. In this modification, patient's legs are placed in lithotomy position. This facilitates

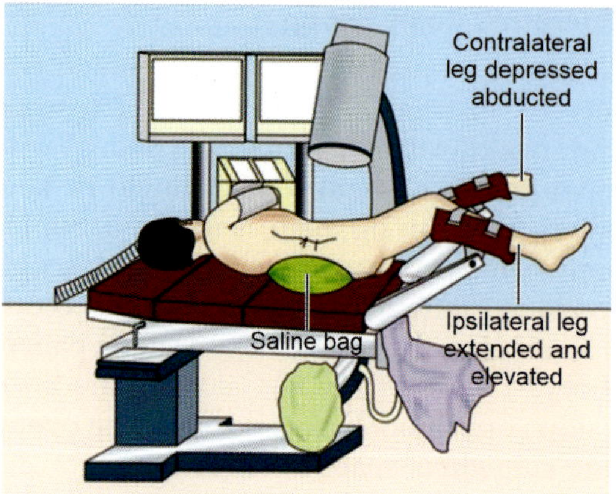

Fig. 12.2: Galdakao-modified Valdivia position

simultaneous access for antegrade and retrograde ECIRS if required.[7]

Further *Giusti's position* came into picture as in Galdakao position it was difficult for manuvering nephroscope in upper calyx from lower calyceal access.

And operating side leg is left straight on half of the operating bed without the stirrup so there is substantial room for another surgeon to perform flexible ureteroscopy simultaneously.[8]

The anaesthesia team works at the head end of the patient, commonly performed puncture is fluoroscopy guided but as and when facilities available ultrasound access should be kept handy in operating room to prevent visceral injury.

For operating surgeon also supine PCNL is ergonomic, as surgeon comfortably can sit and operate with good manuverability of nephroscope in modified Valdivia position without fatigue.

Also if combined ECIRS procedure is needed, it can be performed simultaneously.

Armamentarium Required

- Video trolly, light source, camera
- Puncture needle (IP initial puncture)
- Guidewire (GW)
- Screw dilatator
- Serial metallic telescopic dilator or single step dilator with Amplatz sheath/mini-

PCNL with and without suction (Shah's superperc or Clear Petra sheath)
- Nephroscope: Rigid (flexible, if available)
- *Energy source:* Laser-holmium, thulium fiber laser, LithoClast, shock pulse, etc.

Achieving Access to Target Calyx (Figs 12.3A to C)

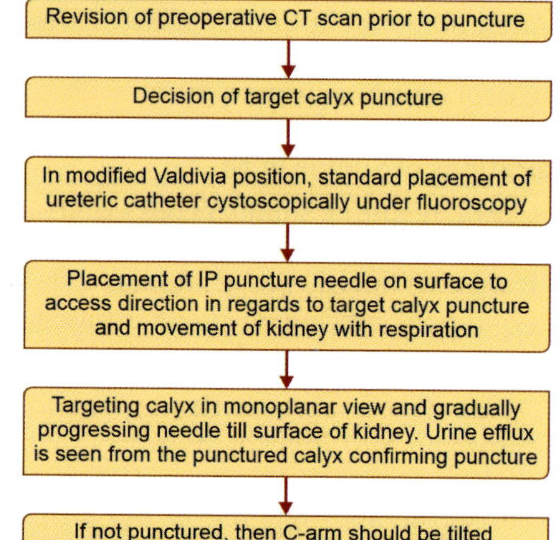

Tract Dilatation

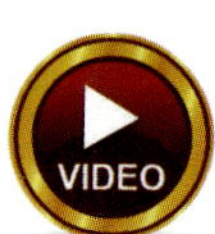

Scan QR Code for Video on
Supine PCNL – Step by Step

Once target puncture achieved and guidewire is placed in position or advanced in ureter below using cobra catheter, then next step would be placement of another safety terumo guidewire over double lumen catheter or Alken canula. Safety guidewire is parked outside in guidewire house and secured in place with towel clip to linen. Then tract dilatation can be done by serial telescoping metal dilator of single step Amplatz dilator followed by Amplatz sheath placement. Placement of safety wire is optional.

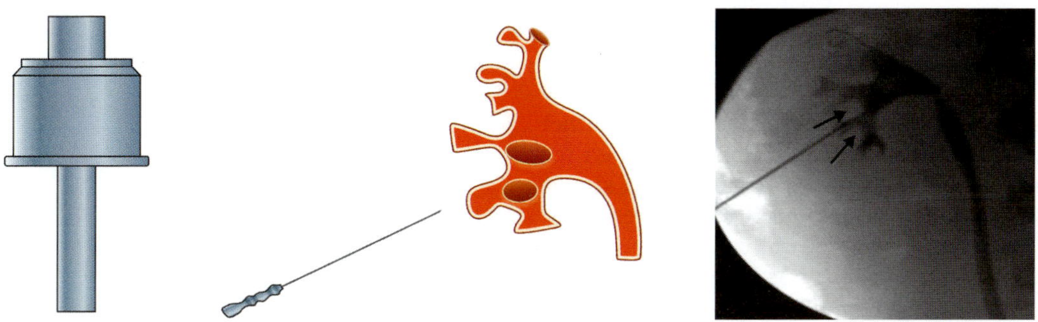

Fig. 12.3A: Initial puncture in zero degree direction of needle is through cup of the calyx

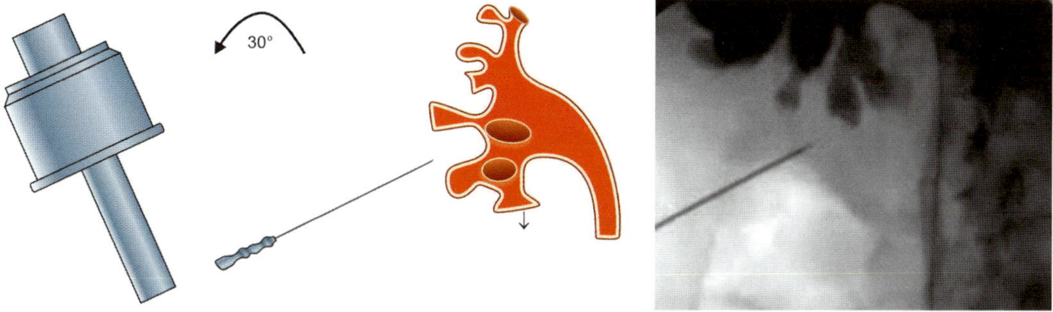

Fig. 12.3B: After rotating C-arm 30 degrees the trajectory is above the target calyx, that means puncture is too posterior, needle is to be withdrawn and readjusted in anterior direction in zero degree

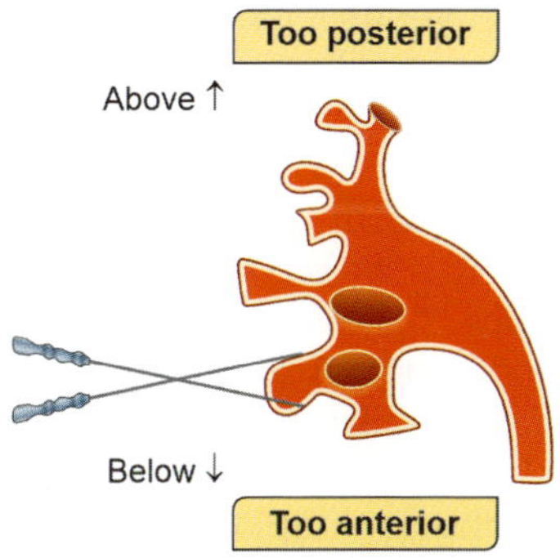

Fig. 12.3C: Diagrammatic presentation if trajectory is below the target calyx in 30 degrees, it means that puncture is too anterior and needle needs to be re-adjusted in posterior direction

Nephroscopy and Intra-Corporeal Lithotripsy

After achieving access and tract dilatation, rigid nephroscope is introduced and collecting system is inspected for stone and after location, lithotripsy performed with choice of lithotripter and availability. Stone, if fragmented, the fragments removed with forceps/suctioned.

At times peripherally placed stones are inaccessible with the help of rigid scope, flexible nephroscopy can help in such situations or second puncture may be required. Also ECIRS can be performed, that is, the main advantage of modified Valdivia position and upper calyceal or peripheraly placed stones can be basketed and repositioned to the nephroscope (passing the ball technique). After complete visual and fluoroscopic clearance, exit strategy can be placement of double J stent antegradely and nephrostomy placement (as per individual case or institute policy). If tubeless, then it should be a habit to inspect the tract while exiting with nephroscope to rule out major bleeding or any inadvertent adjacent organs' injuries.

Postoperative care: Postoperative imaging either X-ray KUB or CT KUB can be performed for confirmation of complete clearance of stones and nephrostomy if placed can be removed on day 1 and per urethral catheter on day 2 and double J stent after 3–4 weeks (as per the institute policy).

Pros and Cons of Supine PCNL

Pros of supine position—for all practical purposes this chapter will restrict to Galdakao modified Valdivia position.

Anaesthesia-wise: No change position of patient required which also reduces operating time, even morbidly obese patients and patients with spinal abnormalities like kyphosis, scoliosis, etc can be managed with supine PCNL.

Surgical advantages: Improved ergonomics of fluoroscopy, decreased radiation exposure simultaneous ECIRS can be performed, access to upper calyx from lower pole calyx puncture can be done, more ergonomic for operating surgeon as surgeon can sit and operate.

Cons of Supine PCNL

Full exposure to flank is not possible in supine position which is main drawback of it that makes initial puncture difficult. Posterior calyx is not always accessible. Supine position is not familiar to most of urologists, difficult to puncture upper calyx.

Pelvi collecting system is collapsed due to low intrarenal pressure—longer PCNL instruments may be needed, restricted mobility of nephroscope.

Troubleshooting supine PCNL and ways to overcome

- *Mobility of kidney:* As oppose to prone position, because of lack of counter pressure, in supine position kidney is more mobile which can make procedure right from puncture difficult.
  Rectification: 1. During puncture counter pressure can be given by assistant of surgeon which can stabilize kidney.
  2. Reduction in caliber of the renal Amplatz sheath—the smaller sheaths (such as < 20 Fr mini PCNL) appear to create less renal mobility during placement than the larger bore renal sheaths.
  3. Through and through guidewire placement—after target calyx puncture wire is deployed in ureter and coiled in bladder then cystoscopically the wire is pulled from per urethra and made taught so the kidney can be stabilized.
  4. Placement of retrograde ureteral access sheath may help sometimes.
- *Longer length tract:* As the puncture is more laterally from skin surface than in prone position, the tract is longer in length from skin to kidney surface and as the entry point of tract on kidney surface acts as a fulcrum, the maneuverable length of nephroscope will be less in collecting system which will be tedious for operating surgeon.
  Rectification – 1. Use of flexible nephroscope along with rigid one if above difficulty occurs as recommended by AUA guidelines.[2]
  2. Long length Amplatz sheath to be used
  3. If not available, then placing a "safety suture" (monofilament as it slides easily) on the plastic Amplatz sheath in obese patients where skin to stone distance is more to avoid inadvertent migration of the sheath beneath the surface of the skin.

Review of Literature

Supine vs prone PCNL—after extensive search in literature the bottom line is both techniques have comparable outcome as far as stone free rates are concerned, only fact that transition from prone to supine position is difficult as surgeons have learnt from their mentors who have been performing PCNL in prone position since year together and are reluctant to take on. Sofer *et al.* demonstrated that changing position is not cumbersome and the learning curve short.[9] Some studies note supine PCNL is feasible, comparable to prone PCNL in respect to operative parameters though statistically insignificant.[10]

Proietti et al in their paper *Tips and Tricks of Supine PCNL* concluded that it is a matter of experience and time to change from standard prone PCNL learned from mentors over years together to supine PCNL.[11]

Take Home Messages/Learning Points

Regarding Position

Recently EUA 2023 guidelines have opined supine is equally safe than prone position for PCNL.[3]

The decision of patient positioning should be multifactorial based on patients' characteristics, i.e. pelvicalyceal anatomy, stone location and stone burden and comorbidities and BMI and surgeon along with anesthetist and assisting nursing team.

The technical skills and knowledge of operating surgeon are the main driving factors for successful outcomes of supine PCNL.

Important take home point would be surgeons should be familiar with supine position along with standard prone position for PCNL.

Regarding Procedure

- Almost all stones can be operated by supine PCNL.
- Situations that preclude prone PCNL like spinal abnormality, morbid obesity etc., supine PCNL is better way out.
- Kidney mobility in supine position can make initial puncture a bit difficult.
- Simultaneous flexible ureteroscopy can be performed for peripherally placed stones and upper calyceal stones in complex calyceal anatomy.

REFERENCES

1. Türk C, Pet ík A, Sarica K, Seitz C, Skolarikos A, Straub M, et al. EAU Guidelines on Interventional Treatment for Urolithiasis. Eur Urol. 2016;69(3):475–82.
2. Assimos D, Krambeck A, Miller NL, Monga M, Murad MH, Nelson CP, et al. Surgical Management of Stones: American Urological Association/Endourological Society Guideline, Part II. J Urol. 2016;196(4):1161–9.
3. Uroweb-European Association of Urology [Internet]. [cited 2023 Sep 6]. EAU Guidelines on Urolithiasis-Introduction-Uroweb. Available from: https://uroweb.org/guidelines/urolithiasis
4. Fernström I, Johansson B. Percutaneous pyelolithotomy. A new extraction technique. Scand J Urol Nephrol. 1976;10(3):257–9.
5. Valdivia Uría JG, Lachares Santamaría E, Villarroya Rodríguez S, Taberner Llop J, Abril Baquero G, Aranda Lassa JM. [Percutaneous nephrolithectomy: simplified technic (preliminary report)]. Arch Esp Urol. 1987;40(3):177–80.
6. Kamphuis GM, Baard J, Westendarp M, de la Rosette JJMCH. Lessons learned from the CROES percutaneous nephrolithotomy global study. World J Urol. 2015;33(2):223–33.
7. Ibarluzea G, Scoffone CM, Cracco CM, Poggio M, Porpiglia F, Terrone C, et al. Supine Valdivia and modified lithotomy position for simultaneous anterograde and retrograde endourological access. BJU Int. 2007;100(1):233–6.
8. Basulto-Martínez M, Proietti S, Yeow Y, Rapallo I, Saitta G, De Coninck V, et al. Technique for supine percutaneous nephrolithotomy. Urol Video J. 2020;7:100042.
9. Sofer M, Tavdi E, Levi O, Mintz I, Bar-Yosef Y, Sidi A, et al. Implementation of supine percutaneous nephrolithotomy: a novel position for an old operation. Cent Eur J Urol. 2017;70(1):60–5.
10. Choudhury S, Talukdar P, Mandal TK, Majhi TK. Supine versus prone PCNL in lower calyceal stone: Comparative study in a tertiary care center. Urologia. 2021;88(2):148–52.
11. Proietti S, Rodríguez-Socarrás ME, Eisner B, De Coninck V, Sofer M, Saitta G, et al. Supine percutaneous nephrolithotomy: tips and tricks. Transl Androl Urol. 2019;8(Suppl 4):S381–8.

MINIATURISED PCNL

Rajesh Kukreja, Arvind P Ganpule, Akshay Nathani

PCNL is a well-established modality for treatment of kidney stones.[1] As with any other procedure, PCNL also has its own set of complications which ranges from pleural injury to the most dreaded one that is bleeding.[2] Bleeding has been the most feared complication of this procedure due to the complexity of the issue at hand. The key factors associated with bleeding during percutaneous renal surgery are tract size, duration of procedure and in some studies the experience of the surgeon.[3,4]

All these factors have to be meticulously taken care by the physician to mitigate the problem.

Evolution of the Technique of Miniperc

In 1997, Helal[5] and Jackman[6] et al, independently described a mini percutaneous nephrostolithotomy. The classical description was a 11Fr peel away sheath. This was the birth of the term "miniperc". Jackman et al, achieved a stone free rate of 85% with an average stone size of 1.2 cm. Chan and Jarrett performed miniperc in an adult population with average stone size of 1.4 cm^2 using 13 Fr ureteroscopy access sheath, the results have been published since then.[7] The success rates in this procedure range between 85 and 90 percent.[8] The peel-away sheaths were found to be too flexible and not suitable for use in adult patients and hence not in vogue now. A balance in between the tract size, vision and the stone clearance should be maintained. Jackman et al[8] defined the 'mini PERC' as a percutaneous nephrolithotomy achieved through a sheath too small to accommodate a standard rigid nephroscope.[8]

Does the Tract Size Correlate with Parenchymal Loss?

The above question was answered by a number of workers. Clayman et al[9] noted that dilatation of a percutaneous nephrostomy tract to 24 versus 36 Fr resulted in a comparable degree of parenchymal fibrosis. Further, the same study noted equal cortical scarring in both degree of dilatation. In a similar porcine model Traxer et al[10] also found no significant difference in parenchymal scarring in standard and mini tracts and, furthermore, the amount of renal scarring was insignificant compared with overall renal volume.[10]

Initial Challenges to Miniaturization

The challenges with Miniperc have already been described in the initial paragraphs of this chapter. Giusti and colleagues[11] performed a retrospective comparison of standard *vs* mini PERC. They demonstrated a lower stone free rates despite longer operative times in the Mini PERC group

The operative time was longer.[11] The reduced sheath diameter caused a decreased flow of irrigation, thus leading to less visibility. Another worker, Low et al, in his study reiterated the fact that higher intrapelvic pressures were associated with nephroscopy sheaths of smaller calibre and greater length.[12]

Overcoming the Problems

The problem of increased intrarenal pressures has been circumvented in the latest inventions. Success of miniaturised PCNL (Mini PERC/mini PCNL) in the last decade can be attributed to a number of modifications which include methods to reduce intrarenal pressures, newer lasers, smaller sheaths, etc.

Success of miniaturised PCNL (mini PERC/ mini PCNL) in the last decade is attributed to the following technological improvisation and advantages:

- Maintaining the intrarenal pressures below the desired limit.

- Stone clearance rates comparable with standard PCNL.
- Reducing the operative time by improved sheath design with improved techniques of fragmentation and retrieval of fragments
- Improvement in stone retrieval techniques
- Holmium laser lithotripsy
- Tubeless procedures
- Newer designed sheaths **(Fig. 12.4A)** and scopes with excellent optics.

Intrarenal Pressures

- In the landmark canine study of Hinman and colleagues, pyelovenous backflow occurred at renal pelvic pressures (RPP) above 30 to 35 mm Hg.[13] The study of Hinman has remained a benchmark in instituting various treatments[14], Zhong et al[15] demonstrated that renal pelvic pressure generally remains lower than the backflow level (30 mm Hg) during mini PERC. Higher pressures might lead to associated

problems. The possible solutions suggested by many to overcome these are:

- Nagele U, et al[16] demonstrated that by using a 12 Fr nephroscope in connection with the new open 18 Fr access sheath, critical renal pressure can be avoided, even if the inflow pressure is as high as 125 cm H_2O **(Fig. 12.4B)**.
- Another technique, the ultra mini PERC has an outer (13 Fr) and inner (6 Fr) sheath. The 3.5 Fr telescope fits into the inner sheath. Saline escapes through the space between the inner sheath and the outer sheath. The whirlpool effect helps in clearance of the stones.[17]

Success Rates

It is imperative that stone clearance rates are not compromised by reducing the tract size. Over the last decade, many series have now established the success of miniaturized PCNL with stone clearance rates at par with standard PCNL.

- Mishra et al[18] and Knoll et al[19] compared mini PCNL (18 Fr) with standard PCNL (26 Fr) for medium-sized stones in prospective studies. Both the studies demonstrated com-parable stone clearance rates between the mini PCNL and standard PCNL groups.
- Cheng et al[20] in a prospective randomized study compared mini PCNL with standard PCNL. The Mini-PCNL group has a higher stone-free rate for multiple calyceal stones than the standard PCNL.[21]
- Kukreja[22] demonstrated that mini-PERC reduced the morbidity of standard PCNL in terms of reduced blood loss without compromising the stone clearance rates or the operative time.
- In a meta-analyses comparing mini PCNL to standard PCNL, operative time was longer in mini PCNL, but overall hospital stay was shorter with similar stone free rates.[23]

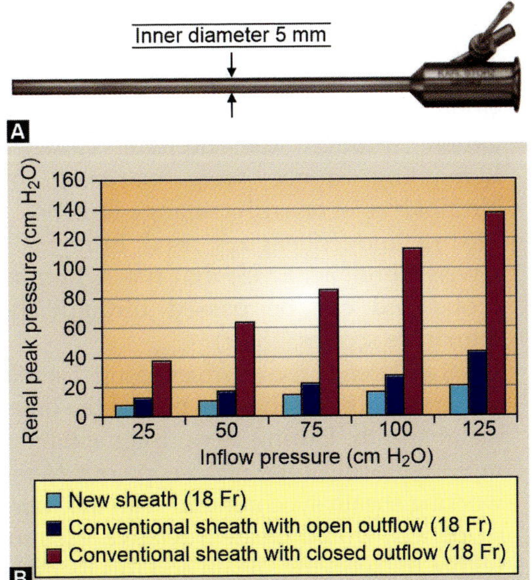

Figs 12.4A and B: (A) The newly designed hydrodynamic sheath with 15 Fr and 16 Fr inner and outer diameters; (B) Comparison of infrarenal pressures. Nagele Udo, et al[13]

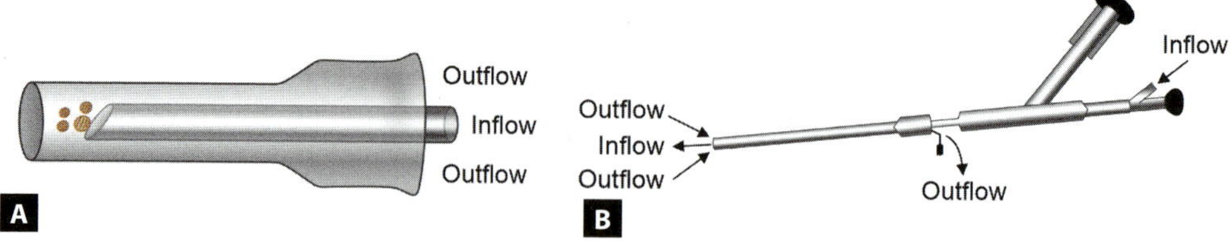

Figs 12.5A and B: Nagele modular MIP system. (A) Hydrodynamic vacuum cleaner effect; (B) Open system without any lock between the telescope and the sheath. Inflow is through the irrigating channel in the telescope and outflow is through the space between the telescope and operating sheath keeping the intrarenal pressure low and also helping in continuous evacuation of the stone dust

Operative Time

As experience increased and stone fragmentation and retrieval techniques were improved, the operative time reduced. Kukreja[22], and Lange and Gutierrez[24] in comparative studies found no significant difference in residual stone burden, operative time, or postoperative analgesic use between standard PCNL and mini PCNL (16.5 Fr).

Stone Retrieval

Stone retrieval posed a big challenge for mini PCNL, the reasons being the small diameter requiring smaller fragments and delicate stone retrieval forceps and baskets. Improvements in fragmentation and retrieval techniques have helped improve the immediate stone clearance rates, reduce the operative or nephroscopy time and reduce the need for delicate and fragile forceps and baskets.

- Pulsatile low pressure perfusion pump by Zeng et al[22] used a pulsatile low-pressure perfusion pump. This helped in fragment clearance.
- Nagele and colleagues demonstrated the "vacuum cleaner effect", allowed the carefully directed extraction of stone fragments without any supplementary tool.[25] The stone extraction depends on the relation between nephroscope diameter and inner sheath diameter. The strongest effect was observed with a 12 Fr nephroscope and an inner sheath diameter of 15 Fr.

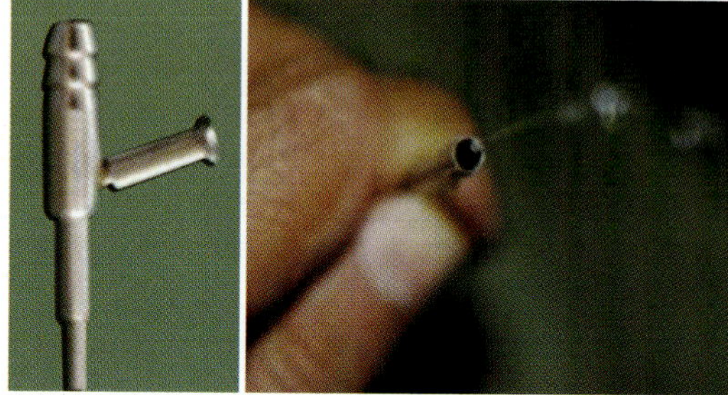

Fig. 12.6: Ultra mini PERC; outer sheath with a side port for saline flushing

- Lezrek and colleagues proposed a technique in which the nephroscope is used as a vacuum cleaner.[26]
- Bhattu and colleagues[26] flushed out the stone fragments from the kidney by irrigation through the ureteral catheter. Remaining stones were extracted by Nitinol basket or with triflange forceps.
- Mishra and colleagues used Lithovac™ (Swiss Lithovac, EMS) that has a 1.6 mm probe and can be passed through the miniature scopes (18 Fr).[27]
- Desai and Zeng[28] use a syringe to inject sterile saline solution via the side port of the outer metal sheath. During stone fragmentation, rapid removal of the endoscope out of the working sheath synchronized with the water jet period, would create a relative vacuum within the working sheath and this together with the recoil of water jets, would flush out the small stone fragment (3 mm) and blood clots **(Fig. 12.6)**.

Intracorporeal Lithotripsy

As the instrument size goes smaller so does the working channel and in effect the energy.

- Reduced shaft size in mini PCNL poses a challenge for fragment retrieval. The stones need to be fragmented into much smaller particles as compared to standard PCNL.
- Ganesamoni, Sabnis and colleagues compared the stone fragmentation characteristics and outcomes of laser lithotripsy and pneumatic lithotripsy in mini PERC for renal calculi.[29]
- Bellman and colleagues[30] compared fragment sizes obtained after different intracorporeal lithotripsy energy devices. Holmium:YAG fragments were significantly smaller than fragments from the other lithotrites for all stone compositions.
- *Laser settings:* Fragment size may be less related to laser lithotripter settings and more dependent on the surgical technique employed, i.e. whether the stone is repeatedly perforated, chipped, or fragmented.[30–32] It is a interplay between the pulse and energy.

Tubeless Procedures

The relative lack of bleeding allows surgeons get the confidence to not insert the nephrostomy tube.[33] Stents and tubes result in symptoms, healthcare cost, decreased quality of life and further procedure to facilitate removal. Multiple series have shown similar results with no nephrostomy tubes.[27]

Armamentarium for Mini PERC (Fig. 12.7 and Table 12.1)

- Schilling et al.[34] have proposed a uniform terminology for PCNL based on the outer sheath size.
- The Storz mini PERC is also called Nagele modular miniature nephroscope system with automatic pressure control and is probably the commonest system used.

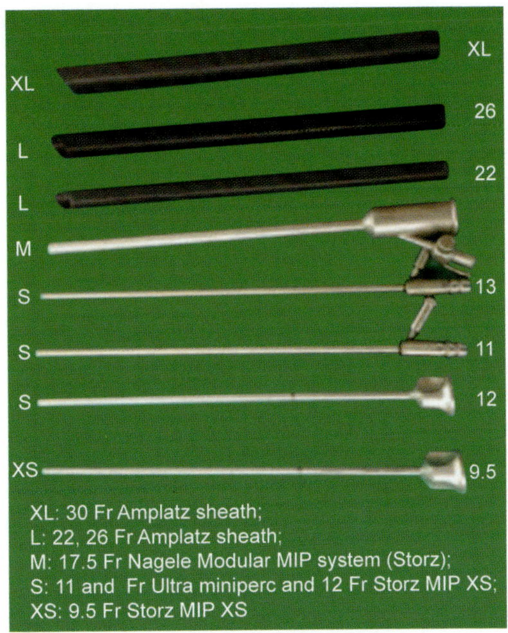

Fig. 12.7: Various sheath sizes

- *Dilatation:* Sheaths have their own one step dilators. Subsequent passage of the metal dilators and sheath becomes easier with reduced risk of kinking of the guidewire or loss of the tract.
- *Optics:* The Storz, Wolf and Olympus have a 12 Fr mini PCNL fiberoptic have fiberoptic telescopes with excellent vision. Storz also has a 7.5 Fr fiberoptic scope for MIP S and XS systems. The Ultra mini PERC has a 3.5 Fr telescope with 17000 pixels resolution, while the Microperc has a flexible 0.9 mm telescope with resolution up to 10,000 pixels.
- *Energy source:* As the sheath and nephroscope dimensions reduce, so does the working channel and energy sources.
- *Optics:* The fiber optic telescope (10,000 pixels) was initially used for endoscopic inspection of the lacrimal duct. The unique feature of this telescope is its flexibility. It consists of micro optics 0.9 mm in diameter with a 120° of view and resolution up to 10,000 pixels.

TABLE 12.1: Comparison of mini PCNL system

	Outer diameter	*Nephroscope size*	*Working channel*	*Instrument size permissible*	*Direction of view*	*Length of sheath*
Storz MIP Mini PERC set	15/16, 16.5/17.5, and 21/22 Fr (inner/outer diameter)	12 Fr	6.7 Fr	5 Fr	12°	18 cm
Wolf mini PERC Olympus Ultra mini PCNL (UMP)	15 and 18 Fr 15 Fr 11 and 13 Fr (with 6 and 7.5 Fr inner sheaths)	14 Fr 11 Fr 3.5 Fr	6 Fr 7.5 Fr 7 Fr	6 Fr 6 Fr 4 Fr	12° 7° 0°	20.5 cm 22 cm 15 and 18 cm
Storz MIP XS Micro PERC Super PERC (Shah sheath)[35]	9.5 and 12 Fr 4.8 and 8 Fr 12,14 and 18 Fr	7.5 Fr 0.9 mm Compatible with Storz/Wolf and UMP nephroscope	2 Fr Absent	1.9 Fr	6°	15 and 18 cm 8–22 cm

- *Energy source:* Laser is the choice for the disintegration of the calculus. The energy source should be set in such a way that the calculus is evaporated in dust rather than having larger fragments. The laser fiber used is 275 micron. If an 8 Fr sheath is used, an ultrasound energy source can be used.

Superperc

These sheaths are developed by Kaushik Shah et al. from India. Multiple sheaths are available with this technology, i.e 10 Fr, 12 Fr and 15 Fr. The sheath has been innovated by Shah et al. and the length of the sheath may vary from 8 to 20 cm (**Fig. 12.8A**).[14] The key feature of this technology is that the master suction is attached to the sheath not to the channel (**Fig. 12.8B**).[35] The suction is controlled using a suction port which is finger controlled. It allows larger fragment size retrieval. A short ureteroscope can be used as nephroscope.

Microperc telescope, micro nephroscope from 18 Apple life sciences, UMP (ultra miniperc) telescope with inner sheath or Karl Storz™ nephroscope can be all used with 10 and 12 Fr sheath. Miniperc nephroscope from

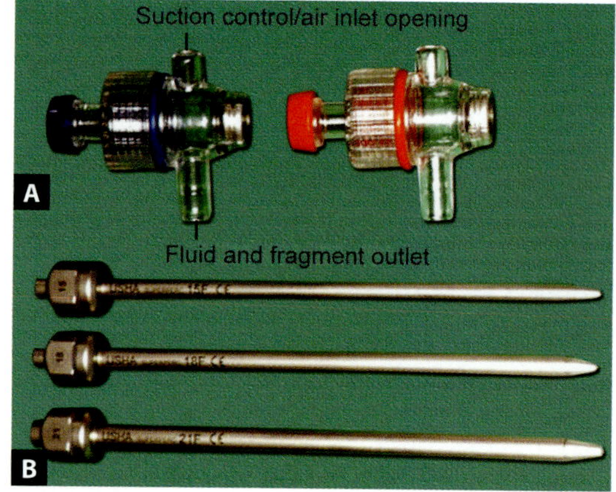

Figs 12.8A and B: Shah Superperc sheaths (autoclavable)

Karl Storz™, Olympus™ or Richard Wolf™ can be used with 15 Fr sheath size.

MICROPERC (Fig. 12.9)

Markus Bader and colleagues presented their work of "see-through needle" for gaining access to the collecting system.[36] The concept was based on the fact that the "see-through needle" helped the surgeon to be sure that the puncture was accurate and into the desired calyx.

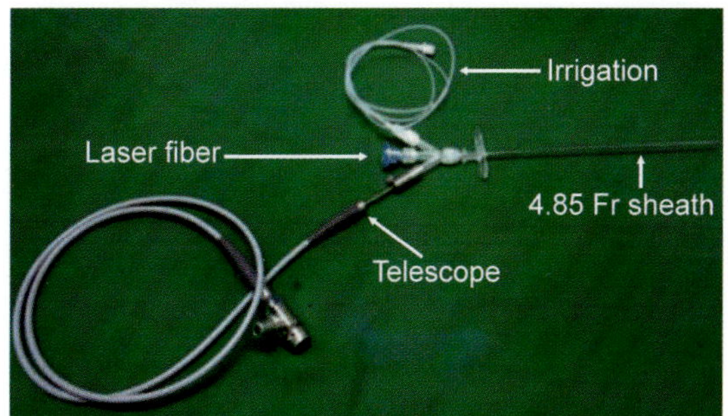

Fig. 12.9: All seeing needle assembled for stone fragmentation

Desai and colleagues further developed the concept wherein the procedure was completed through the needle itself obviating the need to dilate the tract.[37]

The key component of this new technique was excellent optics. This technique was christened as "Microperc". Theoretically, the advantage perceived was limiting and/or obviating the complications of tract dilatation.

- *The needle has three parts:* (a) The outer sheath acts as a conduit for passage of optics and energy source such as laser. (b) The central part comprises a beveled hollow needle. (c) The innermost part is a radiopaque stylet. Deasi et al. in one of their studies concluded that, for the management of small renal calculi, Microperc is as safe as RIRS.[38–40] This study suggested that the RIRS is associated with higher need for the placement of DJ stents, whereas Microperc causes more hemoglobin drop, increased pain and higher analgesic requirements.

- *Intrarenal pressures:* Tepeler et al[41] measured intrarenal pelvic pressure during PNL procedures using 4.8 Fr nephroscopes in comparison to conventional PNL. Intrarenal pressure was significantly lower in the conventional group during all steps of the procedure. Even though there was no difference in outcome in their series, surgeons should be aware of higher pressure.

CONCLUSION

Miniperc has established its role in the management small and medium sizes renal stones (up to 3 cm).[22] It offers success rates comparable to standard PCNL with significantly reduced blood loss and increased incidence of tubeless procedures.[22,33] Single step dilatation and reducing the need for stone retrieval devices are other advantages.

Complex situations such as diverticular stones, stones in ectopic kidneys and pediatric moderate-sized stones would be other suitable indications.

Regardless of how small the tract size is, the key to a successful procedure remains perfect percutaneous renal access.

REFERENCES

1. Turk C, Knoll T, Petrik A. et al. Guidelines on Urolithiasis. European Association of Urology; 2015. http://uroweb.org/wp-content/uploads/22-Urolithiasis_LR_full.pdf.
2. Seitz C, Desai M, Häcker A, et al. Incidence, prevention, and management of complications following percutaneous nephrolitholapaxy. Eur Urol. 2012;61:146–58.
3. Yamaguchi A, Skolarikos A, Buchholz NP, et al. Operating times and bleeding complications in percutaneous nephrolithotomy: a comparison of tract dilation methods in 5,537 patients in the Clinical Research Office of the Endourological Society Percutaneous Nephrolithotomy Global Study. J Endourol. 2011;25:933–39.
4. Kukreja R, Desai M, Patel S, et al. Factors affecting blood loss during percutaneous nephrolithotomy: prospective study. J Endourol 2004; 18:715–22.
5. Helal M, Black T, Lockhart J, Figueroa TE. The Hickman peel-away sheath: alternative for pediatric percutaneous nephrolithotomy. J Endourol. 1997;11:171–72.
6. Jackman SV, Hedican SP, Docimo SG, et al. Miniaturized access for pediatric percutaneous nephrolithotomy. J Endourol 1997 suppl; 11: S133.
7. Chan DY, Jarrett TW: Mini percutaneous nephrolithotomy. J Endourol. 2000;14:269.

8. Jackman SV, Docimo SG, Cadeddu JA, et al. The "mini PERC" technique: a less invasive alternative to percutaneous nephrolithotomy. World J Urol. 1998;16:371.

9. Clayman RV, Elbers J, Miller RP, et al. Percutaneous nephrostomy: assessment of renal damage associated with semi-rigid (24F) and balloon (36F) dilation. J Urol. 1987;138:203.

10. Traxer O, Smith TG, et al. Renal Parenchymal Injury after Standard and mini PCNL. J Urol. 2001;165;1693–95.

11. Giusti G, Piccinelli A, Taverna G, et al. mini PERC? No, thank you! Eur Urol. 2007;51:810–15.

12. Low RK. Nephroscopy sheath characteristics and intrarenal pelvic pressure: Human kidney model. J Endourol. 1999;13:205–08.

13. Hinman F, Redewill FH. Pyelovenous back flow. JAMA. 1926;87:1287–88.

14. Landman J, Venkatesh R, Ragab M, et al. Comparison of intrarenal pressure and irrigant flow during percutaneous nephroscopy with an indwelling ureteral catheter, ureteral occlusion balloon, and ureteral access sheath. Urology 2002;60:584–87.

15. Zhong W, Guohua Z, et al. J Endourol. 2008; 22(9):2147–51.

16. Nagele U, Horstmann M, Sievert KD, et al. A newly designed Amplatz sheath decreases intrapelvic irrigation pressure during mini percutaneous nephrolitholapaxy: An *in vitro* pressure measurement and microscopic study. J Endourol. 2007;21:1113–16.

17. Desai J, Solanki R. Ultra-mini percutaneous nephrolithomy (UMP): one more armamentarium. BJU Int. 2013;112:1046.

18. Mishra S, Sharma R, et al. Prospective comparative study of mini PERC and standard PNL for treatment of 1 to 2 cm size renal stone. BJUI 2011;108:896– 900.

19. Knoll T, Wezel F, Michel MS, et al. Do Patients Benefit from Miniaturized Tubeless Percutaneous Nephrolithotomy? A Comparative Prospective Study. J Endourol. 2010;24(7):1075–79.

20. Cheng F, Yu W, Zhang X, et al. Minimally Invasive Tract in Percutaneous Nephrolithotomy for Renal Stones. J Endourol. 2010;24(10):1579–82.

21. Zeng G, et al. Minimally Invasive PCNL for simple and complex renal calyceal stones: A comparative analysis of more than 10000 cases. J Endourol. 2013;27(10):1203–08.

22. Kukreja RA. Should mini Percutaneous Nephrolithotomy (mini PERC) be the ideal tract for Miniaturization in PCNL 115 medium sized renal calculi (15–30 mm)? World J Urol 2018;36:285. https://doi.org/10.1007/s00345-017-2128-z.

23. Zhu W, Liu Y, Liu L, et al. Minimally invasive versus standard percutaneous nephrolithotomy: a meta-analysis. Urolithiasis. 2015;43(6): 563–70.

24. Lange JN, Gutierrez-Aceves J, Comparative Outcomes of Conventional PCNL and Miniaturized PCNL in the Treatment of Kidney Stones: Does a Miniaturized Tract Improve Quality of Care? Urology Practice (2017), doi: 10.1016/j.urpr. 2017.04.003.

25. Nicklas AP, Schilling D, Bader MJ, Herrmann TRW, Nagele U. The vacuum cleaner effect in minimally invasive percutaneous nephrolitholapaxy. WJU. 2015;33:1847–53.

26. Lezrek M, Qarro A, Bazine K, Najoui M, Asseban M, Benjelloun M, el Kasmaoui H, Beddouch A, Alami M. A vacuum cleaner for the pelvicalyceal system during percutaneous nephrolithotomy. J Endourol. 2010;24(6):949–52.

27. Bhattu AS, Mishra S, Ganpule A, et al. Outcomes in a Large Series of mini PERCS: Analysis of Consecutive 318 Patients. J Endourol 2015;29(3):283–87.

28. Desai J, Zeng G, Zhao Z, Zhong W, Chen W, Wu W. A novel technique of Ultra-mini percutaneous nephrolithotomy: introduction and an initial experience for treatment of upper urinary calculi less than 2 cm. Biomed Res Int. 2013; 490793.

29. Ganesamoni R, Sabnis RB, Mishra S, Parekh N, Ganpule A, Vyas JB, Jagtap J, Desai M. Prospective Randomized Controlled Trial Comparing Laser Lithotripsy with Pneumatic Lithotripsy in mini PERC for Renal Calculi. J Endourol 2013; 27(12):1444–49.

30. Teichman JM, Bellman GC, et al. Holmium:YAG lithotripsy yields smaller fragments than LithoClast, pulsed dye laser or electrohydraulic lithotripsy. J. Urol. 1998;159(1):17–23.

31. Kronenberg P, Traxer O. *In vitro* fragmentation efficiency of holmium:yttrium-aluminum-garnet (YAG) laser lithotripsy: a comprehensive study encompassing different frequencies, pulse energies, total power levels and laser fiber diameters. BJU Int. 2014;114(2):261–67.

32. Traxer O, Kronenberg P. Update on lasers in urology (2014): current assessment on holmium: yttrium-aluminum-garnet (Ho:YAG) laser lithotripter settings and laser fibers. World J Urol. 2015;33:463.

33. Desai J, et al. Prospective Outcomes of Ultra mini Percutaneous Nephrolithotomy: A Consecutive Cohort Study. J Urol. 2016;195:741–46.

34. Schilling D, Hu?sch T, Bader M, et al. Nomenclature in PCNL or the Tower of Babel: a proposal for a uniform terminology. World J Urol. 2015;33:1905.

35. Shah K, Agrawal MS, Mishra DK. Super PERC: A new technique in minimally-invasive percutaneous nephrolithotomy. IJU. 2017;33(1):48–52.

36. Bader M, Christian G, Boris S, et al. The "All Seeing Needle"—an optical puncture system confirming percutaneous access in PCNL. J Urol. 2010;183(4):e734.

37. Desai MR, Sharma R, Mishra S, et al. Single-step percutaneous nephrolithotomy (Microperc): the initial clinical report. J Urol. 2011;186:140–145.

38. Tepeler A, Armagan A, Sancaktutar AA, et al. The role of Microperc in the treatment of symptomatic lower pole renal calculi. J Endourol. 2013;27:13–18.

39. Armagan A, Tepeler A, Silay MS, et al. Micropercutaneous nephrolithotomy in the treatment of moderate-sized renal calculi. J Endourol. 2013;27:177–81.

40. Sabnis RB, Ganesamoni R, Doshi A, et al. Micropercutaneous nephrolithotomy (Microperc) vs retrograde intrarenal surgery for the management of small renal calculi: a randomized controlled trial. BJU Int. 2013;112(3):355–361.

41. Tepeler A, Akman T, Silay MS, et al. Comparison of intrarenal pelvic pressure during micropercutaneous nephrolithotomy and conventional percutaneous nephrolithotomy. Urolithiasis. 2014;42:275–79.

PAEDIATRIC PCNL

Akshay Nathani, Ravindra Sabnis

INTRODUCTION

Incidence of paediatric renal stone disease 1–5% in Asian population[1] and overall children contribute 2–3% of the total population of stone-formers.[2] Etiology in most of the case relates to abnormal anatomy or metabolic or infections. Complete stone clearance remains the mainstay of treatment to avoid recurrence which would not be affordable in poor socio-economic strata. Evolution of endourologic management for stone disease has led for better management of paediatric renal stones with minimal procedural morbidity. Miniaturisation of PCNL armamentarium has contributed to minimize morbidity in children. This chapter will focus on the procedural steps and how paediatric PCNL is different from adult with learning points.

Challenges in paediatric population
- Size of kidneys is small.
- Hypermobility of kidney.
- As kidneys are growing and treatment should not affect its growth.
- Risk of radiation exposure both for preoperative CT scan and intraoperative fluoroscopy.
- Retreatment in children is troublesome.

Preoperative Concerns in Paediatric Population

Challenge starts from history as well as examination, as infants and toddlers are unable to express so it becomes difficult to identify symptomatology. Investigations need to be tailored as challenges start right from collection of blood sample for laboratory examination and urine collection is still challenging in children. Imaging need to be restricted to low dose CT IVU (computed tomography intravenous urography) for which anaesthetist support is required which leads to additional drug administration from anaesthesia point of view. Also urine should be sterile as paediatric age group is more vulnerable to undergo in sepsis and show subtle signs of the same. Therefore, they should be covered with antibiotics prior to procedure. Operating room time of children should also be restricted as they are more prone for hypothermia than adults.

Operatives Steps and Challenges

- Anaesthesia concerns and positioning
  All paediatric PCNLs should be performed under general anaesthesia, special care should be taken to avoid hypothermia like use of warmers, warm irrigation fluids, etc. usually performed in prone position after standard placement of ureteric catheter before turning the patient to prone position **(Fig. 12.10)**.
- Operative concerns
  Avoidance of hypothermia, less space of working in paediatric patients, hypermobile kidneys and subtle clinical signs

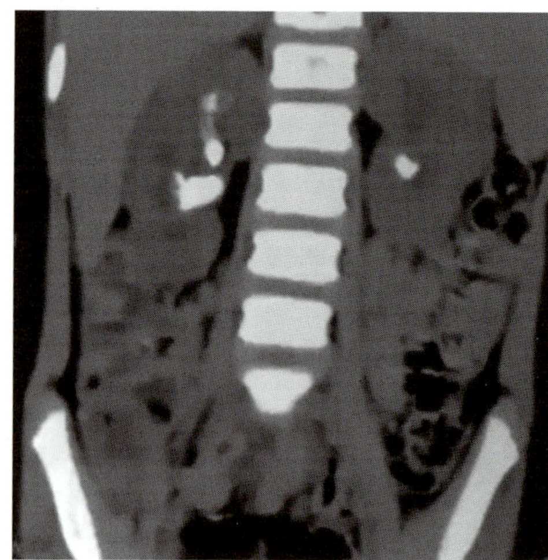

Fig. 12.10: Bilateral renal calculi in a 12-year-old boy

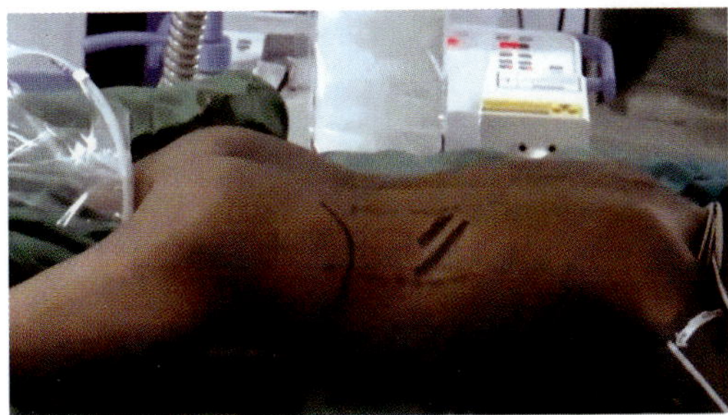

Fig. 12.11: Prone position after insertion of ureteric catheter

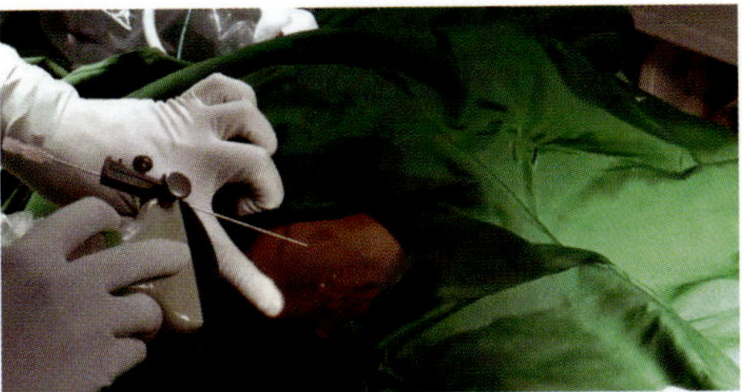

Fig. 12.12A: Ultrasound probe with puncture attachment guide with initial puncture 18 G in position

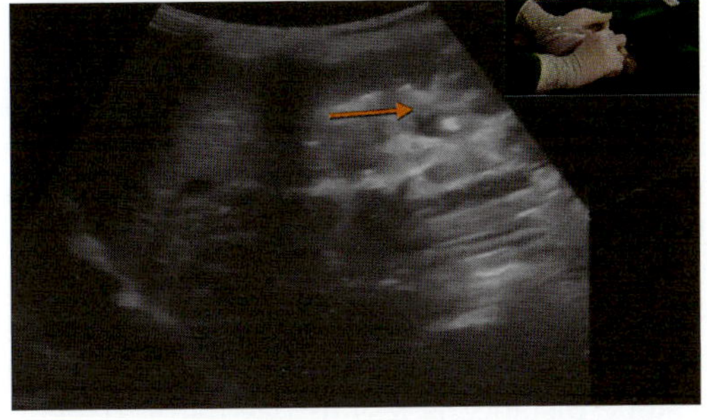

Fig. 12.12B: USG guided initial puncture step with echotip of the needle can be seen with orange arrow

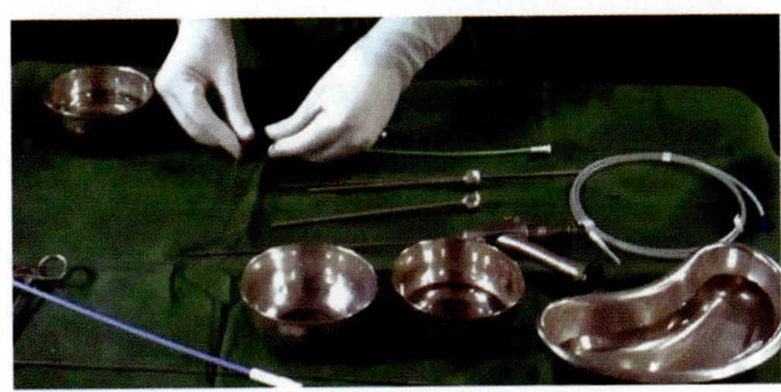

Fig. 12.13: Instrument trolly MIP-S (Minimally invasive PCNL–Small) sheath size 11/12 Fr and scope size 7.5 Fr with 2/3 Fr working channel for laser fiber

of sepsis in paediatric population are the main operative concerns. In prone position in children's soft bolsters can be placed one below chest **(Fig. 12.11)** and second below lower abdomen that makes bowel fall and avoids bowel injury during puncture.

- Access planning
  Preoperative imaging CT IVU guides plan target calyx puncture. Also depending on stone bulk, pelvi calyceal anatomy, dilatation of calyx and infundibular width, that tract dilatation can be planned. Preferred is ultrasound guided puncture so as to avoid radiation exposure with fluoroscopy guided puncture.

- Initial puncture
  USG guided puncture requires 3.5 or 5 MHz probe **(Figs 12.12A and B)**. To start with ultrasound probe is scrolled from posterior axillary line, then anteriorly till the whole of kidney is in frame to decide for target calyx puncture which is the first calyx seen from posteriorly. USG also helps to see whether any overlying bowel, spleen, liver are coming in way of tract or not. Puncture guide attachment is a very useful tool to guide for correct direction of puncture and echotip needle is seen throughout the puncture process entering through the cup of calyx and if not seen jiggling movements can be done. Correct puncture can be confirmed by efflux of clear urine

after removing the stellate if needle and by contrast instillation and checking on fluoroscopy.

Fluoroscopy guided puncture procedure *per se* remains the same as adult, a few differences being short length 18 G puncture needle to be used, 0.025 inch guidewire can be an option after initial puncture if system is not too capacious instead of 0.035 inch **(Fig. 12.13)**.

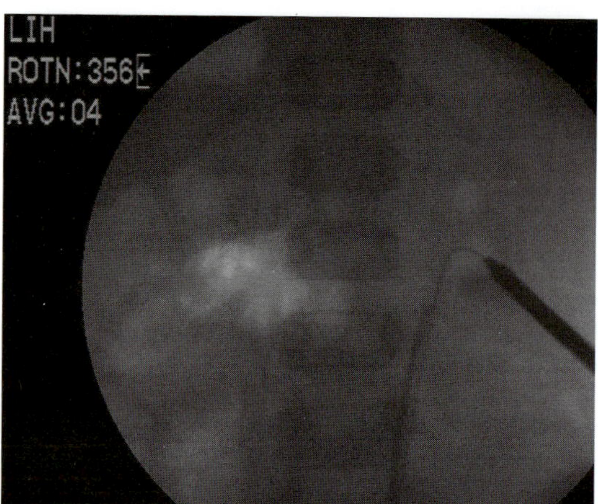

Fig. 12.14: Tract dilatation with single step dilator with metallic 11/12 Fr MPI-S sheath deployed with ureteric and guidewire positioned in ureter

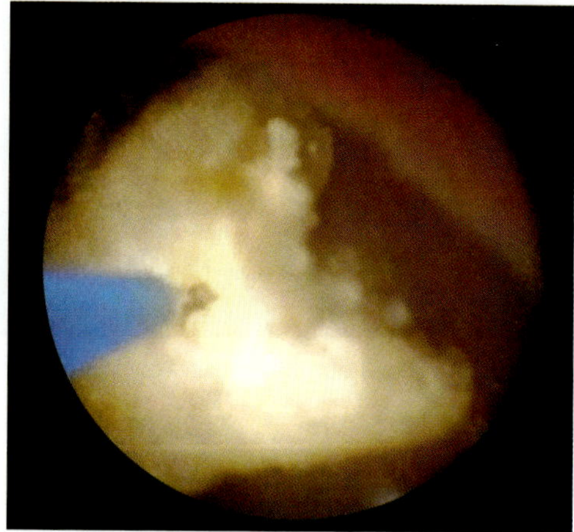

Fig. 12.15: Thulium fiber laser 200 micron in action for lasing stone

6 Fr or 8 Fr screw dilator, good assistance to keep the sheath in place to avoid tract loss as skin to stone distance is less in paediatric patients. Least possible radiation should be used.

- **Tract dilatation**

  Depending on stone bulk PCNL tract dilatation is planned usually in paediatric age group tract size is restricted to < 22 Fr, i.e mini PCNL preferably MIP-M (minimally invasive PCNL medium 15 to 19 Fr) or MIP-S (minimally invasive PCNL small 10–14 Fr) **(Fig. 12.14)**. As the tract dilatation increases, risk of bleeding increases.[3]

- **Lithotripters**

  Depending upon the size of the dilated tract, the energy used should be laser or pneumatic or shock pulse. The later two can be used only if mini PCNL is done or tract is dilated till 20 Fr.

  For smaller tracts preferred energy is laser holmium or thulium fiber laser **(Fig. 12.15)**.

Exit Strategy

Exit strategy of placement of nephrostomy tube, DJ stent or ureteric catheter is individualised **(Fig. 12.16)**. If the PCS is not

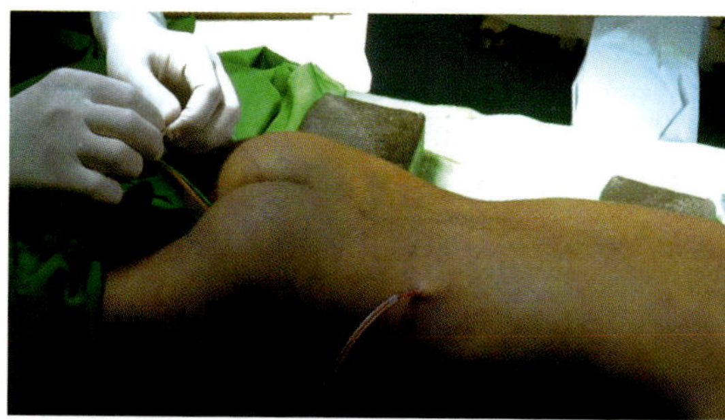

Fig. 12.16: Nephrostomy placement and ureteric catheter being fixed with suture material to Foley's catheter as exit strategy

edematous, procedure is uncomplicated, no or minimal bleeding, non-infected stones and no residual stones, then totally tubeless PCNL can be done. Totally tubeless PCNL means a ureteric catheter is placed for 1–2 days and it is removed if there is no soakage from PCNL site. However, if there are residual fragments, stone is infected, edematous pelvis, then it is advisable to keep a PCN tube with/without DJ stent. If the stones are infective stones, then a PCN with a ureteric catheter can be placed so that antibiotic solution irrigation can be started in postoperative period.

Why such a discussion on tubeless procedure in children?

If not needed preference is not to put in a tube as stent removal requires another set of admission and anaesthesia and urethral instrumentation.

If after the completion of lasing, there are concerns regarding the residual dust or gravel that has been deposited in the pelvicalyceal system, it would be prudent to place a JJ stent of an appropriate size.

The placement of nephrostomy drainage tube depends on presence of any complication like bleeding or significant perforation or infected stones. If the stone bulk is large, then placement of nephrostomy tube will be a good option, so if required relook second check nephroscopy can be done for removal of residual fragments, if any.

Follow-up Protocol

It is usually based on case to case basis and institution policy. Usual trend is to perform X-ray KUB on postoperative day 2 and if clear the nephrotomy tube is removed followed by per urethral catheter.

If any residual fragments seen, the relook nephroscopy can be done.

After complete clearance and stent removal, metabolic work up and blood biochemistry should be done.

Simultaneous Bilateral PCNL (SBPCNL)

3–4 studies were conducted for bilateral simultaneous PCNL and suggested that it is a feasible and safe if carefully selected cases and concluded children with bilateral renal stones undergoing SBPCNL. Advantages of SBPCNL reported were reduced psychological stress, one cystoscopy and anesthesia, less medication, and a shorter hospital stay and convalescence, with considerable savings in costs.[4–6]

CONCLUSION

Complete stone clearance should be the aim as paediatric population are at high risk of stone recurrence with increased amount of predisposing factors.

Complete metabolic evaluation should be done as paediatric renal stones recur frequently.

Efforts should be made to reduce the number of procedures performed to a minimum and to save the developing kidney from the deleterious effects of the repeated interventions.

A urine culture before PCNL is required and prophylactic antibiotics 3 to 5 days before the procedure are recommended despite a negative preoperative culture to minimize bacteriuria.

The key to success in PCNL in these small patients is staging the procedure if required, miniaturization of instruments, and using ultrasound as the method of achieving access.

REFERENCES

1. Ramello A, Vitale C, Marangella M. Epidemiology of nephrolithiasis. J Nephrol. 2000;13(Suppl 3):S45–50.
2. Schwarz RD, Dwyer NT. Pediatric kidney stones: long-term outcomes. Urology. 2006;67(4):812–6.
3. Kukreja R, Desai M, Patel S, Bapat S, Desai M. Factors affecting blood loss during percutaneous nephrolithotomy: prospective study. J Endourol. 2004;18(8):715–22.
4. Samad L, Aquil S, Zaidi Z. Paediatric percutaneous nephrolithotomy: setting new frontiers. BJU Int. 2006;97(2):359–63.
5. Salah MA, Tállai B, Holman E, Khan MA, Tóth G, Tóth C. Simultaneous bilateral percutaneous nephrolithotomy in children. BJU Int. 2005;95(1):137–9.
6. Guven S, Ozturk A, Arslan M, Istanbulluoglu O, Piskin M, Kilinc M. Simultaneous bilateral percutaneous nephrolithotomy in children: no need to delay. J Endourol. 2011;25(3):437–40.

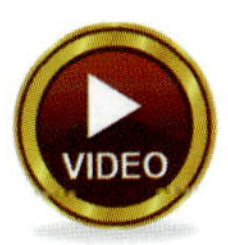

Scan QR Code for Video on
Pediatric PCNL

ENDOSCOPIC COMBINED INTRARENAL SURGERY (ECIRS)

Akshay Nathani, Abhishek Singh

In 2008, the acronym ECIRS was first used for endoscopic combined intrarenal surgery with an effort to standardize the management of complex large renal stones by addition of retrograde flexible ureteroscope to antegrade PCNL.[1] The existence of ECIRS was after the invention of Galdakao-modified supine position. Its advantages being both PCNL and simultaneous retrograde intrarenal surgery for aiding complete stone clearance as well as limiting the complications of PCNL. In initial period, ECIRS was not a standard terminology but eventually in the last decade it has been included in EUA guidelines.[2]

Why ECIRS ??

Rationale behind development of ECIRS was to completely clear the complex renal stones with multiple peripheral calculi in single sitting without much of morbidity. With the advent of modified Valdivia position ECIRS got invented and feasible.

To avoid multiple tracts for complex renal stones, ECIRS is an excellent operation provided with the availability of armamentarium.

Indications of ECIRS:
- Complex renal stones.
- Staghorn calculi with multiple peripherally placed calculi.
- Multiple renal calculi with complex renal anatomy like malrotated, ectopic kidneys.

Preoperative Preparations

Clinical history, examination and investigations, i.e laboratory hemogram, renal function test, coagulation profile and imaging in the form of X-ray KUB (kidney ureter bladder), CT IVU (intravenous urography) if renal parameters are normal or else plain CT KUB for preoperative planning for stone size, location, stone burden and Hounsfield unit (Biorad™Flexible ureterorenoscope). The preoperative culture should be checked, if it shows evidence of infection, the infection should be treated preoperatively as per hospital antibiogram policy.

Operative technique will be divided into the following steps:
1. Operating room set up
2. Patient positioning and ergonomics
3. Armamentarium required
4. Flexible ureteroscopy
5. Puncture of target calyx
6. Dilatation of tract
7. Nephroscopy and intracorporeal lithotripters and passing the ball
8. Exit strategy.

1. Operating Room Set up and Armamentarium

Operating room should be capacious enough to comfortably accommodate simultaneous set of RIRS and supine PCNL set up along with surgeons, healthcare personnel. RIRS set up will include retrograde surgeon and its armamentarium, carm, video trolly, laser as energy source **(Fig. 12.17)**.

Antegrade supine PCNL surgeon and its armamentarium video trolly, C-arm energy source.

Picture demonstrating two surgeons, one performing PCNL and the second surgeon performing RIRS **(Fig. 12.18)**.

2. Patient Positioning and Ergonomics

Galdakao modification of valdivia position which is most commonly used position for simultaneous access from retrograde manner. In this modification, patient's legs are placed in a modified lithotomy position with both legs on stirrups. The side to be operated is oblique with leg extended and straight while contralateral leg is depressed and abducted

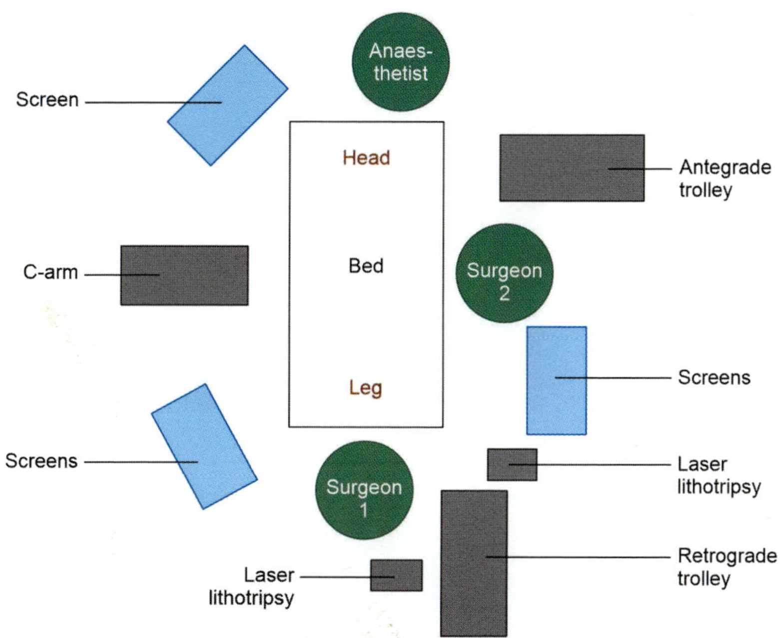

Fig. 12.17: Operating room setup

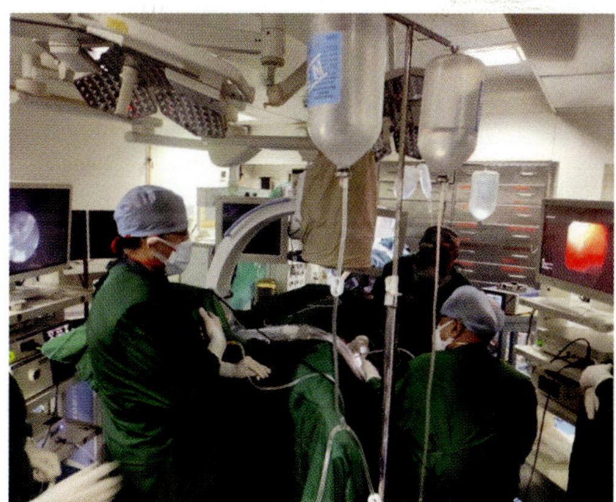

Fig. 12.18: Position of surgeons for the ECIRS

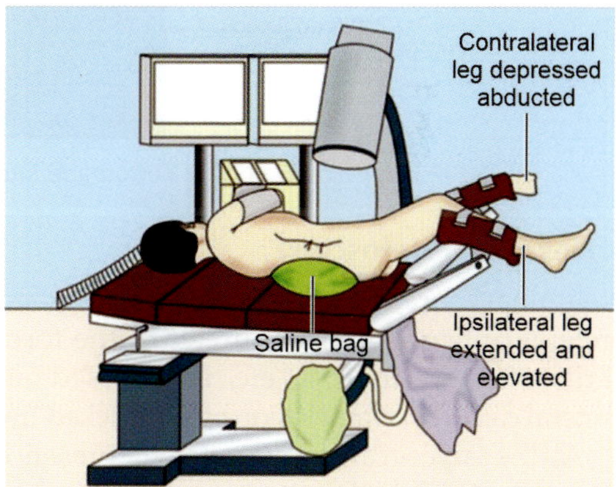

Fig. 12.19: Galdakao–modified Valdivia position

(Fig. 12.19). This facilitates simultaneous access for antegrade and retrograde ECIRS if required.[3]

The working area is marked by skin markings, i.e. iliac crest, costal margins and posterior axillary line.

3. Armamentarium Required

Two sets each in two different trolleys, one for supine PCNL **(Fig. 12.20)** and another for RIRS **(Fig. 12.21)**.

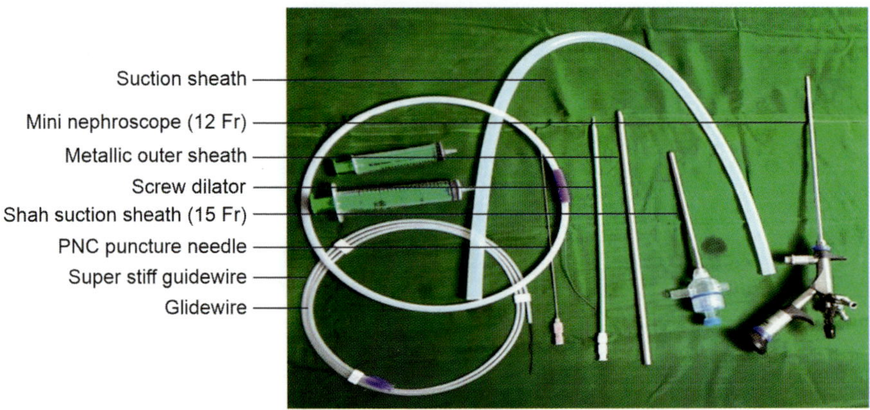

Fig. 12.20: PCNL armamentarium

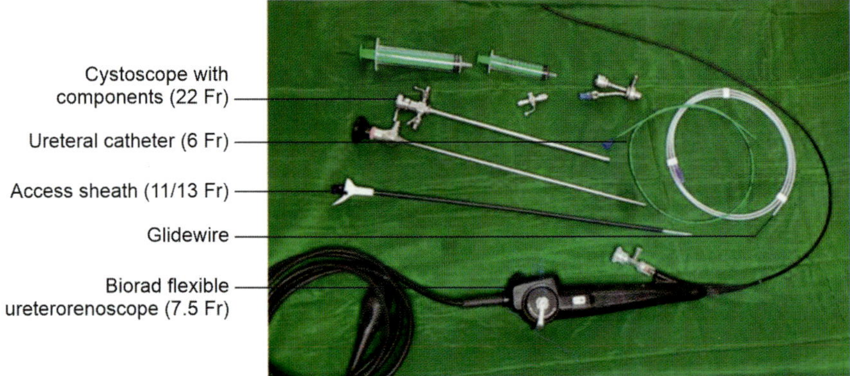

Fig. 12.21: Retrograde intrarenal surgery armamentarium

4. Flexible Ureteroscopy

Preliminary ureteroscopy helps understand ureteral orifices, nature of ureter in the form of distensibility, mucosa, etc., any missed out ureteral calculus or any lesion can be picked up.

All the calyces can be inspected for presence of stones and whether its infundibulum can admit removal of basketed calulus or not.

The preferred target calyx for puncture can be identified under vision and its accessibility to maximize stone clearance.

5. Puncture of Target Calyx

Initial puncture can be achieved fluoroscopy guided or ultrasound guided and supported by endoscopy (RIRS), the tip of retrograde scope can be visualized on ultrasound.

The target calyx for puncture would be shortest and straight tract and through which maximum stone bulk can be removed. 18 Gauge needle is used for initial puncture and 0.035" terumo guidewire is placed in the system. The wire can be pulled with the help of basket through RIRS. This through and through placement of wire reduces the mobility of kidney and that aids initial access to pelvicalyceal system.

6. Dilatation of Tract

Dilatation of tract is next step after initial puncture which is subjective, options being serial telescopic metal dilators, single step Amplatz dilator, balloon dilatation, etc. Advantage of ECIRS being all steps, i.e start from initial puncture, tract dilatation and lithotripsy and stone removal can be done under vision of endoscope from below. This also helps reduce radiation exposure to patient and healthcare personnels.

7. Nephroscopy and Intracorporeal Lithotripters and Passing the Ball

Rigid nephroscope is used for visualizing the pelvicalyceal system and to approach the stone with a back up of flexible nephroscope as well. Lithoclast (ballistic) or ultrasonic energy is used with the latest available shock pulse or trilogy for stone disintegration and suction at tip of handpiece. While doing so retrograde scope is withdrawn into upper ureter so that it does not gets damaged and fragments do not migrate to ureter. The stones in parallelly placed calyces are picked up if basket able or fragmented with laser and basketed and with the help of RIRS scope passed to the nephroscope (passing the ball technique).

Also retrograde irrigation helps to improve vision while performing nephroscopy and improvises the stone lithotripsy.

8. Exit Strategy

JJ stent is usually placed after ECIRS in majority of the cases but it should be individualized, also nephrostomy tube is placed if in doubt of tract bleeding for tamponade effect which can be decided intraoperatively by visually inspecting the calyx through RIRS.

Troubleshooting

- Hypermobility of kidney—this can be circumvented by placing through and through guidewire (urethra to pelvicalyceal system) to stabilize the kidney and requesting the anaesthetist for Valsalva manoeuvre while gaining access.
- Double armamentarium and two surgeons—it increases the cost of the procedure but to balance the cost, it can act as one stop procedure of complex renal calculi and can avoid additional auxillary procedures for residual fragments.

Technical Considerations of ECIRS

- Preliminary flexible ureteroscopy—volume of contrast instilled can be reduced as the ureteroscope will be in upper ureter itself and which acts like a balloon for retaining contrast (if no access sheath is placed) maintaining a closed circuit and target calyx can be focused for fluoroscopy guided puncture.
- Ureteral access sheath placement—preferable as it helps lower intrarenal pressure and flow of irrigation fluid can be bidirectional from RIRS to nephroscope and vice versa.
- *Impacted calyceal calculus:* To create water path by selectively filling the target calyx from RIRS scope and making a bit of a purchase for deployment of guidewire in the desired calyx.

Advantages of ECIRS

- *High stone free rates:* One step for complex renal stones as compared to staged PCNL/multitract PCNL.[1] Multiple tracts can be avoided as the peripherally placed stones can be passed to antegrade surgeon with the help of basketing through RIRS. Also reduces need for postoperative CT scan and need for auxillary procedures.
- Position related: Galdakao modified supine Valdivia position is anaethesia friendly, also reduces the procedural time of changing the position and with redution in manpower required for the same.
- *The endovision control:* Practically all steps start from intial puncture till nephroscopy is under direct endovision control which adds to benefits like under or overdilatation apart from correct direction of puncture, reduces the risk of perforation,

bleeding and minimizing the radiation exposure.

- Improved vision – irrigation fluids, both antegrade and retrograde, help improve vision and stone extraction.
- Stabilizes kidney by through and through placement of guidewire.

Review of Literature

In 2008, Scoffone et al prospectively analyzed the safety and efficacy of endoscopic combined intrarenal surgery (ECIRS) in GMSV (Galdakao modified supine Valdivia) position for the treatment of large and/or complex urolithiasis and concluded to be a safe, effective, and versatile procedure with a high one-step stone-free rate, unquestionable anaesthesiological advantages, and no additional procedure-related complications.[1]

In 2022 Yung-Hao Liu et al performed a systematic review and meta analysis of ECIRS Vs PCNL, they concluded that ECIRS is more effective and safer than PCNL. When treating complex renal stones, ECIRS has better initial/final SFR, fewer overall/severe complications, and requires fewer blood transfusions than PCNL.[4]

In July 2023 Gauhar et al., systematically reviewed the evolution of techniques, technology, clinical utility, limitations and possible future applications of endoscopic combined intrarenal surgery (ECIRS) for ureteral and kidney stones and concluded that ECIRS is ready for primetime in endourology and can be considered the next gold-standard for a personalized stone approach in complex kidney stones.[5]

Learning Points

- ECIRS should be considered as one of the priority-based treatment options vis-à-vis PCNL for complex renal stones.

- If there is availability of armamentarium, then definitely ECIRS should be treatment of choice for complex renal calculi.
- Advantages of ECIRS are under vision initial puncture and all steps of PCNL are under endovision minimising chances of under or over dilatation, perforation, blood loss, reduced radiation exposure.
- Drawbacks of ECIRS are dual set of instruments and two surgeons and cost of treatment.

REFERENCES

1. Scoffone CM, Cracco CM, Cossu M, Grande S, Poggio M, Scarpa RM. Endoscopic combined intrarenal surgery in Galdakao-modified supine Valdivia position: a new standard for percutaneous nephrolithotomy? Eur Urol. 2008; 54(6):1393–403.
2. Uroweb-European Association of Urology [Internet]. [cited 2023 Sep 20]. Uroweb - European Association of Urology. Available from: https://uroweb.org/wp-content/uploads/EAU-Guidelines-on-Urolithiasis-2020.pdf
3. Ibarluzea G, Scoffone CM, Cracco CM, Poggio M, Porpiglia F, Terrone C, et al. Supine Valdivia and modified lithotomy position for simultaneous anterograde and retrograde endourological access. BJU Int. 2007;100(1):233–6.
4. Liu YH, Jhou HJ, Chou MH, Wu ST, Cha TL, Yu DS, et al. Endoscopic Combined Intrarenal Surgery Versus Percutaneous Nephrolithotomy for Complex Renal Stones: A Systematic Review and Meta-Analysis. J Pers Med. 2022;12(4):532.
5. Gauhar V, Traxer O, Fuligni D, Brocca C, Galosi AB, Teoh JYC, et al. Evolution and current applications of endoscopic combined intrarenal surgery: a scoping review from back to the future. Curr Opin Urol. 2023;33(4):324.

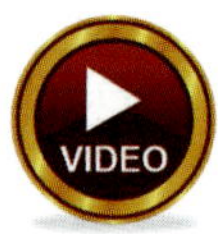

Scan QR Code for Video on
ECIRS

13

How do I do it

Akshay Nathani, Aruj Shah, Chandramohan Vaddi

RETROGRADE INTRARENAL SURGERY (RIRS)

Operating Room Setup

- C-arm to the left of the patient
- Endoscope tower to the right of the patient
- Surgeon chair in between the legs
- Instrument trolley behind the surgeon to the patient's left

Instrument Tray

- Surgeon gowns
- Drapes
- Camera cover
- Lignocaine jelly
- Gauze pieces
- Cystoscope with bridge and sheath
- Light cable
- Irrigation set
- Ureteric catheter
- Guidewire
- Contrast medium
- Double lumen catheter
- Ureteral dilators
- Ureteric access sheath
- Flexible ureteroscope
- Double J stent
- Foley catheter
- Kidney tray
- Normal saline

Anesthesia

General Anesthesia

- Most commonly used method
- Spontaneous breathing using LMA can be done
- Muscle relaxation especially to control respiratory motion of kidney
- Modulating tidal volume, apnea

Spinal Anesthesia

- Prilocaine—around 1.5 h (full regression by 4 h)
- Bupivacaine—around 3 h (slow regression—6 h, risk of urinary retention)
- Can be combined with conscious sedation for patient comfort

Local Anesthesia

The local anaesthesia can be administered either by Lidocaine gel™, penile blocks in males or conscious sedation. Reserved for unfit patients only.

Patient Positioning

- Lithotomy position
- Contralateral leg is relatively more abducted and placed at a lower level—this helps

the surgeon align himself to the ipsilateral ureter without clashing with the contralateral leg of the patient
- Do not flex hips or knees beyond 90 degrees
- Leg—slightly extended and abduction of hip to decrease angulation
- Proper padding to prevent nerve injuries

Painting and Draping

- Iodine less irritative as compared to alcohol-based agents for genitalia
- Draping—one sheet under the buttocks, leg covers on each leg, hole towel around the genitalia and one sheet over the abdomen

Ergonomics

- The flexible ureteroscope has 3 main movements:
    1. Inside out—controlled by the thumb and index finger of non-dominant hand
    2. Lateral—controlled by the wrist movements of the dominant hand
    3. Deflection—controlled by the dominant thumb by moving the lever up and down
  Additionally, the entire scope may be moved by movement at the shoulder joint.
- Standing or sitting—we prefer the standing position
- The neck and body in the same line
- Right foot forward on laser foot paddle
- The dominant hand should be flexed at the elbow by 60–70.

Cystoscopy

- *Purpose:*
    - Assess the anatomy of lower tract
    - Size and shape of ureteric orifices
- We use 19 Fr cystoscope in males and 22 Fr cystoscope in females
- After identifying the ureteric orifice, advance a 5/6 Fr ureteric catheter into the cystoscope and place it next to the orifice
- Performing a retrograde dye study helps in the following ways:
    - Delineates the anatomy of the ureter
    - Delineates the anatomy of the pelvicalyceal system
    - Provides a baseline to which post-lithotripsy RGP can be compared to see if there is any extravasation
- Advance the guidewire slightly beyond the ureteric orifice to resemble a pencil tip
- The ureteric catheter is then placed flush at the ureteric orifice and the guidewire is then advanced further.
- Advancing guidewire directly without ureteric catheter may lead to a false passage
- After placing the guidewire in the PCS and confirming its position under fluoroscopy, the cystoscope is dismantled and removed while simultaneously pushing the guidewire to ensure it stays in place.
- The cystoscope is dismantled and only the sheath is kept so that it allows the passage of ureteral dilators to dilate the ureter.
- For dilatation, one can choose between serial Teflon dilators/single step Nottingham dilator or balloon dilatation.
- We prefer dilating the ureter up to 14 Fr so that 9/11 or 10/12 Ureteral Access Sheath (UAS) can be comfortably placed.
- Align the sheath in the axis of the ureteric orifice to allow easy passage of the dilators.
- Use adequate lubrication. Use gentle rotatory movements and never use excessive force.
- Never use excessive force. In case of doubt, stent the patient and return after 2 weeks.
- EAU and AUA guidelines recommend placing a safety guidewire using a double lumen catheter. However, as Indian ureters are narrow, they do not accommodate UAS and safety guidewire together in many cases.

Ureteral Access Sheath (UAS)

- Need for routine use is debatable—arguments on both sides
- We place in all cases whenever feasible

- *Size:* 9.5/11.5 or 10/12
- Lubricate both outer and inner sheaths with saline before placement
- It is to be placed under fluoroscopic guidance
- Advance in a gentle rotating fashion
- Do not force under any circumstance
- We place it at the level of the upper ureter as it allows for complete deflection of the scope and it avoids PUJ injury associated with PCS placement.

Flexible Ureteroscopy

- Infant feeding tube should be used to drain the urinary bladder during the procedure.
- Before introduction of the flexible ureteroscope, check the proper functioning of the scope
- Depending on the preoperative imaging, choose appropriate scope with proper laser position (e.g. 11 o'clock)
- We use 7.5 Fr sized scope: 1. Indian ureters are narrow 2. We perform RIRS in unstented patients
- Keep the shaft and the tip of the scope in a straight line at all times
- Use any of the suitable irrigation methods.

Lithotripsy

- Tuohy Borst adapter is an useful tool—it prevents unwanted movement of the laser fiber during movement of the scope by fixing it in place
- Introduce the laser fiber only when the scope is straight to prevent damage to the scope
- Do not force the laser fiber
- While navigating through calyces it is recommended to withdraw the fiber and then navigate
- It is recommended to keep the laser fiber such that it occupies 25% of the screen
- Use active flexion first—passive flexion as and when needed

- Keep the laser machine in 'standby mode' whenever not in use
- It is recommended to start at the lowest possible settings initially and then change as per stone composition
- We use unstrapped 200 µm laser fiber
- Our recommended TFL settings: 1 J/10 Hz (Max 1 J/15 Hz)
- Watch for the return flow of irrigating solution via the access sheath to ensure adequacy of drainage
- Whenever possible, reposition the stone from lower calyx to a favorable one. This reduces the damage to the scope, increases the efficiency of lasing and ensures proper gravity dependent drainage after the procedure
- If there are fragments left, we perform popcorning. This helps create a whirlpool effect and break them into even smaller fragments
- *End point of lithotripsy:* Golden dust sized less than the size of the laser fiber.

Exit Strategy

- At the end of lithotripsy, check RGP should be performed through the UAS to see if there is extravasation of contrast.
- UAS should be removed only after placing the obturator inside to prevent ureteric damage.
- Place a guidewire through UAS and remove the UAS after confirming the position of the guidewire on fluoroscopy.
- Place DJ stent over guidewire and confirm its position under fluoroscopy guidance.
- Foley's catheter placed at the end of the procedure.

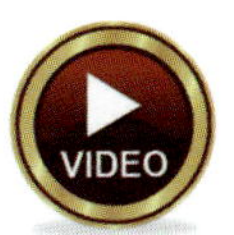

Scan QR Code for Video on
RIRS

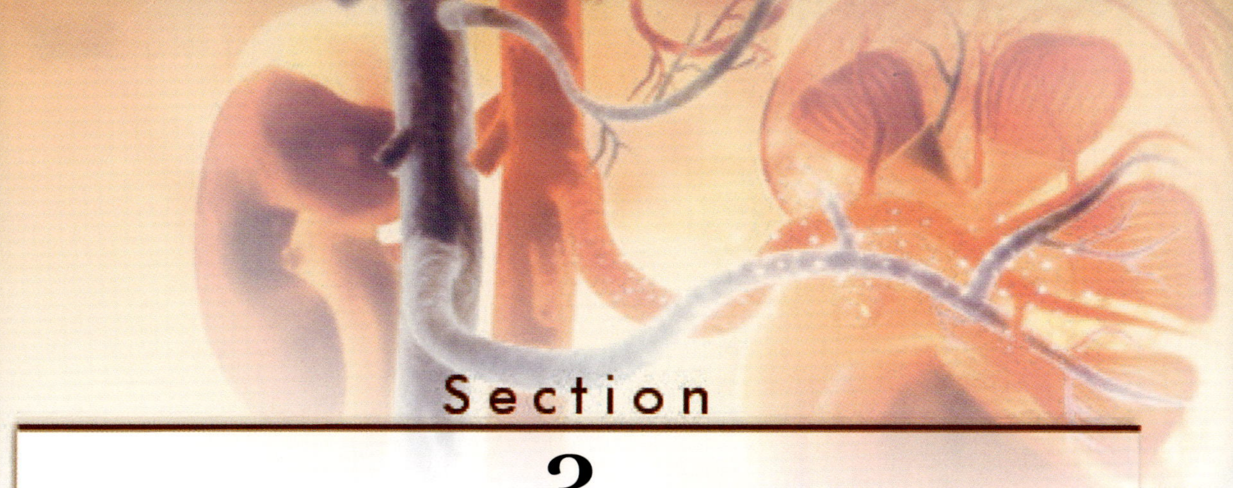

3

Practical Tips and Tricks in General Urology

Part 1

AV Fistula

CHAPTERS

14

Introduction

Abhishek Singh

In India, 151 patients per million population suffer from chronic kidney disease (CKD) stage 5, all of whom require renal replacement therapy.[1] With limited number of cadaver and living donor the access to renal transplantation is limited to a handful of patients. A large number of these patients rely on vascular access for hemodialysis, this number is estimated to be more than 3,00,000 in the United States.[2] Vascular access is one of the major causes for hospital admission and morbidity in CKD stage 5 patients.[3] An ideal access should be able to deliver ideal dialysis prescription for as long as possible and should be free of any complications. From the options available for hemodialysis, surgically created fistula seems to come closest to the ideal. Arteriovenous fistula (AVF) requires the least number of intervention and is most likely to lasts for 4–5 years when compared to other forms of access.[3–5]

It was James Cimino, who made the observation that arteriovenous fistula (AVF) in Korean war survivors did not cause any adverse health effects. From here originated the idea of construction of AVF for hemodialysis.[6–8] Since then AVF has been the cheapest and most effective form of vascular access. In late 1990s and early 2000s grafts became very popular in the United States as they were easy to use and cannulate. This upsurge in the use of grafts was also attributed to the market forces which were pushing its use.

Aim of Construction of AVF and What is Ideal Fistula

An ideal fistula should be easy to construct and maintain, should give adequate blood flow for dialysis , should be easy to cannulate, should allow rotation of cannulation sites, should last long, should be comfortable for the patient and should be free of complications. A normal radial artery has a flow of about 21.6 to 20.8 ml/min, this flow increases immediately after construction of fistula to 175 to 208 ml/min and is about 600 to 1200 ml/min at maturation.

Rule of Six

- Greater than 600 ml/min flow
- Matured vein should be greater than 6 mm in diameter
- The vein should be less than 6 mm deep from skin surface
- All fistulas should be examined 6 weeks postoperatively
- There should be a 6 cm straight segment of vein for cannulation.

Indications of AVF Creation

- Hemodialysis
- Patient requiring lifelong treatment with some injectable drug-like calcium.
- Patient requiring lifelong parenteral nutrition.

Preoperative Work up

Once the vascular surgeon has overcome his initial learning curve, it is the preoperative work up and choice of the site of creation of fistula as per the preoperative work up, which will determine the outcome of AVF.

REFERENCES

1. Jha V. Current status of end-stage renal disease care in India and Pakistan. Kidney International Supplements 2013;3(2):157–60.
2. Eknoyan G, Levin NW. Impact of the new K/DOQI guidelines. Blood purification 2002;20(1):103–8.
3. Pisoni RL, Young EW, Dykstra DM, et al. Vascular access use in Europe and the United States: Results from the DOPPS. Kidney Int 2002;61:305–16.
4. Mehta S. Statistical summary of clinical results of vascular access procedures for haemodialysis. In: Sommer BG, Henry ML (eds). Vascular Access for Hemodialysis-II (ed 2). Chicago, IL, Gore, 1991; pp 145–57.
5. Kaufman JL. The decline of the autogenous hemodialysis access site. Semin Dial 1995;8:59–61.
6. Quinton WE, Dillard DH, Scribner BH. Cannulation of blood vessels for prolonged hemodialysis. Trans Am Soc Artif Intern Organs 1960;6:104–13.
7. Konner K. History of vascular access for haemodialysis. Nephrol Dial Transplant 2005;20:2629–35.
8. Allon M. Current management of vascular access. Clin J Am Soc Nephrol. 2007;2:786–800.

15
Instruments for Vascular Access Surgery

Aruj Shah, Raisa Shetty, Pavan Jain, Arvind P Ganpule

BARD-PARKER HANDLE

Description

It is a reusable flat instrument with a slot on either side of one end for attaching the scalpel blade.

In scalpel handle no. 4, the site for attachment of the blade is a little wider than the handle number 3, 5 and 7 where it is a little narrower **(Fig. 15.1)**.

Use

It is used to make skin incisions **(Fig. 15.2)**.

SURGICAL BLADES

Description

Blades number 10, 11, 12 and 15 fit in BP handle number 3, 5 and 7 **(Fig. 15.1)**.

Use

Surgical blade number 11 is used for making precise 'stab' incisions as in case of arteriotomy and venotomy.

Surgical blade number 15 is used for making narrow incisions **(Figs 15.3 and 15.4)**.

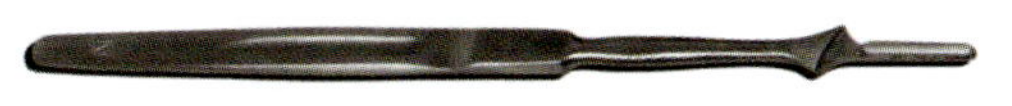

Fig. 15.1: Bard-Parker handle

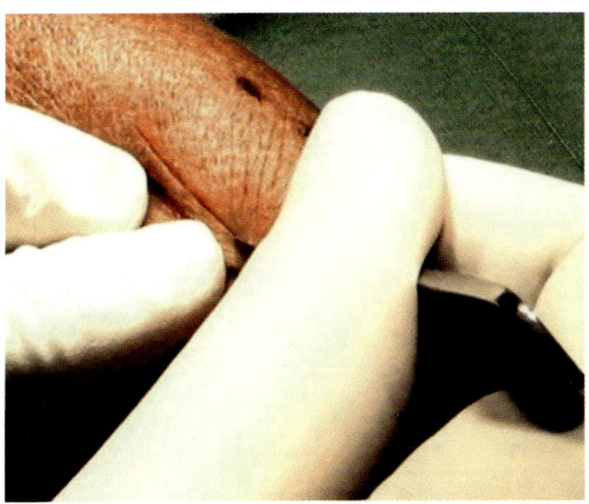

Fig. 15.2: Skin incision

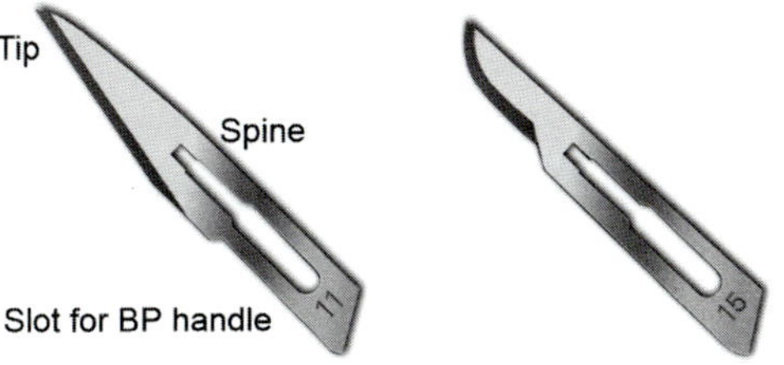

Fig. 15.3: Surgical blade (no. 11 and no. 15)

SCISSORS

Mayo Dissecting Scissor

General purpose scissors used for cutting sutures, dressing materials, drains and

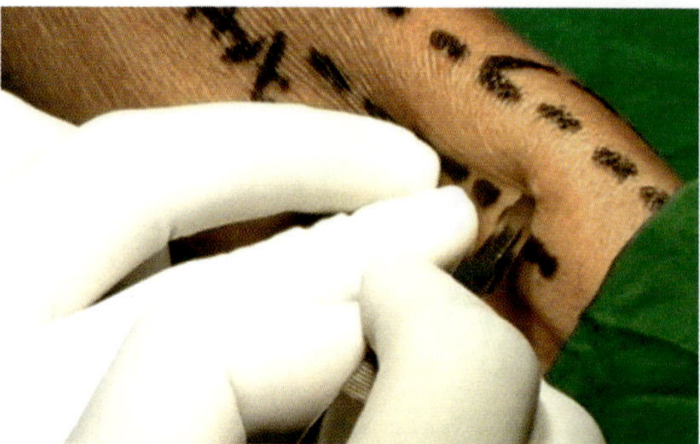

Fig. 15.4: The 15 number blade for narrow incisions

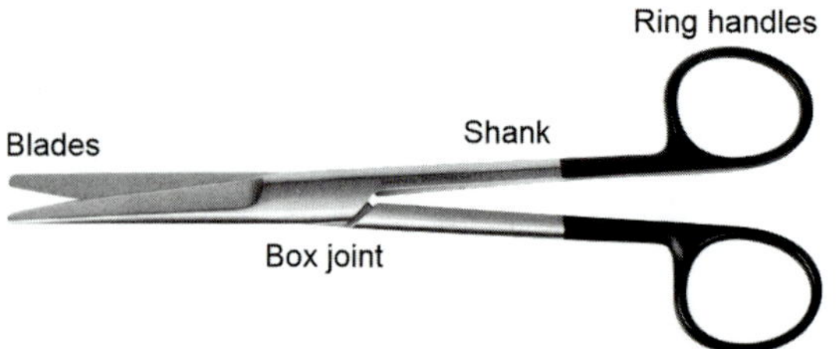

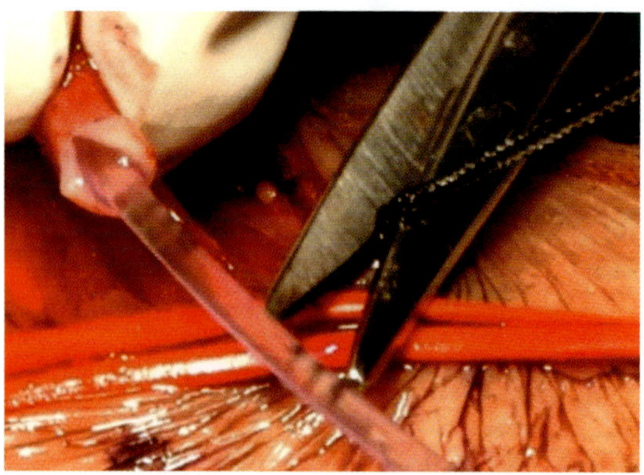

Fig. 15.5: Mayo dissecting scissors

occasionally tough structures during surgery **(Fig. 15.5)**.

Metzenbaum-Lahey Scissors

Description

This is a long fine scissors with long blades in comparison to the shaft of the instrument. This instrument may be straight or curved **(Fig. 15.6)**.

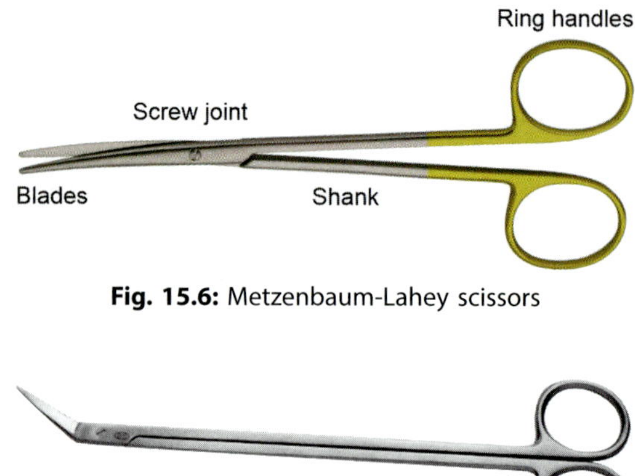

Fig. 15.6: Metzenbaum-Lahey scissors

Fig. 15.7: Potts-Smith scissors

Use

It is used for dissection at the depth.

Potts-Smith Scissors

Description

This instrument features pointed angled tips that are used for sharp dissection and cutting of tissues.

It has long shanks and short blades that helps increase accuracy of dissection by providing better control. The blades are beveled and angled to ensure clean dissection with minimal effort by providing a better view for the surgeon.

Use

It is commonly used to dissect vessels and enlarge vascular incisions **(Figs 15.7 and 15.8)**. It can also be used to dissect fascia as well as organ sheaths and tissues during surgery.

Stevens Tenotomy Scissors

Description

Tenotomy scissors have characteristically long handles and small skin incision, sharp blades with sharp or blunt wedge-shaped tips **(Fig. 15.9)**. The long shanks provide the surgeon with

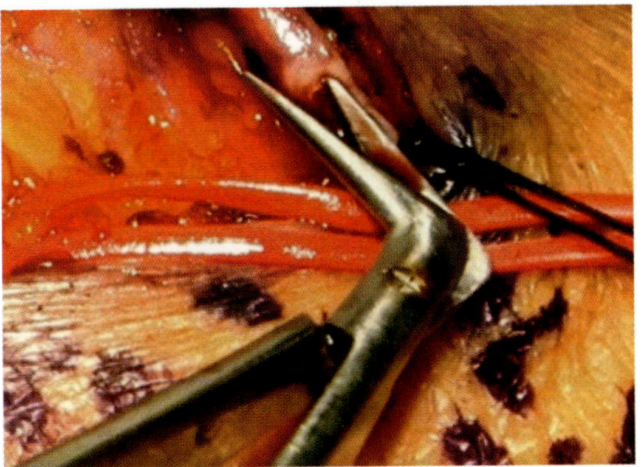

Fig. 15.8: Potts scissors

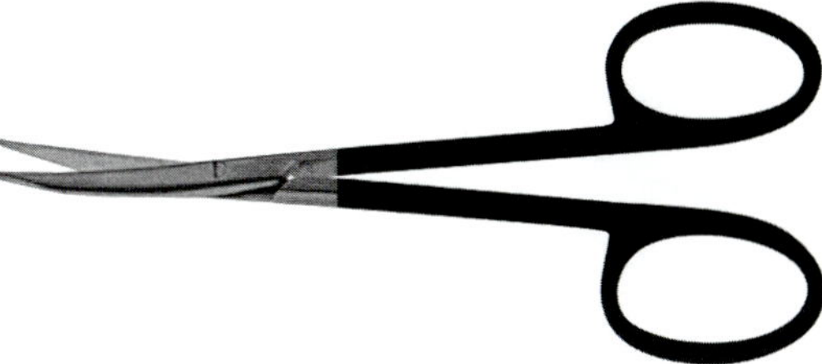

Fig. 15.9: Stevens tenotomy scissors

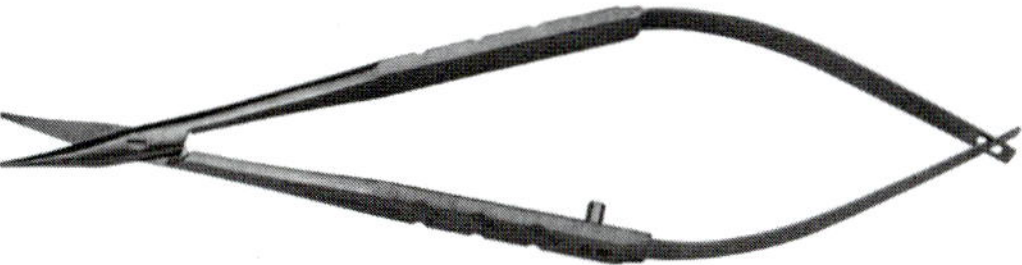

Fig. 15.10: Westcott tenotomy scissors

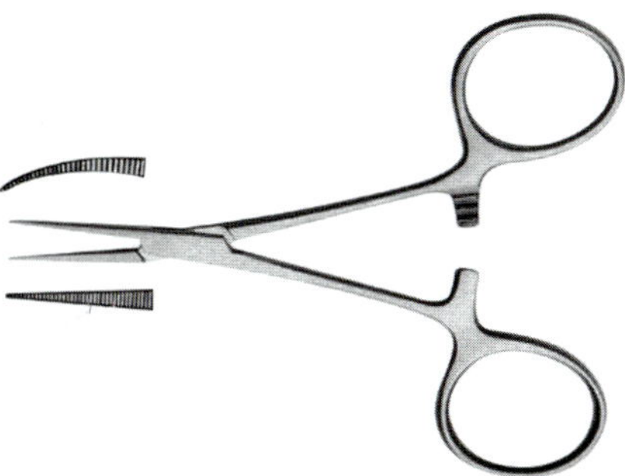

Fig. 15.11: Halsted mosquito forceps

a firm grip and control while operating in narrow and deep areas.

Use

They are used for dissection and cutting.

Westcott Tenotomy Scissors

These versatile spring-handle thumb scissors are designed for cutting delicate tissues, and come in both blunt and sharp-tip forms.

The instrument has narrow blades which increase precision **(Fig. 15.10)**. They may have curved blades that contort to the surface for increased accuracy.

It has a small blades-to-shank ratio for better control.

HALSTED MOSQUITO FORCEPS

They are versatile, ratcheted, finger ring forceps used for clamping small bleeding vessels.

The blades are smaller in comparison to Spencer Wells type of hemostatic forceps and there are fine transverse serrations in the blades **(Fig. 15.11)**. The tip of the blades are conical and are non-toothed.

ROCHESTER OCHSNER FORCEPS

Description

They feature a 1 × 2 toothed profile for enhanced clamping. The pair of jaws have a tapered design to easily traverse narrow

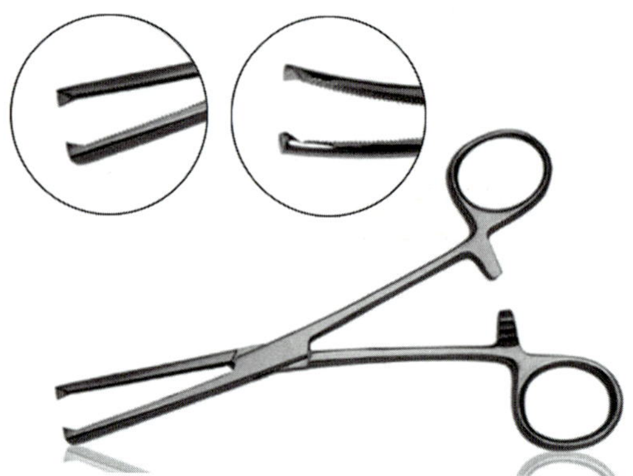

Fig. 15.12: Rochester Ochsner forceps

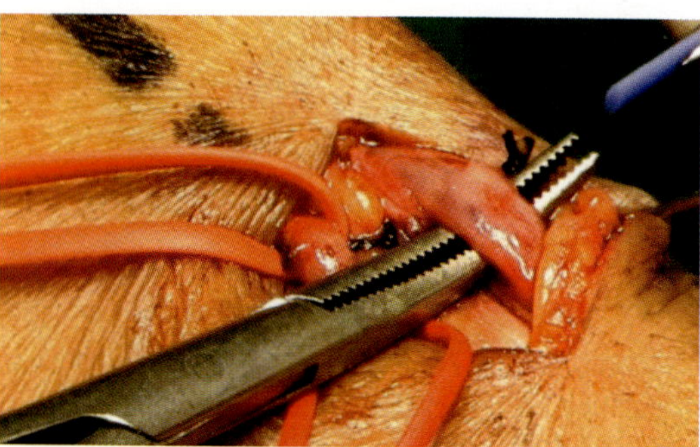

Fig. 15.14: Crile forceps

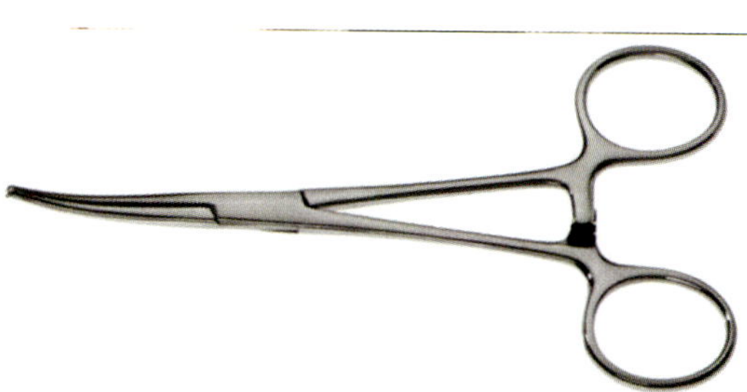

Fig. 15.13: Crile forceps

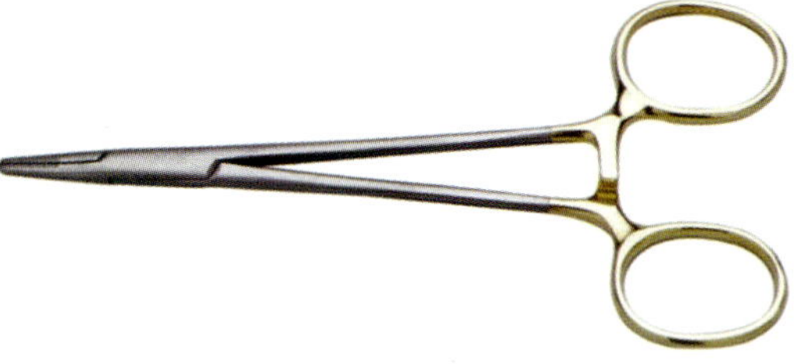

Fig. 15.15: Halsey needle holder

passages **(Fig. 15.12)**. In addition, the opposing surfaces of the jaws have transverse serrations to obtain a strong but atraumatic grip while preventing endothelial damage.

Use

They are used to clamp blood vessels, especially small arteries, during a variety of surgical scenarios. The instrument is also useful to grasp disposable materials, tissues and sutures.

CRILE FORCEPS

Description

They are larger and heavier hemostats with a locking ratchet on the ring-handles **(Figs 15.13 and 15.14)**. They have transverse inter-digitating striations present along the entire jaw length (as opposed to the Kelly hemostats which have the striations only on the tips).

Use

They are primarily used to grasp larger vessels or tissue **(Fig. 15.14)**.

NEEDLE HOLDERS

The blades of the needle holder are smaller in comparison to the shaft of the instrument. There are criss cross serrations in the blade and there is a longitudinal groove in the center of the criss-cross serration which allows firm gripping of the needle.

Halsey Needle Holder

Halsey needle holders are used for holding small needles during surgical procedures. Its strong jaws ensure a firm grip over the needle **(Figs 15.15 and 15.16)**.

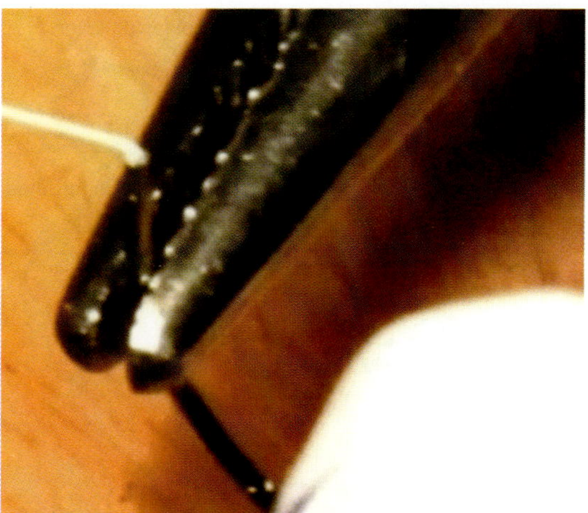

Fig. 15.16: Halsey needle holder

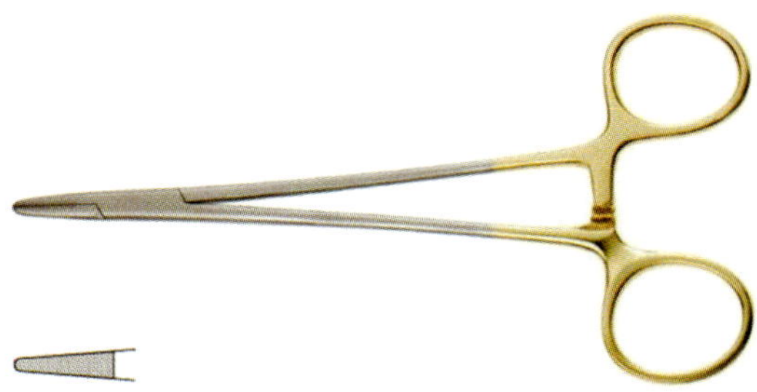

Fig. 15.17: Crile-Wood needle holder

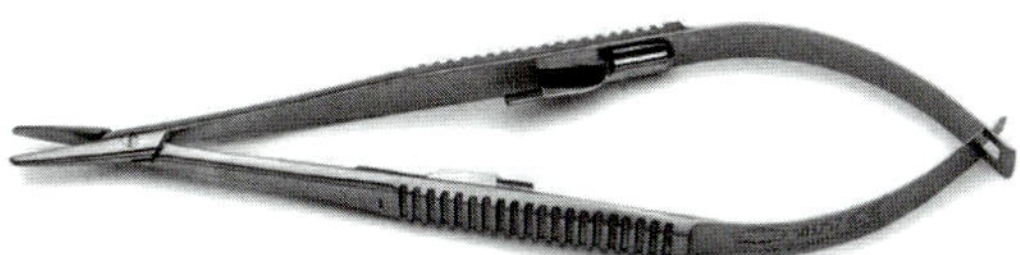

Fig. 15.18: Castroviejo needle holder

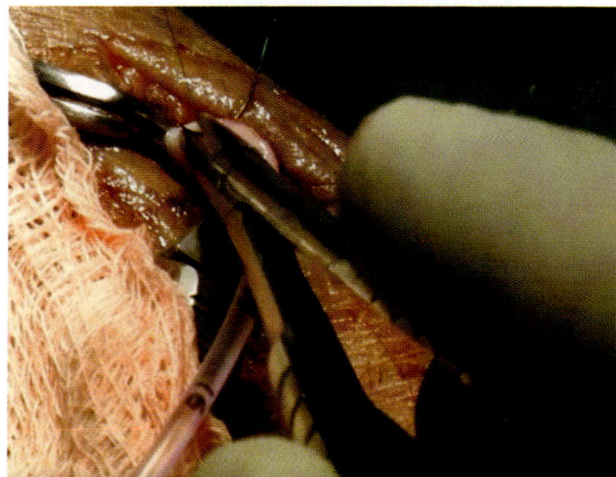

Fig. 15.19: Castroviejo needle holder

Crile-Wood Needle Holder (Serrated, Narrow Jaw)

It has a narrow jaw with cross serrations **(Fig. 15.17)**. It is similar to the Mayo-Hegar needle holder but the end tip is finer and gently tapered. It is used to grasp and guide the needle when suturing.

Castroviejo Needle Holder

They are distinguished from other needle holders by their slender tip and the mechanism of their handle which allows the jaws to be activated without effort.

They feature a spring-loaded lock with "ratchet" system: Without grip rings, this instrument works via a spring that curves inwards to lock/unlock the needle holder **(Figs 15.18 and 15.19)**. Unlike other needle holders, the surgeon does not need to gauge the tightness of the needle, a single press on the arms with the palm of the hand engages the mechanism.

They help to reduce repetitive movements during lengthy surgeries, thus relieving the practitioner. The unique design features allow them to suture wounds and incisions very precisely and smoothly, with minimal trauma, thus reducing the risk of damaging peripheral tissue **(Fig. 15.19)**.

These so-called microsurgical needle holders are used to hold very small needles for sutures with a gauge of 5–0 to 8–0.

DeBakey Needle Holder

They have straight serrated DeBakey style jaws and are used for holding fine suture needles **(Fig. 15.20)**.

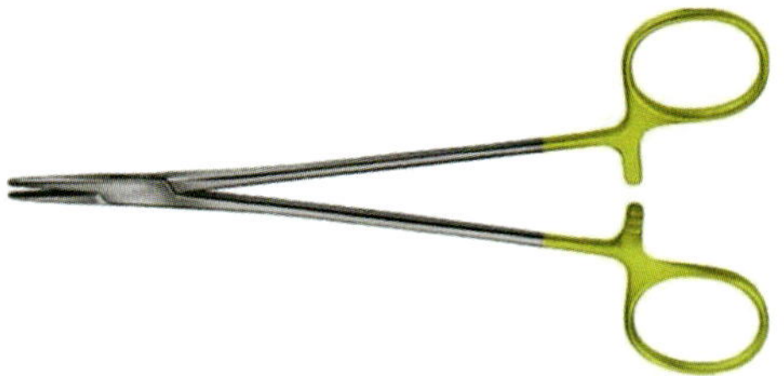

Fig. 15.20: DeBakey needle holder

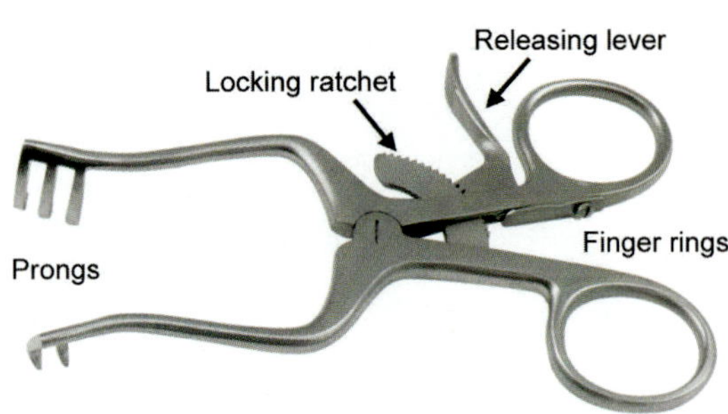

Fig. 15.22: Weitlaner retractor

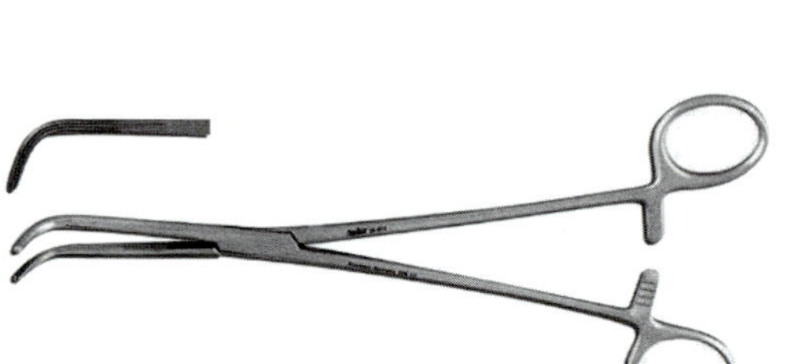

Fig. 15.21: Mixter right angled forceps

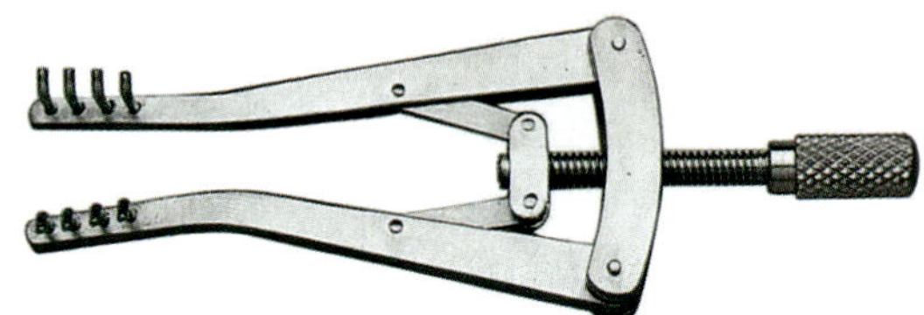

Fig. 15.23: ALM self-retaining retractor

MIXTER RIGHT ANGLED FORCEPS

Description

These forceps feature a pair of right-angled jaws that ensure access into hard-reaching cavities **(Fig. 15.21)**. In addition, the fully-serrated working end profile enhances gripping and minimizes clamping injury. Moreover, they have a ratchet to self-lock the jaws. As a result, surgeons can apply different levels of pressure when clamping vessels and tissues.

Use

They are used to grasp tissues, mobilize and clamp blood vessels, pass ligature and perform blunt dissection to divide soft layers of tissue.

WEITLANER RETRACTORS

Description

This self-retaining retractor features 3 by 3 hooked prongs to ensure secure grip on incision edges **(Fig. 15.22)**.

Use

It helps secure and separate delicate incision planes and wounds to enlarge surgical planes for better visualization.

ALM SELF-RETAINING RETRACTOR

Description

This retractor features 4 × 4 prongs which are available in sharp and blunt profiles, in order to protect local tissues **(Fig. 15.23)**.

It has a compound action joint for spreading the tips with comfort. The adjustable screw mechanism permits to self-retain the prongs at the desired width.

Use

It is used to pull back the margins of large wounds.

ALLIS TISSUE FORCEPS

Description

The blades of this instrument are longer and there is a gap between the blades which can accommodate some amount of tissue **(Fig. 15.24)**.

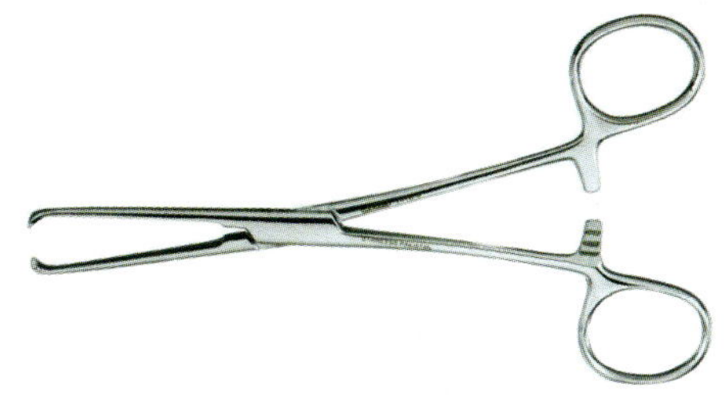

Fig. 15.24: Allis tissue forceps

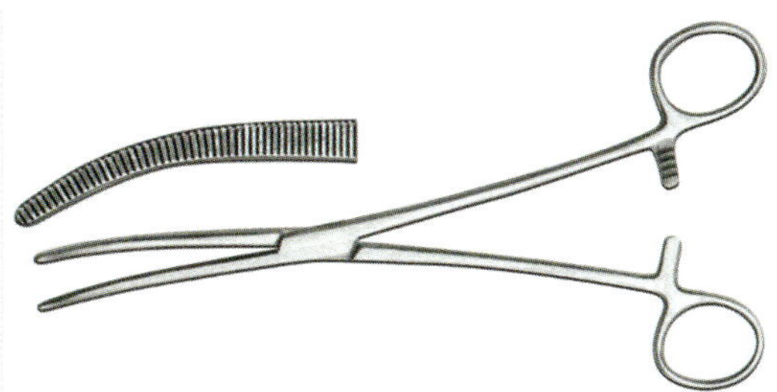

Fig. 15.25: Rochester-Pean forceps

The tip of the blades are provided with sharp teeth with grooves in between. When the ratchet is closed, the teeth of the one blade fits in the groove of the other blade and vice versa.

Use

It is used to hold tough structures only as it can be traumatic to the tissue. It may be used to hold skin flaps during surgery.

ROCHESTER-PEAN FORCEPS

Description

This sturdy, versatile ratchet forceps has full horizontal jaw serrations **(Fig. 15.25)**.

Use

It is designed to clamp larger blood vessels and control blood flow.

GILLIES SKIN HOOK

Description

This instrument has a shaft with handle. There is a single or double hook at the tip **(Fig. 15.26)**. The tip of the hook may be sharp or blunt.

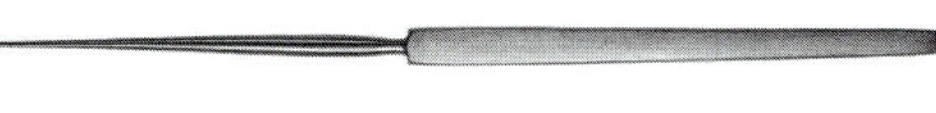

Fig. 15.26: Gillies skin hook

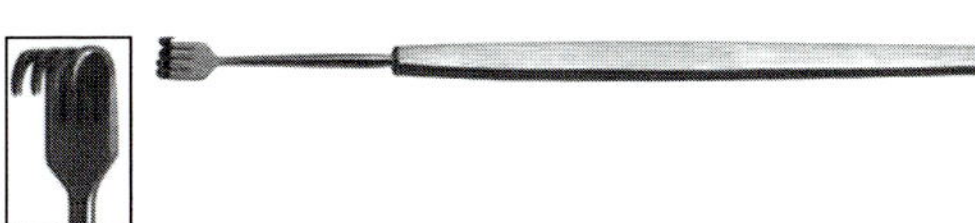

Fig. 15.27: Blair (Rollet) retractor

Use

It is commonly used for retraction of skin flaps.

BLAIR ROLLET RETRACTOR (CAT PAW)

Description

There are multiple hooks with pointed edges **(Fig. 15.27)**. The pointed edges are helpful for firm retraction.

Use

This is used for retraction of skin flaps or fascia for operation at the surface.

FRANZIER SUCTION TUBE

Description

This suction tube has a slim profile for easily traversing narrow spaces. Its length allows it to reach deep cavities **(Fig. 15.28)**. It features a finger cut-off valve for controlled aspiration.

Use

It is used to aspire fluids, debris and blood from multiple cavities, in order to achieve a greater view of the operating field.

FORCEPS

Adson Tissue Forceps

The design is the same as the plain dissecting forceps but there is a tooth at the tip of one

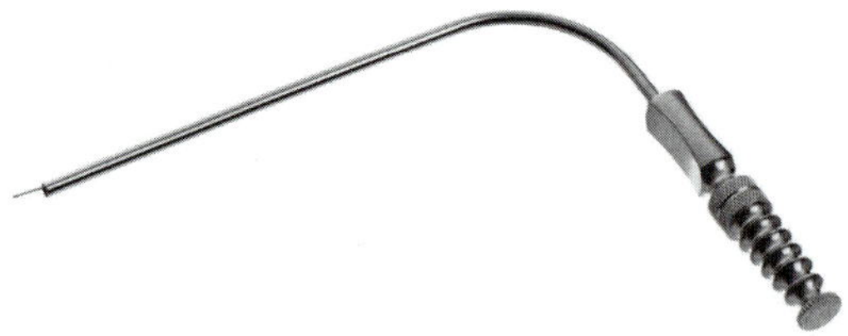

Fig. 15.28: Franzier suction tube

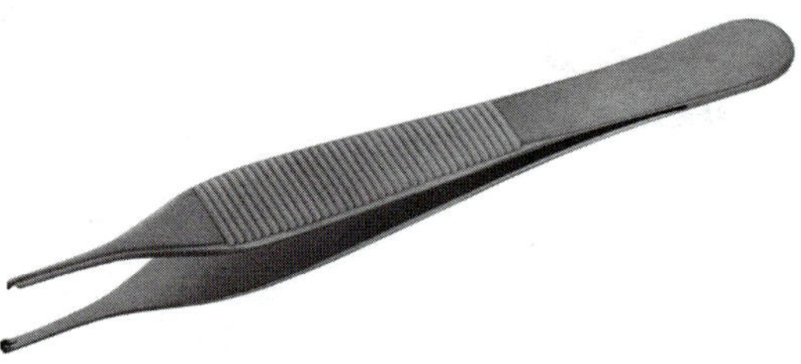

Fig. 15.29: Adson tissue forceps

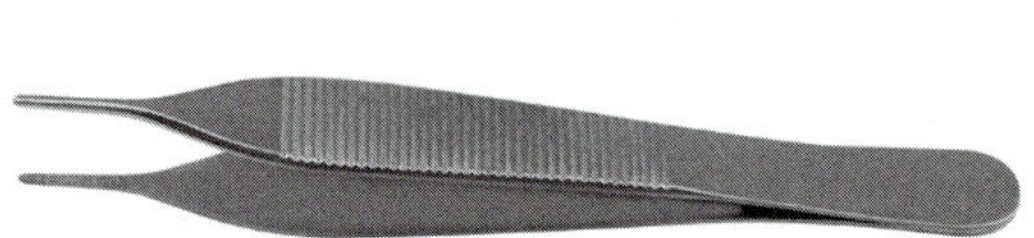

Fig. 15.30: Adson dressing forceps

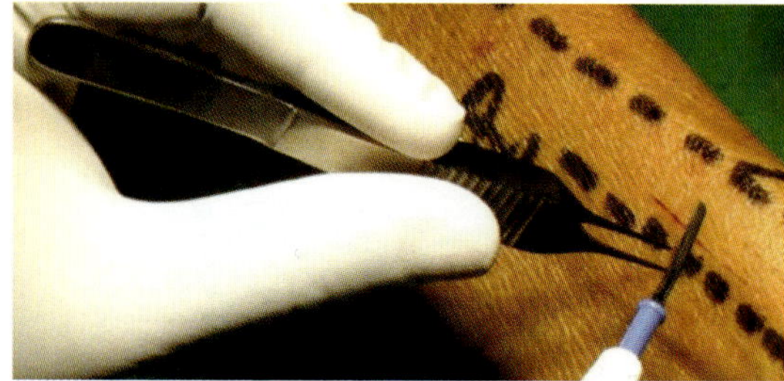

Fig. 15.31: Adson plain forceps

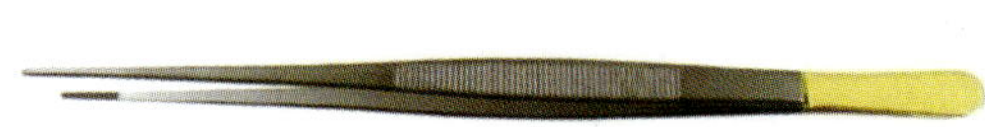

Fig. 15.32: Potts Smith dressing forceps

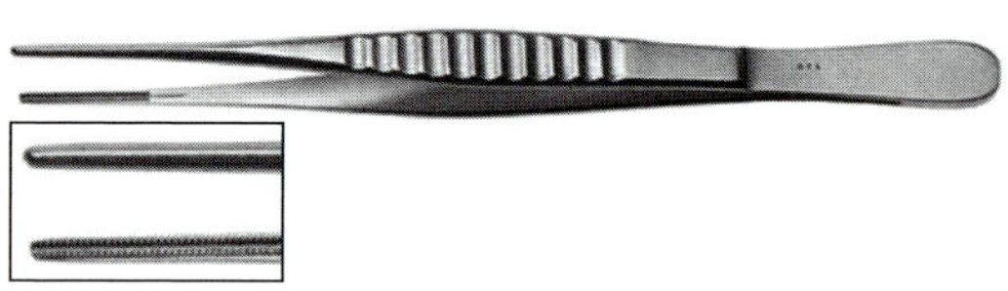

Fig. 15.33: DeBakey atraumatic forceps

blade and a groove at the tip of the other blade. When the blades are approximated, the toothed tip fits into the groove **(Fig. 15.29)**. Because of the presence of the tooth, the tissues may be better gripped and there is less chance of slipping.

Adson Dressing Forceps (Serrated)

There are grooves on the shaft of the instrument which allows easy gripping. The two limbs of the shaft are so designed that it provides a spring action and the blades are kept apart. Pressing the two limbs of the shaft of the instruments brings the two blades closer and helps in gripping the tissues **(Figs 15.30 and 15.31)**. There are transverse serrations at the tip of the blades which help in lifting the tissues and the needle during suturing. There are no tooth at the tip.

Potts Smith Dressing Forceps

This thumb-type, clamping instrument features straight, tapering tips that easily pass into narrow cavities **(Fig. 15.32)**. The handle has outer horizontal ridges that facilitate gripping. The handle's stems feature a flat outline and form a spring system, which results in a smooth tip closure movement.

Its principal use is to maintain a clear view of the operating site by manipulating swabs and sterile gauzes.

DeBakey Atraumatic Forceps

The instrument features a pair of tapered jaws with 1×2 serrations that ensure a steady grip **(Fig. 15.33)**. It may come with straight or angled working end patterns. As a result, the device conforms to the anatomy of different narrow cavities of the body.

It features a spring-action handle with a flat design. The outer surfaces of the handle

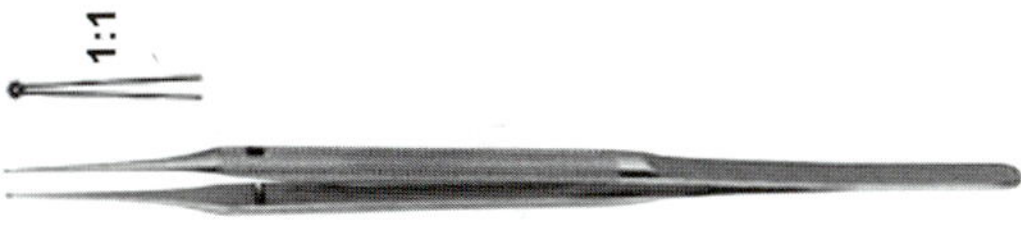

Fig. 15.34: Micro ring forceps

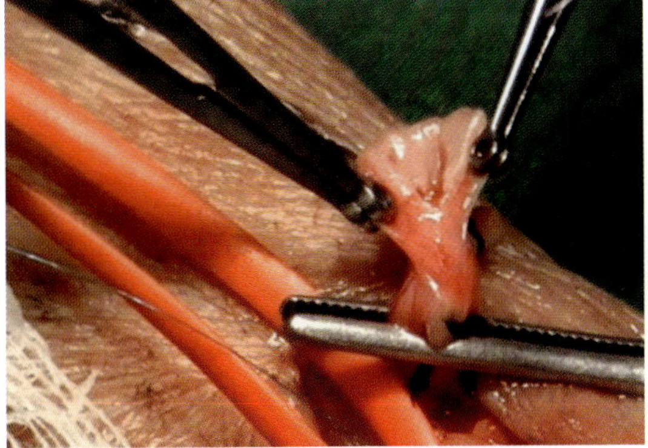

Fig. 15.35: Micro ring forceps

include transverse ridges that prevent accidental slippage and provide comfort.

Micro Ring Forceps

The instrument features a pair of small, ring-shaped tips designed to reach minute surgical targets **(Figs 15.34 and 15.35)**.

They have a spring-action handle with semi-round shanks for optimal control. The outer surfaces of the shanks include a knurled style pattern that provides comfort and prevent finger strain.

Its principal use is to manipulate arteries, veins and small tissues within small operating sites **(Fig. 15.35)**.

VASCULAR DILATOR SET

The instrument features a long probe supplied with a blunt tip **(Fig. 15.36)**. Moreover, the device is available in multiple probe widths.

The idea is to dilate small-sized vessels to allow more distal AVF and to increase the maturation rate.

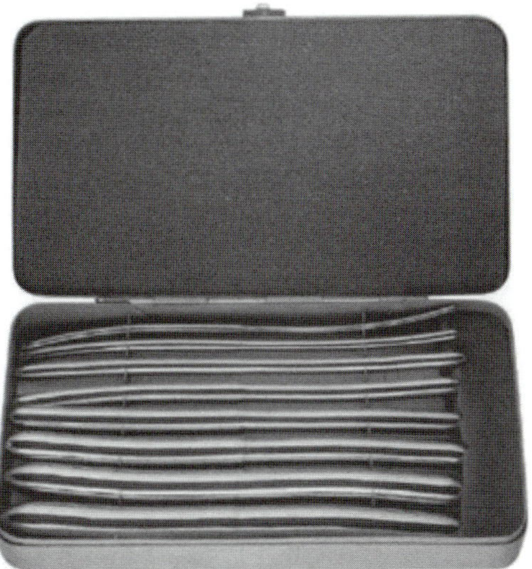

Fig. 15.36: Vascular dilator set

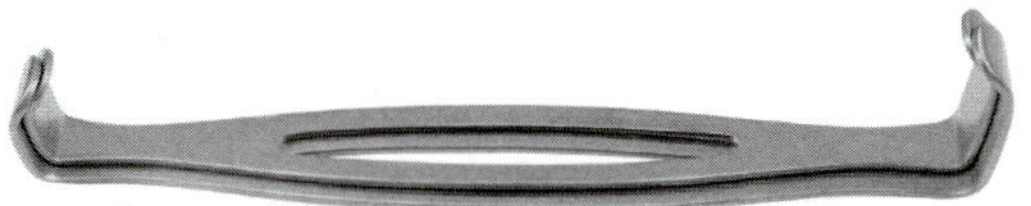

Fig. 15.37: Parker Langenback retractor

RETRACTORS

Parker Langenback Retractor

The central handle has an oval fenestration for improving gripping **(Fig. 15.37)**. In addition, two small, flat shafts arise from the handle, afterwards turning into L-shaped blades.

The retractor's blades have terminal descending lips for locking onto the retracted tissues. The blunted borders help avoid accidental puncture and local injury.

Richardson with Handle

The retractor has a crescent-shaped blade with a slight terminal curvature **(Figs 15.38 and 15.39)**. It ensures an atraumatic blade insertion and grants deep retractions.

The retractor has a wide neck with a flat design for sliding over the skin.

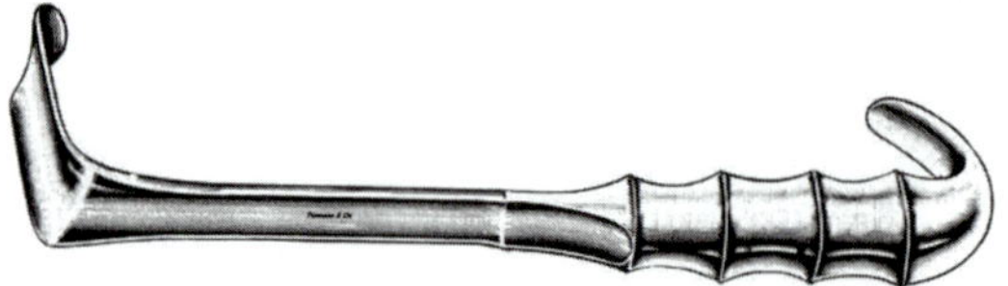

Fig. 15.38: Richardson with handle

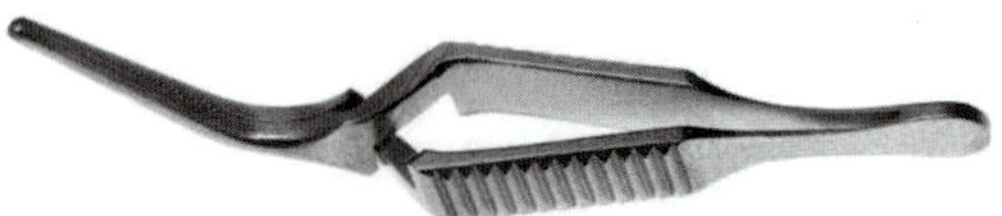

Fig. 15.41: Diethrich Bulldog clamp

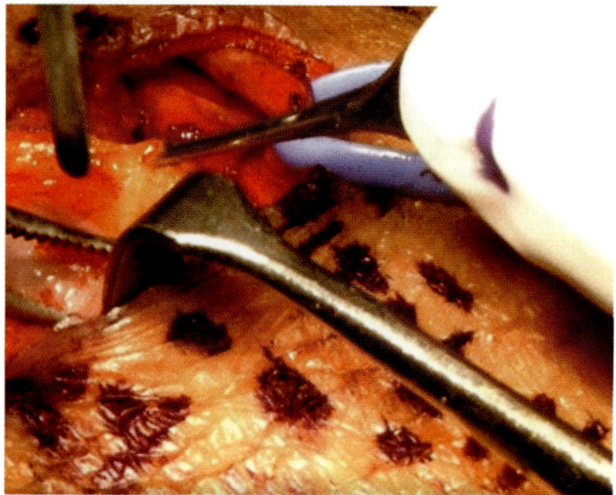

Fig. 15.39: Right angle retractor

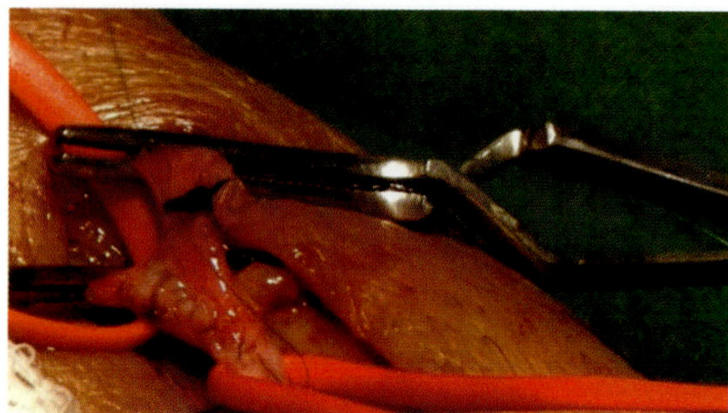

Fig. 15.42: Bulldog clamps

Use

It is used to probe and flush heparin saline into arteries and veins.

DIETHRICH BULLDOG CLAMPS

Description

Diethrich Bulldog clamps are hemostatic thumb devices with a couple of horizontally serrated atraumatic jaws to avoid endothelial damage **(Figs 15.41 and 15.42)**. The jaws can be curved or straight for reaching different cavities. The clamps have a resilient cross action spring handle. As a result, surgeons can control the aperture degree by pressing the handle with the thumb and the index finger.

Use

They are used to block the blood flow in small arteries and veins **(Fig. 15.42)**.

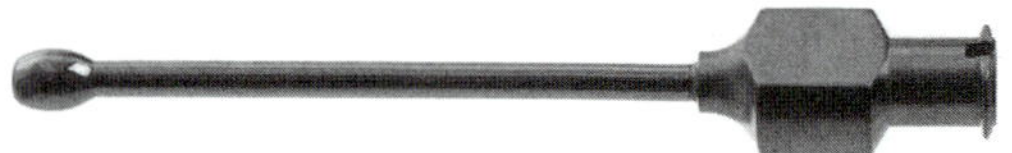

Fig. 15.40: Zanger-DeBakey heparin needle

ZANGER-DEBAKEY HEPARIN NEEDLE

Description

The instrument features a small, straight needle. The Luer lock connection ensures safe attachment and permits a smooth flow of fluids between the irrigation system and the needle **(Fig. 15.40)**.

16
History and Examination

Abhishek Singh

It is very important to take a detailed history of these patients; it would give surgeon a great deal of insight on AVF creation. Some of the important question that a surgeon must ask the patient is as follows:

- *Which is dominant arm?*
  AVF should be constructed in his non-dominant arm as far as possible. Quality of life is improved by doing so, as the dominant limb is safeguarded from the complications of AVF. Also, the patient spends a lot of time in the dialysis unit, during this time he or she can do some activity like reading a book or using a computer with the dominant arm.
- *Does the patient have central venous stenosis?*
  No AVF is going to be functional in an upper limb with central venous stenosis unless the stenosis is treated by angioplasty or stenting.
- *History of peripheral vascular disease (PVD)*
  The quality of the vessel wall may be poor in PVD and surgeon may have to consider brachial instead of radial fistula.
- *History of pacemaker insertion*
  It is associated with high risk of central venous stenosis.
- *History of congestive cardiac failure (CCF)*
  CCF may worsen after creation of AVF.
- *Recent history of peripheral arterial and venous cannulation*
  Both of which can cause damage to intima of the vessels.
- *History of diabetes mellitus*
  Peripheral vessels may have atherosclerotic changes.
- *History of taking anticoagulant and antiplatelet medication:* It is good if the patient is taking 75–150 mg of aspirin before construction of fistula but if the patient is taking clopidogrel or newer antiplatelet drugs they should be stopped prior to fistula creation. Patient on warfarin or low molecular weight heparin should either be stopped or shifted to conventional heparin.
- *Patient with severe coronary artery disease or malignancy:* The AVF creation may not be justified.
- History of heart valve disease or prosthesis may be at a higher risk of vascular-borne infections.
- A history of previous arm, neck or chest surgery may limit the feasibility of fistula construction. Axillary lymph node dissection is a classic example which may limit fistula creation.
- *Anticipated renal transplant in near future*
  Venous catheters may alone be enough for short-term management of these patients.

Preservation of Venous Network

Veins must be preserved in all patients with declining renal function and those planned for renal replacement in near future. Patients must be sensitized about its importance. The sites of venipunctures must be rotated and preferably dorsum of hand should be used, avoiding the cephalic vein. Low plasmatic consumption techniques should be used. Avoid using jugular and subclavian catheters.

PHYSICAL EXAMINATION

General Examination

Surgeon must look for edema of the extremity and the comparative sizes of both the arms. Also, examine the chest wall and neck, look for dilated veins suggesting central venous stenosis.

Examination of Arterial System

Start from distal to proximal, radial artery and ulnar artery, followed by brachial, axillary and subclavian arteries. Arterial pulsation should be felt, vessel wall condition examined.

Allen's test: The hand is elevated and patient is asked to clench his fist for 30 seconds. The radial and ulnar arteries are occluded using examiners fingers. The patient is then asked to open his hand, which at this stage should appear blanched. Now the finger occluding the ulnar artery is released, the palm should turn pink in 5 to 15 seconds suggesting a normal flow from ulnar artery. The test is repeated but this time the pressure on radial

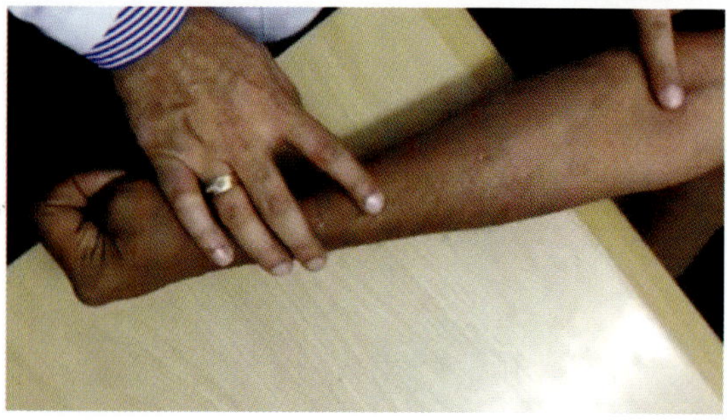

Fig. 16.1: Tap test, vein is tapped at wrist and impulse felt at elbow

artery is released and if palm turns pink in 5–15 seconds, it is suggestive of normal flow from radial artery.

Blood pressure should be measured in both the limbs and a difference of <10 mm of Hg should be considered normal.

Venous Examination

Veins should be examined distal to proximal, both cephalic and basilic system should be evaluated. A tourniquet is applied in the upper arm and all the veins are allowed to dilate, a pressure of 40 mm of Hg is required for venous dilation. Veins are assessed for caliber, course and distance from skin. Veins should be collapsible and supple to palpate. Thrombosed veins are cord-like and tender.

Tap test or Schwartz test **(Fig. 16.1):** The venous segment over the wrist is tapped and the impulse is palpated at the level of elbow. An impulse palpated is suggestive of a continuous column of blood without interruption.

17
Imaging in AVF

Abhishek Singh

USE OF ULTRASOUND AND DOPPLER IN PREOPERATIVE EVALUATION

Ultrasound helps in imaging the limb vessels and identifying vessel wall condition which may affect fistula outcome. It can identify anatomical variations and help surgeon choose an appropriate access. Surgeon can be prepared of a "Plan B" in case of a primary failure on the operation table itself. It makes a surgeon more confident and is a wonderful follow-up tool.

CONCEPT OF VASCULAR MAPPING

Both arteries and veins are mapped from wrist to axilla, this can be done by physical examination or by Doppler ultrasound examination. It gives surgeon a road map as to which AVF is to be created and once this fails which is the next option to be used.

VASCULAR MAPPING USING A DOPPLER ULTRASOUND

Doppler is surgeon's stethoscope and is best done by the operating surgeon **(Fig. 17.1)**. Vascular mapping substantially increases the number of patients dialyzing with a fistula.[1-4] Preoperative vascular mapping can potentially change surgical management with resultant increased in the number of

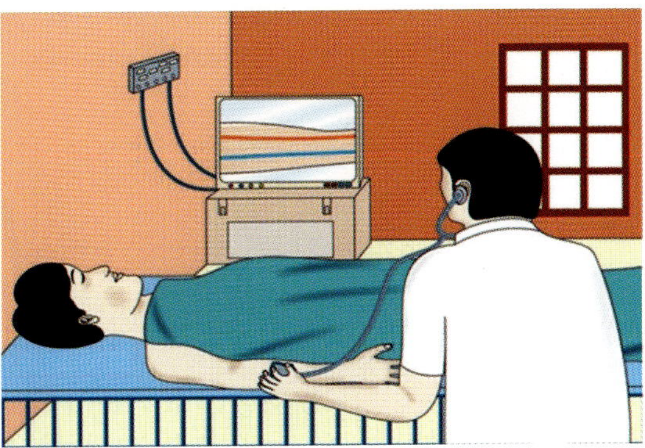

Fig. 17.1: Doppler being surgeon's stethoscope

AVF construction and appropriate selection of the best available vessels.[5]

ARTERIAL DOPPLER EXAMINATION

It is done from distal to proximal, internal diameters of all the vessels are recorded, presence or absence of vessel wall calcification is noted and also thickening of the arterial wall is noted. Normal artery is identified as a pulsatile non-compressible structure, with surrounding venae comitantes. Arterial waveforms are observed and normally a triphasic flow should be present. Laminar flow should be seen in all the vessels. Doppler can be used to do Allen's test, to check the integrity of palmar arch.

In Doppler examination surgeon should look for arterial hyperemic response. For this the patient is asked to clench his fist for 2–3 minutes and waveform in the radial artery is recorded, it should be a normal triphasic flow. When the patient is asked to open his fist and the flow is recorded, it should suddenly become monophasic and the resistive index should be less than 0.70. If the patient does not have normal hyperemic response, creation of AVF in the limb may decreased blood supply to the limb and hence it is a contraindication to AVF creation. Resistive index is a measure of potential of a vessel to dilate, as diastolic flow increases in a hyperemic state, the resistive index should fall.

VENOUS DOPPLER EXAMINATION (Fig. 17.2)

Role of venous Doppler is to assess the size of the vein, to know the condition of vessel wall,

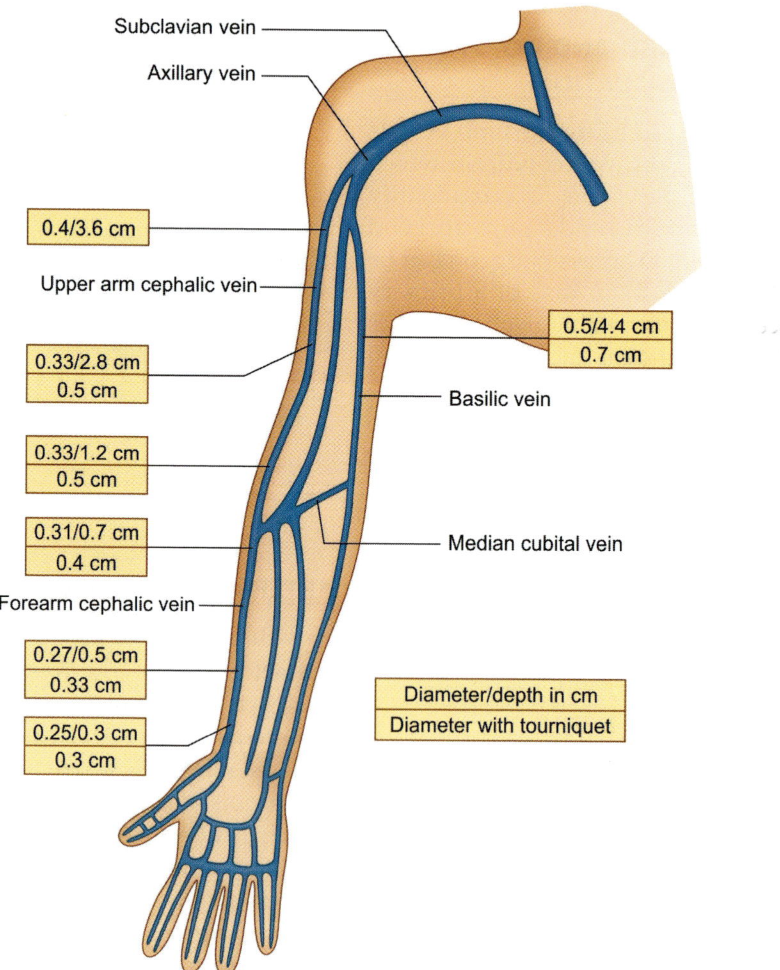

Fig. 17.2: Venous mapping

to look for stenosis or thrombosis. Doppler also gives functional information like flow through the vein and venous distensibility. Venous Doppler can help delineate continuation with central veins and rule out central venous stenosis.

Normal vein is identified as a compressible structure, which has spontaneous flow, phasic variation with respiration and augmentation is noted by applying pressure above or below the vein. The lumen should be an echoic and the walls thin and smooth.

Silva et al. in a study concluded that with venous mapping there was an increase in native AVF creation from 14 to 63%, early failure rates also decreased from 36 to 8.3% and primary patency rates at one year increased from 48 to 83%.[4]

VENOUS AND ARTERIAL SELECTION FOR AVF

A venous diameter should be 2 mm or more, for a radiocephalic fistula, a venous diameter of <2 mm has a primary patency rate of 16% at three months as compared to a venous diameter of >2 mm which has a 3-month patency rate of 76%.[6] Similarly, optimal arterial diameter should be 2 mm, with a diameter >1.6 mm patency rate is 93% as compared to 32% with a diameter of <1.6 mm.

CHOOSING A SURGICAL SITE FOR AVF CREATION

All the AVFs are compared against the standard of Brescia-Cimino fistula (2-year patency: 55 to 89%). There has been no randomized trial comparing the proximal to the distal fistulas, but the general consensus is to start with the most distal AVF which is feasible.

The order of creation of autologous fistulas is as follows **(Flowchart 17.1)**:
- Snuff box fistula
- Brescia-Cimino fistula (radiocephalic)

Flowchart 17.1: The chronology in which AVF should be created

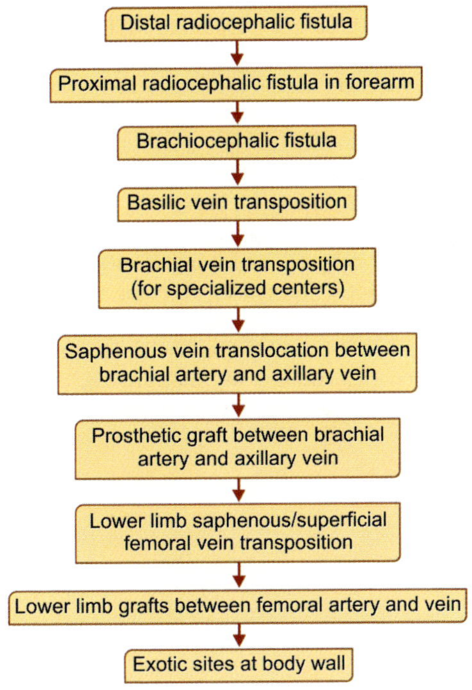

- Mid-forearm or high radiocephalic
- Proximal radial artery to cephalic vein fistula—high forearm fistula
- Radiobasilic transposed fistula
- Brachiocephalic fistula
- Brachiobasilic transposed fistula

TIMING OF AVF CREATION

There is no consensus on timing of creation of AVF but the guiding principle is that, at the time when the patient need hemodialysis (HD), he should have a matured fistula. As per the kidney disease outcomes quality initiative (KDOQI) guidelines fistula should be created when serum creatinine is >4 mg% or glomerular filtration rate (GFR) drops to <25 ml/min and 6 months before HD is required.

REFERENCES

1. Allon M, Lockhart ME, Lilly RZ, Gallichio MH, Young CJ, Barker J, Deierhoi MH, Robbin ML. Effect of preoperative sonographic mapping on vascular access outcomes in hemodialysis patients. Kidney international 2001 Nov 30; 60(5):2013– 20.
2. Ascher E, Gade P, Hingorani A, Mazzariol F, Gunduz Y, Fodera M, Yorkovich W. Changes in the practice of angioaccess surgery: impact of dialysis outcome and quality initiative recommendations. Journal of vascular surgery 2000 Jan 31;31(1):84–92.
3. Gibson KD, Caps MT, Kohler TR, Hatsukami TS, Gillen DL, Aldassy M, Sherrard DJ, Stehman-Breen CO. Assessment of a policy to reduce placement of prosthetic hemodialysis access. Kidney international 2001 Jun 30;59(6):2335–45.
4. Silva Jr MB, Hobson II RW, Pappas PJ, Jamil Z, Araki CT, Goldberg MC, Gwertzman G, Padberg Jr FT. A strategy for increasing use of autogenous hemodialysis access procedures: impact of preoperative noninvasive evaluation. Journal of Vascular Surgery 1998 Feb 28;27(2):302–8.
5. Robbin ML, Gallichio MH, Deierhoi MH, Young CJ, Weber TM, Allon M. US Vascular Mapping before Hemodialysis Access Placement 1. Radiology 2000 Oct;217(1):83–8.
6. Mendes RR, Farber MA, Marston WA, Dinwiddie LC, Keagy BA, Burnham SJ. Prediction of wrist arteriovenous fistula maturation with preoperative vein mapping with ultrasonography. Journal of vascular surgery 2002 Sep 1;36(3): 460–63.

18
Technique of Vascular Anastomosis

Abhishek Singh

BASIC PRINCIPLE OF VASCULAR ANASTOMOSIS

Dissection and Exposure

- Surgeon should have sound anatomical knowledge of the arterial and venous anatomy of the limbs.
- The operative field should have a good exposure, so that the vascular bulldogs and the slings can be comfortably placed, incision should be planned accordingly.
- The plane of dissection should be exactly on the vessels, leaving the adventitia intact.
- It is ideal to do a sharp dissection with scissors on the vessels.
- Side branches of the arteries should not be ligated unless they interfere with the anastomosis and all the venous side branches should be ligated.

Vascular Control

- Distal and proximal control of the artery and vein must be taken with the help of slings. In case of side to side anastomosis they can be controlled with same sling and bulldog clamps. In case of end to side anastomosis artery is controlled separately, distal end of the vein is ligated and proximal end controlled.
- Bulldog clamps should be atraumatic and not cause any intimal injury.

- Clamps should be placed in such a way that they do not interfere with the anastomosis.

Arteriotomy

Arteriotomy should be planned on the anterior wall in midline, it should be done with tip of 11 number surgical blade held on a Bard Parker's handle, arteriotomy should be just enough for the Potts angled scissors to enter. After flushing with saline, site should be inspected and then opened with Potts scissors. Arteriotomy should be 7–9 mm on radial artery and 5–7 mm on brachial artery. While doing arteriotomy care should be taken not to injure the posterior wall of the artery and at the same time all the three layers of the vessel should be traversed, this can be done by guarding the knife by your fingers.

Vascular Anastomosis

- Use of vascular forceps (ring tip, diamond tip) is recommended. Do not hold the vessel wall tightly, just support the vessel wall or give countertraction for the needle to pass.
- A double-armed monofilament suture should be used (6–0/7–0 polypropylene). Suturing can be done using "open (parachute)" or "closed" technique. In

the open method, first the sutures are passed through the angles (heel) and then continued on sides up to opposite angle (toe), none of the sutures are tightened and at the end of the anastomosis both the ends are pulled to tighten the entire suture line. In closed technique first angle is secured by tying a knot and both the walls are taken one after the other and sutures are tightened as the throws are passed.

In the closed technique both the angle can be first secured and knots tied. The suturing of the walls can then be completed in quadrants.

- The direction of suturing should be inside-out on artery and outside-in on the vein. Place the anastomosis is such a way that forehand suturing is possible for the maximum length.
- Continuous suturing is advocated unless the vessels are very friable in which case interrupted sutures can be used.
- Sutures should traverse all the three layers of the vessels and all the bites should be evenly placed.
- Edges of the anastomosis should be everted. Inverted edges or intima will increase the chances of thrombosis.
- Needle and suture should be pulled out in the direction of the throw, with the turn of the wrist. This will prevent cutting through suture and laceration of the vessel edge.

- Inflow and outflow should be irrigated with heparinized saline before completion of anastomosis. Heparin can be injected in the venous limb directly or can be given systemically.
- While tying the knot a minimum of 6 throws are required for a monofilament suture.

Declamping

Vessel clamps should be opened gently, just released to look for bleeding and then remove completely if there is no or minimal bleeding. First the distal clamp followed by proximal one is removed. Needle hole bleeding would stop by itself, so surgeon should wait patiently. If pulsatile bleeding is there and one requires suturing, a suture smaller than what was used for initial anastomosis should be used. At this stage one should check for the thrill and flow across the anastomosis.

Warm saline and injection papaverine can be applied locally, these maneuvers help in local vasodilatation.

Types of Vascular Anastomosis (Figs 18.1A and B)

End to Side

End of the vein to side of the artery: This is the most commonly performed fistula anastomosis. The end of the vein is sutured to the side of the artery. It is useful when the artery and vein are far from each other.

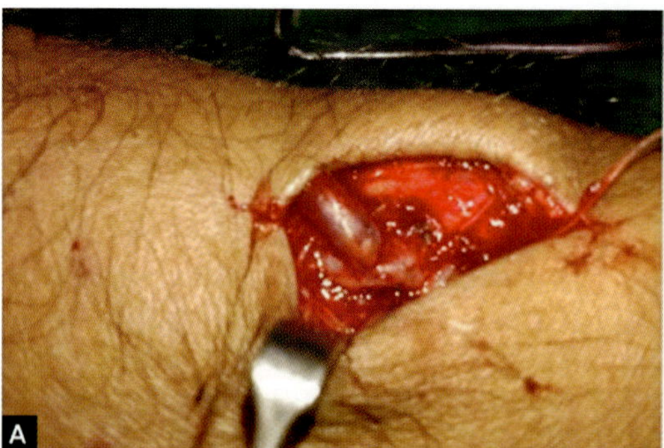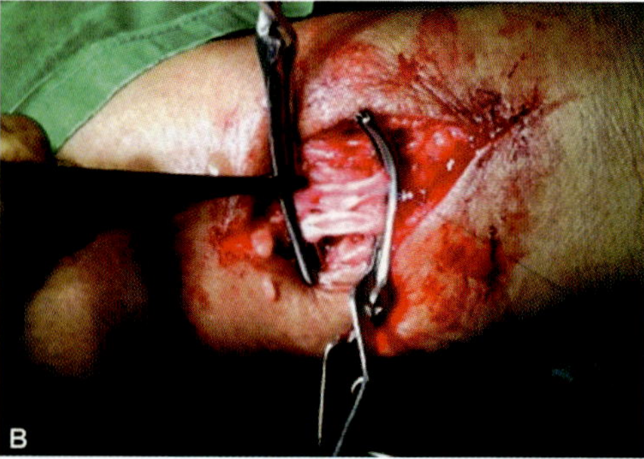

Figs 18.1A and B: (A) End to side anastomosis; (B) Side to side anastomosis

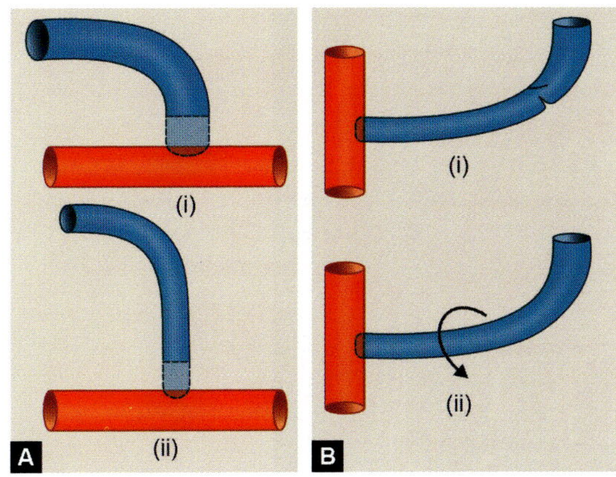

Figs 18.2A and B: (A) Angle of vein when the vein meets the artery; (B) Kink in vein which gets released on outward rotation of vein

Advantage of this technique is that fistula can be created even when the vein is far away from the artery, like a venous branch from the dorsum of the hand can be transposed to the wrist. All transposed fistulae require an end to side anastomosis. Angle at which vein meets the artery is very critical, it should be an obtuse angle and should have a gentle curve **(Fig. 18.2A)**. Also, rotation of the vein should be considered, outward rotation of 60–120 is helpful **(Fig. 18.2B)**.

If thrombosis affects this anastomosis it generally affects only the venous limb. Creation of a higher fistula is possible if this fails. This technique is difficult to learn as compared to side to side technique.

Side to Side Anastomosis

It can be done when the artery and vein are close to each other. The operation is easy to perform and has a shallow learning curve. After completion of the anastomosis the distal limb can be ligated to convert it into an end to side anastomosis.

End to End Anastomosis

It is the rarest of the type of anastomosis as it requires transection of artery. When an AVF anastomotic site aneurysm is excised, the cut end of the artery can be anastomosed with the proximal venous segment in an end to end fashion. It gives rise to limited flow without any hypercirculatory changes.

Disadvantages of end to end anastomosis is that it is technically demanding, especially with regards to maintaining the lie of the vessels. Surgeon also has to be cognizant of the luminal discrepancies. Limb ischemia may occur as the artery is transected. If there is a thrombus in the venous limb, it would progress to the arterial limb in end to end anastomosis.

Preoperative measures to improve venous diameter are before construction of AVF (all these maneuvers of questionable significance):
- Arm exercises with or without tourniquet (isometric exercise, soft ball exercise)
- Thrombolytic ointment for local application
- Locally acting vasodilators like nifedipine can be applied
- Nitroglycerine and diltiazem can be applied locally
- Isometric exercises have shown to increase the venous diameter and should be started before surgery and continued later.[1]

Armamentarium Required

All the AVFs should be constructed under magnification, surgeon should use surgical loupe of power 2.5X to 3.5X. A use of headlight is also suggested **(Fig. 18.3)**.

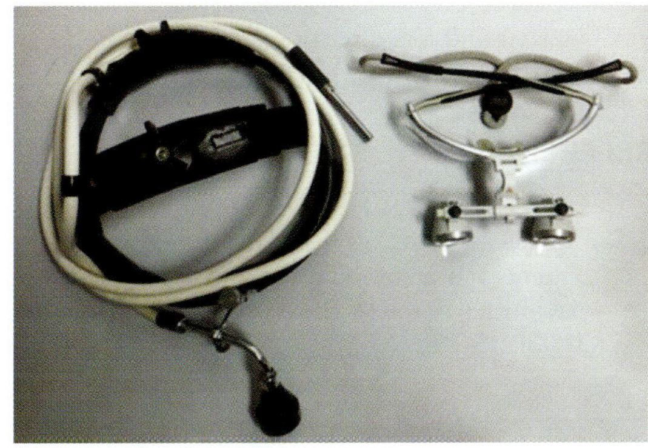

Fig. 18.3: Loupe and headlight

Note: Disadvantage of this anastomosis is that it can cause venous hypertension and painful thumb syndrome.

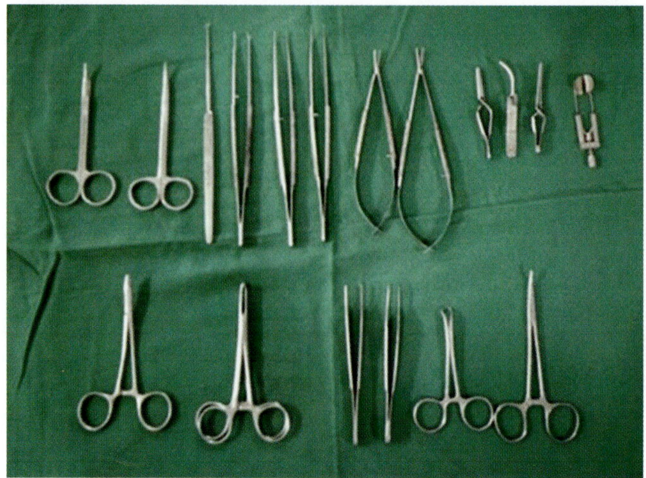

Fig. 18.4: Instrument tray

AVF surgical tray consists of **(Fig. 18.4)**:

- Surgical blade numbers 11 and 15 on Bard-Parker handle.
- Monopolar and bipolar diathermy on low energy settings.
- Fine curved mosquito forceps also known as baby mosquito forceps.
- Adson's tissue forceps both tooth and plain
- Small Allis tissue forceps
- Small dissecting dolphin scissors
- DeBakey atraumatic vascular forceps
- Bulldog clamps, curved and straight
- Angled micro-Potts scissors
- Gerald micro-ring tip forceps
- Castroviejo's micro-needle holder
- Small conventional needle holder.

REFERENCE

1. Leaf DA, MacRae HS, Grant E, Kraut J. Isometric exercise increases the size of forearm veins in patients with chronic renal failure. The American Journal of the Medical Sciences 2003 Mar 31; 325(3):115–19.

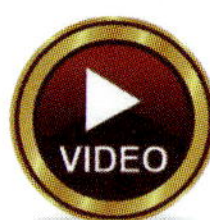

Scan QR Code for Video on
Radio-cephalic Fistula-1

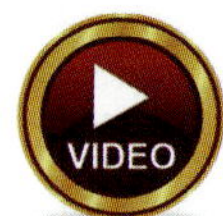

Scan QR Code for Video on
Radio-cephalic Fistula-2 (Parachute Technique)

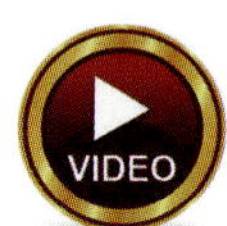

Scan QR Code for Video on
Brachio-cephalic Fistula-3 (Parachute Technique)

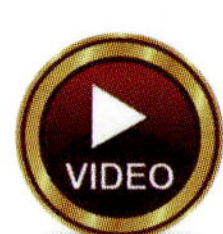

Scan QR Code for Video on
Radio-cephalic Fistula-4

19
Wrist Fistula

Abhishek Singh

Wrist fistula is shown in **Figs 19.1A to D**.
- Snuff box AVF
- Brescia-Cimino fistula

RELEVANT SURGICAL ANATOMY OF FOREARM

Forearm is drained by two major veins: Cephalic and basilic veins. The cephalic vein begins in the anatomical snuffbox at the posterolateral aspect of the forearm. It gradually turns along the forearm to become the lateral vein of forearm. At the level of antecubital fossa, it meets the basilic vein via the median cubital vein. Basilic vein starts from the posterior (dorsal) aspect of the forearm and turns onto the volar aspect.

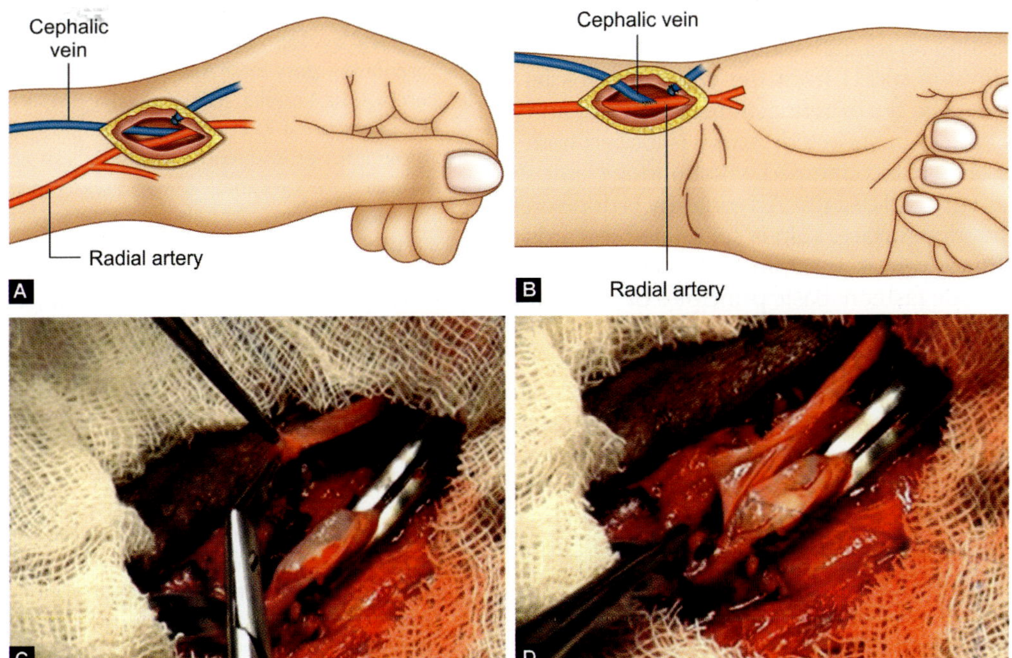

Figs 19.1A to D: (A) Snuffbox fistula; (B) RC fistula; (C) Arteriotomy in RC AVF; (D) Arteriovenous anastomosis

About an inch above the medial epicondyle of humerus it pierces the deep fascia to become deep vein of arm. Radial artery is the non-dominant or the smaller branch of brachial artery, it arises just below the elbow flexion crease. In its upper part, it is covered by brachioradialis muscle, in the distal third of forearm it lies below the deep fascia and is easily palpable against the lower third of radius. Ulnar artery is a deeper artery of the arm and is seldom used for fistula creation. Superficial radial nerve lies in close association to radial artery in its distal course. It should be protected as injury to the nerve, can give rise to parasthesia to the base of the thumb causing painful thumb syndrome.

SURGICAL STEPS

A longitudinal incision is shown in **Fig. 19.2**, it is taken midway between the artery and the vein. Some surgeons prefer to take a transverse incision over the artery and vein. Cephalic vein is first dissected. Cephalic vein is ligated distally and transected. Patency of the vein is checked by passing an infant feeding tube into the vein. Backflow of blood from the vein confirms its patency. The flexor retinaculum is opened and radial artery is dissected. Artery is looped with a vessel loop and clamped with bulldog clamps proximally and distally. Arteriotomy is done on the anterior surface. Vein is spatulated towards the artery. Vein is anastomosed to artery in an end to side fashion. Basic principles of vascular surgery are followed as described earlier.

It is a low impact surgery and can be done under local anesthesia.[1,2] It is usually done as an outpatient procedure. It can be constructed as end to side (recommended) or side to side fashion. It takes about 6 weeks to mature. This type of fistula preserves proximal veins future access placement. It has least fistula complication rates like steal, infection and aneurysm development.[3-5] One major disadvantage of wrist fistula is lower blood flow as compared to other fistulas. Primary

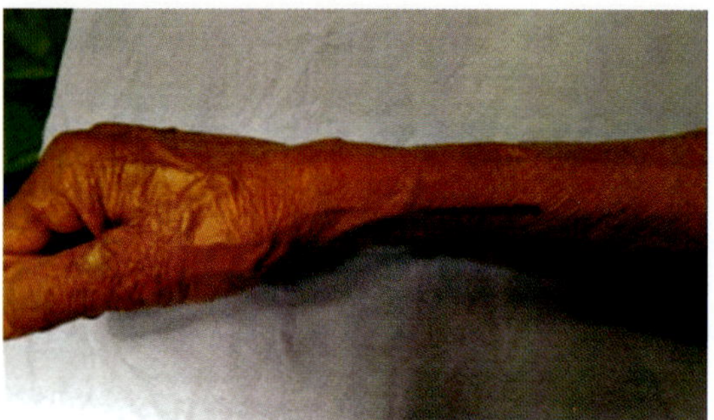

Fig. 19.2: An incision for RC AVF

and secondary patency rate of this fistula at 1 year is 67.6% and 89.2%, respectively.[6]

REFERENCES

1. Brescia MJ, Cimino JE, Appel K, Hurwich BJ. Chronic hemodialysis using venipuncture and a surgically created arteriovenous fistula. New England Journal of Medicine 1966;275(20):1089–92.
2. Bagolan P, Spagnoli A, Ciprandi G, Picca S, Leozappa G, Nahom A, Trucchi A, Rizzoni G, Fabbrini G. A ten-year experience of Brescia-Cimino arteriovenous fistula in children: technical evolution and refinements. Journal of vascular surgery 1998 Apr 30;27(4):640–44.
3. Perera GB, Mueller MP, Kubaska SM, Wilson SE, Lawrence PF, Fujitani RM. Superiority of autogenous arteriovenous hemodialysis access: maintenance of function with fewer secondary interventions. Annals of vascular surgery 2004;18(1):66–73.
4. Huber TS, Carter JW, Carter RL, Seeger JM. Patency of autogenous and polytetrafluoroethylene upper extremity arteriovenous hemodialysis accesses: a systematic review. Journal of vascular surgery 2003;38(5):1005–11.
5. Kinnaert P, Vereerstraeten P, Toussaint C, Van Geertruyden J. Nine years' experience with internal arteriovenous fistulas for haemodialysis: a study of some factors influencing the results. British Journal of Surgery 1977;64(4):242–46.
6. Srivastava A, Sharma S. Hemodialysis vascular access options after failed Brescia-Cimino arteriovenous fistula. Indian Journal of Urology (IJU): Journal of the Urological Society of India 2011;27(2):163.

20

Elbow Fistula

Abhishek Singh

- Brachiocephalic AVF
- Proximal radial artery to cephalic vein

RELEVANT SURGICAL ANATOMY

Antecubital fossa is a triangular space; its base is formed by an imaginary line joining the two epicondyles of humerus. The lateral edge is formed by brachioradialis muscle and the medial edge by pronator teres muscle. Apex is formed by the point where brachioradialis overlaps the pronator teres muscle. Floor of the fossa is formed by brachialis muscle which is covered by the deep fascia. The fossa contains the median cubital vein; it is a continuation of cephalic vein and courses medially from apex of the antecubital fossa to join the basilic vein. Cephalic vein of the forearm traverses the fossa laterally and ascend through the anterolateral aspect of arm. The deep veins of the arm are the brachial veins which accompany the brachial artery. Communicating veins or the perforating veins connect the deep and the superficial system.

Bicipital aponeurosis is a flat tendinous insertion of the tendon of biceps muscle which fuses with the deep fascia of the arm. It lies below the veins and covers the brachial artery. Brachial artery can be exposed by incising the bicipital aponeurosis. It courses medially to the apex of antecubital fossa where it divides into superficial radial and deep ulnar branches. Medial nerve lies medial to the brachial artery in the fossa.

SURGICAL STEPS

A transverse incision below the skin creases at the level of elbow is taken, incision is deepened in layers till the cephalic vein/median cubital vein is identified **(Figs 20.1A to D)**. The vein is dissected along its length for a sufficient length so that it can reach up to the brachial artery. Vein is transected distally and proximal end is spatulated towards the artery.

Once vein is dissected, bicipital aponeurosis is identified and brachial artery pulsations are palpated. Bicipital aponeurosis is opened over the brachial artery and brachial artery is identified, it is closely accompanied by venae comitantes **(Figs 20.1A to D)**. Brachial artery is dissected off the veins and looped proximally and distally. Bulldog clamps are applied proximally and distally **(Figs 20.1A to D)**. Arteriotomy is made on anterior surface and vein is anastomosed to brachial artery in an end to side fashion **(Figs 20.2A to C)**. General principles of vascular anastomosis are followed. If the perforating vein is anastomosed with brachial artery, it is called the Gracz fistula.

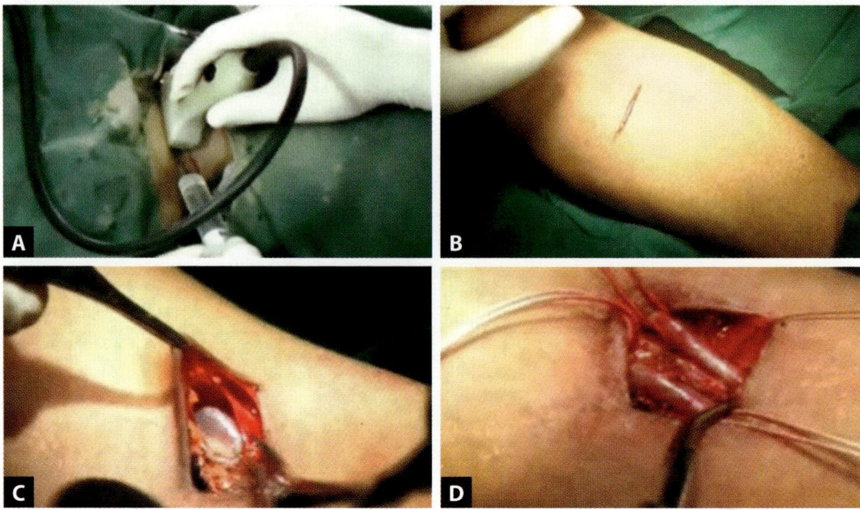

Figs 20.1A to D: (A) Supraclavicular block being given; (B) Incision for BC AVF; (C) Cephalic vein dissection; (D) Brachial artery dissection

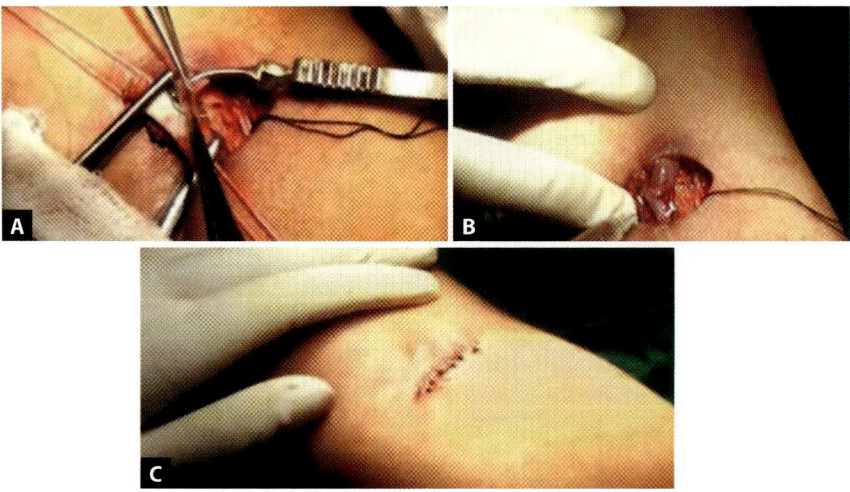

Figs 20.2A to C: (A and B) Arteriovenous anastomosis; (C) Completed surgery

Fistula can also be constructed between proximal radial artery and cephalic vein, but less commonly created by vascular surgeons.

These fistulas are high flow, initially a visible vein is helpful in making decision of construction but not critical. Tough superficial fascia of upper arm may make cannulation difficult. Deltopectoral groove is a trouble spot where the outflow tract may get stenosed. One and four-year patency rate of BC AVF is reported to be 74.1% and 61.3%.[1]

REFERENCE

1. Elcheroth J, de Pauw L, Kinnaert P. Elbow arteriovenous fistulas for chronic hemodialysis. Br J Surg 1994;81:982–84.

21

Brachiobasilic Fistula

Abhishek Singh

SURGICAL ANATOMY

Brachial artery begins at the lower border of the teres major muscle and terminates at the apex of cubital fossa by dividing into radial and ulnar artery. Brachial artery travels along the bicipital groove till it goes under bicipital aponeurosis. Brachial artery has three branches in arm, profunda brachii, superior and inferior ulnar collateral. Artery is associated with medial and lateral brachial veins throughout its course.

The basilic vein traverses the antecubital fossa medially, it ascends in the arm and pierces the deep fascia 1 inch above the medial epicondyle of humerus. As this vein lies deep in arm it is almost always protected from venipunctures and remains patent. Also as this vein is deep to the deep fascia it always had to be transposed so that a AVF is created which can be cannulated. Basilic vein ascends in arm medial to the brachial artery, in the upper arm it is joined by brachial veins to form axillary vein at the level of teres major muscle. Medial cutaneous nerve of arm and ulnar nerve lie medial to brachial artery and separate it from the basilic vein. Median nerve is closely associated with brachial artery, it crosses the brachial artery from lateral to medial in the middle arm. In the lower third median nerve is medial to brachial artery.

SURGICAL STEPS

This surgery is done under supraclavicular block or general anesthesia **(Fig. 21.1A)**. A J-shaped incision is taken starting from the antecubital fossa and extending along the course of the basilic vein. The incision is extended till a point where it joins brachial vein to become axillary vein. Incision is deepened till the deep fascia and deep fascia is opened. Basilic vein is circumferentially dissected all along its length, multiple tributaries are encountered and serially ligated **(Fig. 21.1A)**. The vein is dissected off the branches of medial cutaneous nerve, ulnar and median nerve. All the branches should be meticulously ligated, once the vein is in subcutaneous tunnel there is no way that bleeding can be controlled without taking down the anastomosis. The basilic vein is dissected till it is seen joining the brachial vein. Now the lateral edge of the vein is marked with methylene blue **(Fig. 21.1B)**, so that the lie of the vein can be identified. The vein is now transected at the level of the elbow and cannulated with infant feeding tube to check patency and back flow. A leak test is performed by injecting saline in the vein, if any leak is found it is sutured with polypropylene 7–0.

Brachial artery is dissected at the elbow and looped **(Fig. 21.1A)**. Basilic vein is now

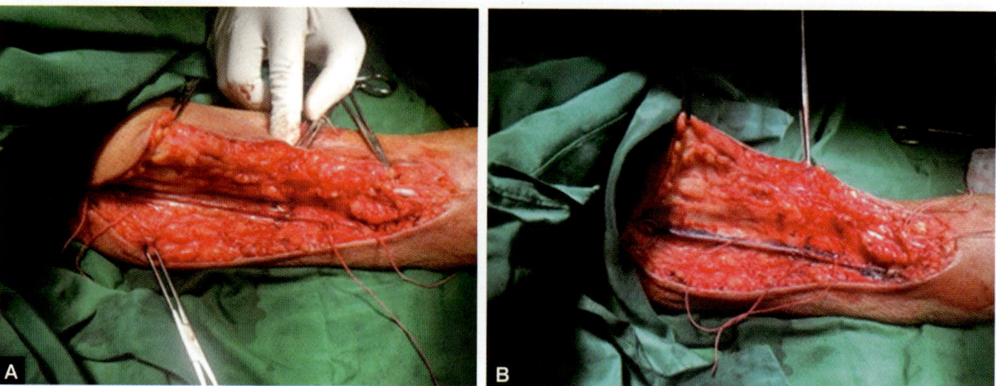

Figs 21.1A and B: (A) Dissected basilic vein and brachial artery; (B) The basilic vein marked with methylene blue (to maintain the lie of the vein)

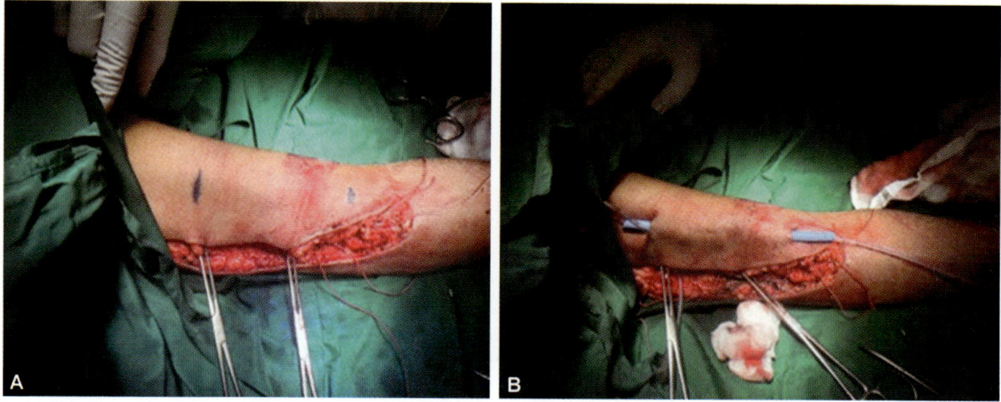

Figs 21.2A and B: (A) Marking of the tunnel; (B) Use of an Amplatz sheath to make a tunnel

tunneled from the medial aspect of the arm onto the anterior aspect of the arm just below the skin and brought down to the level of brachial artery **(Figs 21.2A and B)**. Methods of tunneling include dissecting the subcutaneous tissue using a long artery and pulling the vein through it or vein can be tied to a tunneler used in ventriculoperitoneal shunt or Amplatz sheath can be placed below the skin and vein passed through it **(Figs 21.2A and B)**. Care should be taken to check and recheck for any twist, this can be done by passing an infant feeding tube into the vein, this can also be done by injecting saline into vein, if the lie is abnormal, the vein will appear twisted at the point where it becomes axillary vein. Bulldog clamps are applied on the brachial artery proximally and distally and arteriotomy is made on the anterior aspect. End to side anastomosis is done using polypropylene 6–0. Wound is closed in layers over a suction drain.

Many authors have tried decreasing the morbidity of basilic vein dissection by using multiple skip skin incisions instead of a large single incision[1] **(Figs 21.3A and B)**. Surgeons have used vein inverters to dissect the vein, endoscopic vein dissection has also been

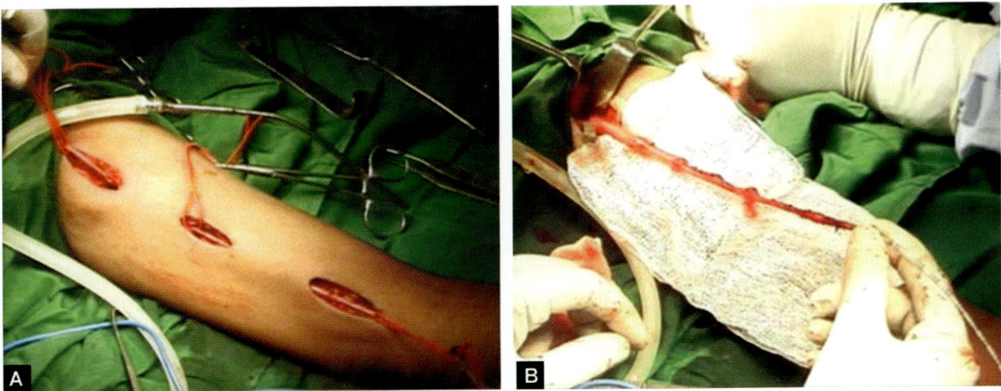

Figs 21.3A and B: (A) Multiple skip incision taken for BBT; (B) Basilic vein being tested for leak

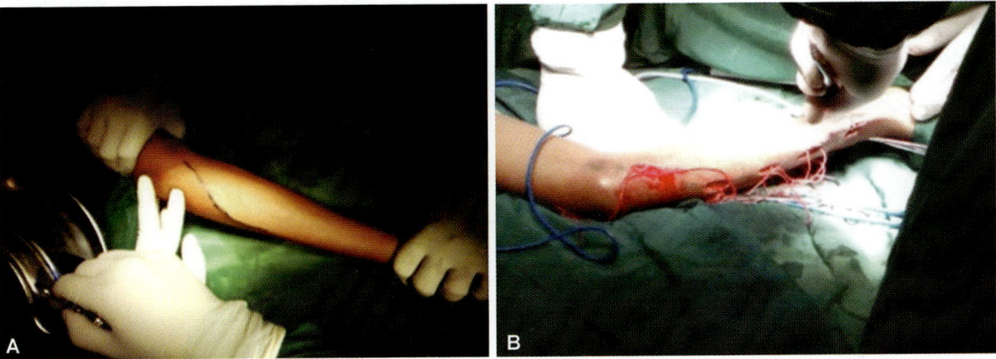

Figs 21.4A and B: (A) Incision for forearm radiobasilic transposition; (B) Multiple skip incision taken for forearm transposition

described.[2,3] Basilic vein transposition can be done in single stage or in first stage only, a brachiobasilic anastomosis is done and once the AVF matures, it is transposed.

BBT has a one year fistula patency rate of 84%, 73% at 3 years.[4] Some authors have reported patency rates for staged procedures as compared to a single-staged procedure.[5]

Forearm Basilic Vein to Radial Artery Transposition (Figs 21.4 and 21.5)

Basilic vein in forearm is not deep but postero-medial in location, hence has to be transposed across the forearm, so that a segment for cannulation is available. The incision is taken

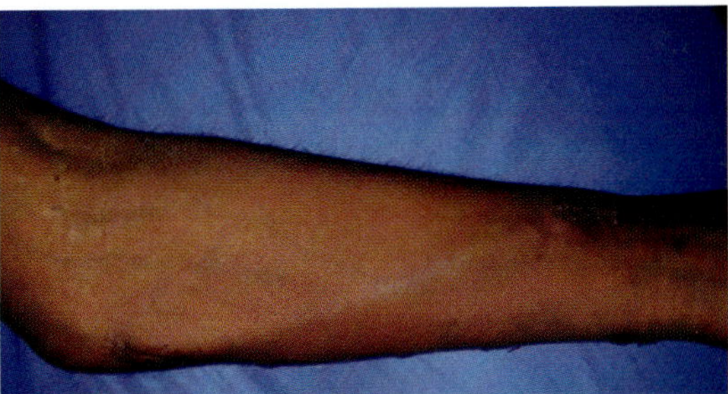

Fig. 21.5: Mature forearm transposed fistula

on the medial aspect of the forearm overlying the basilic vein, this is to ensure an optimal dissection from the wrist to the elbow **(Figs 21.4A and B)**. Vein is then transposed by creating a subcutaneous tunnel under the skin, across the forearm and anastomosed to radial artery **(Fig. 21.5)**. Principle of anastomosis and transposition remain the same. The primary and secondary patency rates at one year for this fistula is 41.5% and 79.1%, respectively.[6]

AVF using Brachial Vein

Brachial vein fistula has been reported by Bazan et al.[7] On most of the occasions it is done in two stages. Dissection of brachial vein is difficult, also due to its limited length it is difficult to transpose this vein. Many patients develop temporary edema after this fistula. Not much experience has been reported with this fistula.

REFERENCES

1. Veeramani M, Vyas J, Sabnis R, Desai M. Small incision basilic vein transposition technique: A good alternative to standard method. Indian J Urol. 2010;26:145–47.
2. Hill BB, Chan AK, Faruqi RM, Arko FR, Zarins CK, Fogarty TJ. Keyhole technique of autologous brachiobasilic transposition arteriovenous fistula. J Vasc Surg. 2005;42:945–50.
3. Tordoir JH, Dammers R, de Brauw M. Video-assisted basilic vein transposition for haemodialysis vascular access: Preliminary experience with a new technique. Nephrol Dial Transplant 2001;16:391–94.
4. Humphries AL Jr, Colborn GL, Wynn JJ. Elevated basilic vein arteriovenous fistula. Am J Surg. 1999;177:489–91.
5. El Mallah S. Staged basilic vein transposition for dialysis angioaccess. Int Angiol. 1998;17:65–68.
6. Srivastava A, Sharma S. Hemodialysis vascular access options after failed Brescia-Cimino arteriovenous fistula. Indian Journal of Urology (IJU): Journal of the Urological Society of India 2011;27(2):163.
7. Bazan HA, Schanzer H. Transposition of the brachial vein: A new source for autologous arteriovenous fistulas. J Vasc Surg. 2004;40:184–86.

22

Lower Limb Fistula

Abhishek Singh

They are undertaken when the upper limb options have been exhausted. These AVFs are more complex and technically more challenging. For creating thigh fistula transposition is always required.

In thigh either the saphenous or superficial femoral vein is used. Saphenous vein is anastomosed in a straight or loop configuration to common femoral or superficial femoral arteries. The saphenous vein is quite muscular and there is a high incidence of secondary intervention about 3 angioplasties per fistula. In one series mean primary patency of this AVF was 7 months.[1] In general, straight configuration has a better outcome than loop configuration.

Saphenous vein can be used as an autologous interposition graft for the upper limb AVF.

Superficial femoral vein can also be transposed in a straight or loop configuration. In a series by Gradman the secondary patency rate at 12 months was 86%.[2] There is a high risk of ischemic complications. Many patients require revision surgery for steal syndrome.

This can be avoided by tapering the end of the femoral vein to 4.5–5 mm. There are no studies comparing the two thigh fistulas.

AVF can be created at the level of ankle using tibial arteries and saphenous vein, the results are not encouraging and literature scant.[3]

After all the autologous options are exhausted grafts should be used, discussion on grafts is beyond the scope of this text.

ANTICOAGULATION AFTER AVF CREATION

There is limited evidence to suggest routine use of heparin, but a single dose of low molecular weight or conventional heparin 5000 IU can be given. Use on antiplatelet prevents early thrombosis in perioperative period, they can be started on clopidogrel 100 mg daily from postoperative day one. Alternately, ecosprin 75–150 mg can be started before surgery and continued. Anti-platelet drugs have shown to decrease AVF thrombosis in the first 6 weeks.[4]

REFERENCES

1. Pierre-Paul D, Williams S, Lee T, Gahtan V. Saphenous vein loop to femoral artery arteriovenous fistula: A practical alternative. Ann Vasc Surg 2004;18:223–27.
2. Gradman WS, Laub J, Cohen W. Femoral vein transposition for arteriovenous hemodialysis access: Improved patient selection and intraoperative measures reduce postoperative ischemia. J Vasc Surg 2005;41:279–84.
3. Srivastava A, Sharma S. Hemodialysis vascular access options after failed Brescia-Cimino arteriovenous fistula. Indian Journal of Urology (IJU): Journal of the Urological Society of India 2011 Apr;27(2):163.
4. Stolic R. Most important chronic complications of arteriovenous fistulas for hemodialysis. Medical principles and practice 2013;22(3): 220–28.

23

Cannulation of AVF

Abhishek Singh

Cannulation is done using a sharp needle with bevel facing the anterior wall of vein. It should be done under all aseptic precautions. It has to be 1.5 inches away from the anastomosis and distance between the two needles should be 1.5 inches. Infiltration may occur due to improper cannulation and if it occurs, fistula should be allowed to rest for a few weeks.

Techniques used for AVF cannulation are as follows

- *Point puncture technique:* Two points for arterial and venous puncture are marked and repeatedly punctured with sharp needles. Over a period of time this area of the vein develops aneurysmal dilatation which may bleed or thrombosis may develop. This technique is easy to replicate, but associated with complications.
- *Rope ladder cannulation:* Using a sharp needle AVF is cannulated and sites are rotated every time along the length of vein.
- *Button hole cannulation:* AVF is cannulated at the same site and with same angle using a sharp needle. The scab over the puncture area is removed. Over weeks a scared tract develops which is now punctured with a blunt needle. It is a method of choice for home cannulation, for precious fistula and when there is a limited area for cannulation.

24
Management of Difficult Situations in AVF Creation

Abhishek Singh

Immediately postprocedure no palpable thrill (Flowchart 24.1)

If the thrill is not palpable, it is suggestive of decreased flow. Surgeon should auscultate for bruit, if bruit is present it is advisable to wait for some time and the thrill may pick up. If no bruit and pulsations are present, examine the fistula carefully, look for fullness of vein. If vein is not full, then the inflow is obstructed. If the vein is full, dissect the vein and release the fascia all around and up to 4–5 cm above the vein. Look for any twist and turns in vein, rotate the vein outwards 60–120. Palpate the vein for any thrombus, if strong pulsations are present it is suggestive of outflow obstruction, a clot or thrombus may be present. Do a venotomy, insert a Fogarty balloon and do a thombectomy. An on-table Doppler if available can be done, spiral laminar flow is suggestive of flow across the fistula. If the vein is collapsed, anastomosis should be taken down to check if the flow is present there from distal arterial end, proximal arterial end and venous end. Once the problem is addressed, re-anastomosis should be done.

A day after the surgery patient has absence of thrill on clinical examination, what next (Fig. 24.1).

Flowchart 24.1: Algorithm of management if no thrill is palpable on operating table

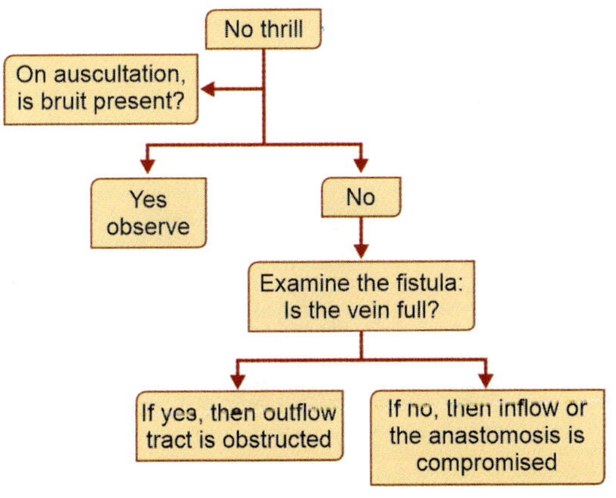

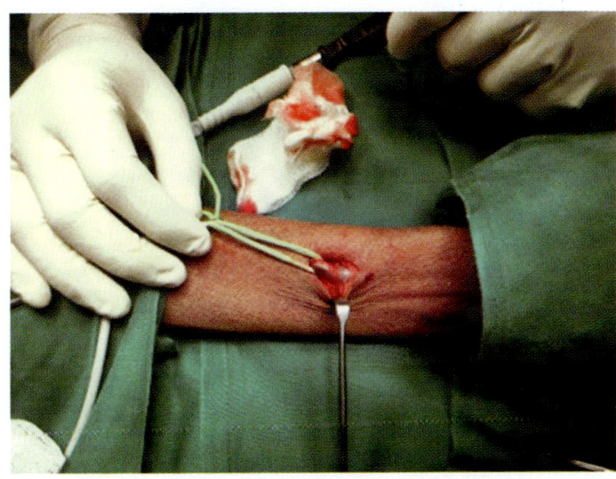

Fig. 24.1: A thrombus is juxta-anastomotic site

A thorough general examination of the patient should be done, blood pressure should be noted, hypotension may be responsible for sluggish flow. Examine the fistula, look for hematoma, edema or swelling around the operative site. Acute thrombosis will give rise to some pain and tenderness can be elicited. Look for a palpable thrombus and a Doppler should be done. If thrombus is suspected, exploration and thombectomy should be done.

Patient comes with loss of thrill in fistula which was being used for dialysis for some time.

This occurs mostly with acute thrombosis of fistula. It is important to ask the patient when was the last dialysis done, when did he/she last feel the thrill? Was there any hypotension during dialysis or were there any symptoms of the same? Clinically, examine the course of the vein and palpate for any thrombus, and a Doppler examination should be done **(Figs 24.2A and B).**

Surgical steps of fistula exploration (Figs 24.3A to C and 24.4):

Before exploration general work up of the patient including the hemogram, blood group should be available, as these patients may bleed during the procedure.

- It should be preferably done under supraclavicular block.
- An incision should be made at the level of thrombus if diagnosed or just proximal to the previous suture site in case of old AVF. If AVF was constructed only a few days back, then suture line can be opened.
- Take proximal and distal control of the vein, if the thrombus is juxta-anastomotic, then proximal and distal control of artery should be taken.

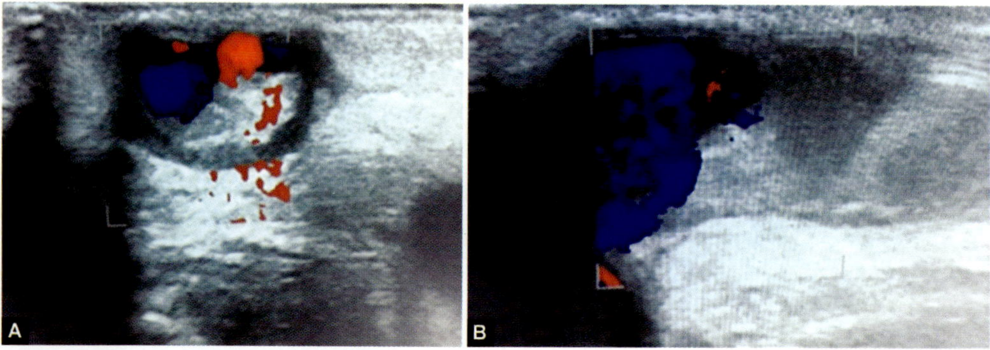

Figs 24.2A and B: (A) Transverse section of a thrombus in AVF; (B) Longitudinal section of a thrombus in AVF

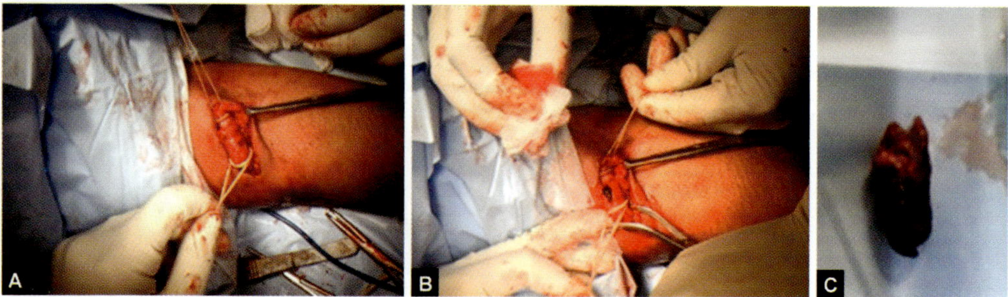

Figs 24.3A to C: (A) Controlled venous limb with thrombus *in situ*; (B) Arteriotomy with thrombus *in situ*; (C) Thrombus remove from fistula

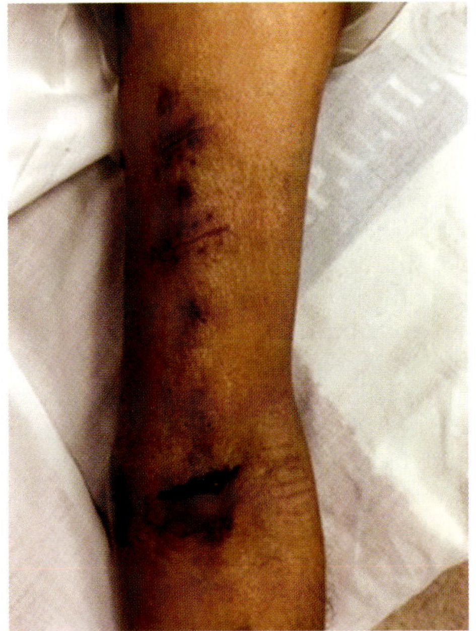

Fig. 24.4: Post-thrombectomy fistula at 3 weeks

- Bulldog clamps are applied proximally and distally.
- Vein is opened along its length (longitudinally) for about 0.5–1 cm, thrombus if seen is delivered using a dura elevator.
- If thrombus is not seen, a Fogarty balloon catheter is introduced proximally, balloon inflated and catheter is pulled out. Procedure is repeated distally. A good inflow and a backflow should be achieved. Incision should be closed transversely, this will prevent incision site stenosis.
- Thrill is palpated, a bruit auscultated, it may be weak initially but picks up in some time. Heparin infusion should be started 50–70 units/kg, 6 hourly.

Non-maturation of AVF

A fistula is said to not mature if it does not have adequate flow or it cannot be cannulated for dialysis 6 weeks after creation. If this situation is encountered, clinically examine the fistula, look for any collateral branches of vein which are diverting significant blood away from the outflow tract. A bounding tense vein may suggest upstream stenosis and weak thrill may suggest inflow obstruction. A Doppler examination should be done, skin to vein distance should be measured. Some deep vein with good flow can be assumed as non-mature. If Doppler shows decrease flow <300 ml/min or increase peak systolic velocity of >400 m/s, it is an indication for fistulogram.

Role of Ultrasound and Doppler in Assessment of Maturation

- *Assessment of flow rate:* Area × velocity × 60
- Assessment of inflow
- Measuring the size of fistula
- Pattern of flow—spiral lamellar flow suggestive to flow.
- Measurement of venous diameter
- Length of venous segment
- Depth of vein
- Evaluation of outflow tract to rule out stenosis.

Managing Different Situation in a Non-maturation Scenario

Deep Vein with Good Flow

One must access how deep is the vein and is the thrill palpable clearly, if it >6 mm but <10 mm deep, it can still be punctured. The vein should be marked in its course and thickness and the dialysis technician should be asked to puncture it in presence of the surgeon. Ultrasound-guided puncture is also very helpful technique. Punctures can be done in rope ladder fashion till the puncture sites get established and then the ultrasound would no longer be required.

If the vein is >10 mm deep and thrill is diffuse at the level of skin. A superficialization of vein should be done. The vein is dissected from a few centimeters above the anastomosis to at least 10 cm proximally. The vein is disconnected above the anastomosis and the superficialized by creating a subcutaneous tunnel and re-anastomosed with the stump of vein near the anastomosis of AVF.

Juxta-anastomotic/Anastomotic Narrowing on Fistulogram (Figs 24.5A and B)

An interventional radiological approach can be used. The brachial artery is cannulated at the level of cubital fossa and wire is passed across the fistula and angioplasty is done.

Surgical revision is possible and is very effective in anastomotic and juxta-anastomotic narrowing. The venous limb is disconnected and anastomosed 2–3 cm above on the artery. This method is very helpful in cases radio-cephalic AVF stenosis and not so much with BC AVF.

Venous Stenosis

Venous stenosis usually occurs at distance away from the fistula, it can also be a central venous stenosis. It is managed by radiological intervention and an angioplasty is done. Focal stenosis can be managed surgically by excision and repair or by opening the stenosed segment longitudinally and closing it transversely.

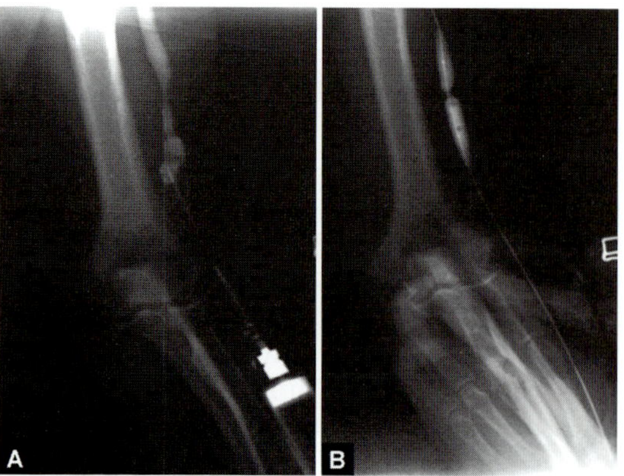

Figs 24.5A and B: (A) Fistulogram; (B) Angioplasty being done

Complications of AVF and their Management

Immediately Post-operative Hemorrhage (Figs 24.6A and B)

In the postoperative period, there may be hemorrhage from the AVF. If it is mild ooze, surgeon should just observe it and good palpable thrill is present. It there is a persistent ooze with development of swelling (hematoma) and thrill decreases or disappears, a re-exploration should be done. It is possible to find anastomotic leak, but generally ooze is and no bleeder is found, but hematoma should be evacuated, this will re-establish the flow. All suspicious areas coagulated and wound closed.

Infection (Figs 24.7A and B)

Infection accounts for 20% of all the complications of AVF.[1] Most common type of the infection is perivascular cellulitis; this presents pain, swelling around the anastomosis or puncture site. Management for the same is antibiotics, glycerin and magnesium sulphate dressing can be used. All most all of them subside with conservative management.

Infection can manifest as infected hematoma at the site of surgery postoperatively. This requires drainage and on most occasions closure of fistula. Abscess can also be formed at the puncture site and require drainage.

Infected pseudoaneurysm is one of the most dreaded complications of AVF. It can harbor fungal infection. It requires surgical excision and taking the fistula down.

Aneurysmal Dilatation (Figs 24.8 and 24.9A and B)

Aneurysmal dilatation can occur at the anastomotic site or in the venous limb. It can be true aneurysm or pseudoaneurysm. True aneurysm involves dilatation of all the three layers of wall of vessels. Pseudoaneurysm is

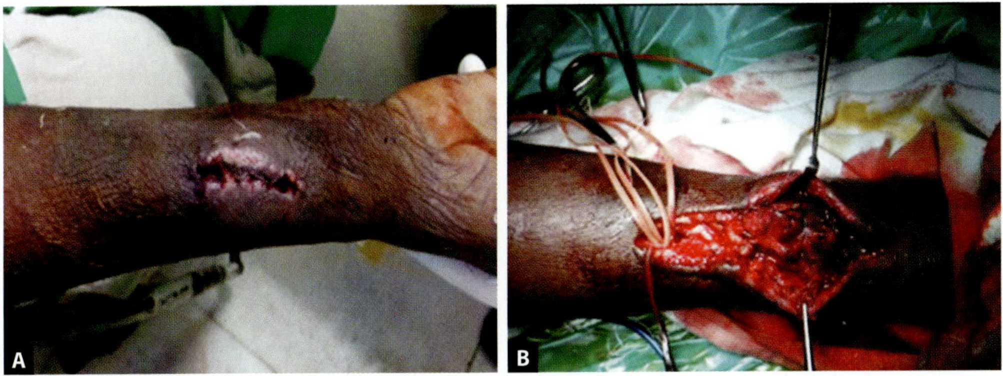

Figs 24.6A and B: (A) Swelling at AVF site with sentinel bleed; (B) Infected ruptured aneurysm

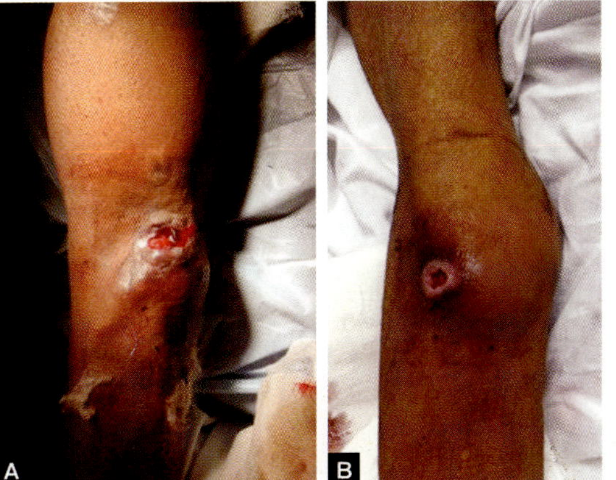

Figs 24.7A and B: Infected aneurysm

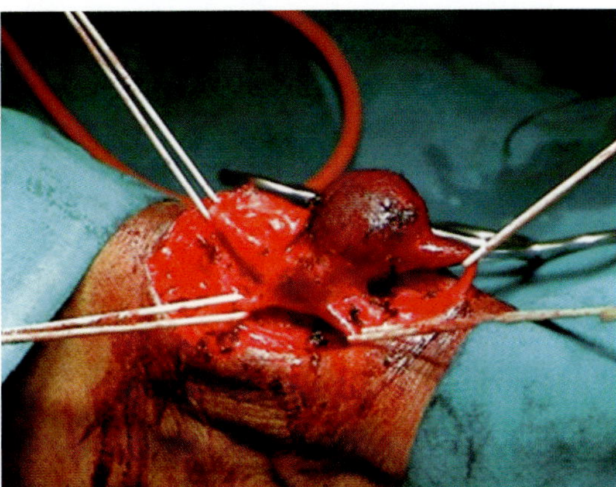

Fig. 24.8: Four-quadrant ligation of fistula

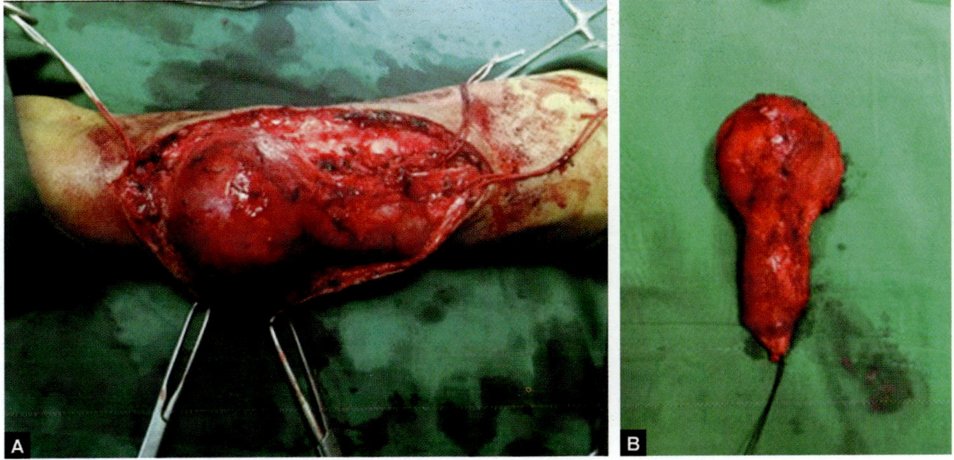

Figs 24.9A and B: Excision of aneurysm of fistula

hematoma outside the vessel which is caused by collection of blood leaking from the artery due to repeated punctures.

A true aneurysm of the AVF has to be managed surgically. In case of RC AVF, a surgical exploration with all quadrant ligation and excision of aneurysm should be done. The fistula should be explored, proximal and distal arterial control and venous control should be taken and artery ligated and cut. Venous limb is also disconnected and the aneurysm excised. If the proximal arterial and venous segment are healthy and there is no evidence of infection, an end-to-end arteriovenous anastomosis can be done at this stage to create a new fistula (only in cases of radiocephalic fistula). Hand should be evaluated for signs of ischemia.

In case of a BC AVF flow is very high and potentially larger blood loss may occur. The brachial artery should be controlled proximally and distally, aneurysm should be dissected all around, venous limb should be dissected and ligated. Aneurysm should be excised, circulation around the elbow is adequate on many occasions to maintain circulation to the limb, but a primary repair of artery should be attempted, if there is no evidence of infection. A jump graft can be used at a later date if vascular flow is compromised.

Managing a Ruptured Aneurysm (Figs 24.10A to D)

Principles
- Compress the bleeding site with a tourniquet.
- Arrange blood.
- Do not explore the site of bleeding
- Explore the feeding artery proximally and distally at a distance away from aneurysm

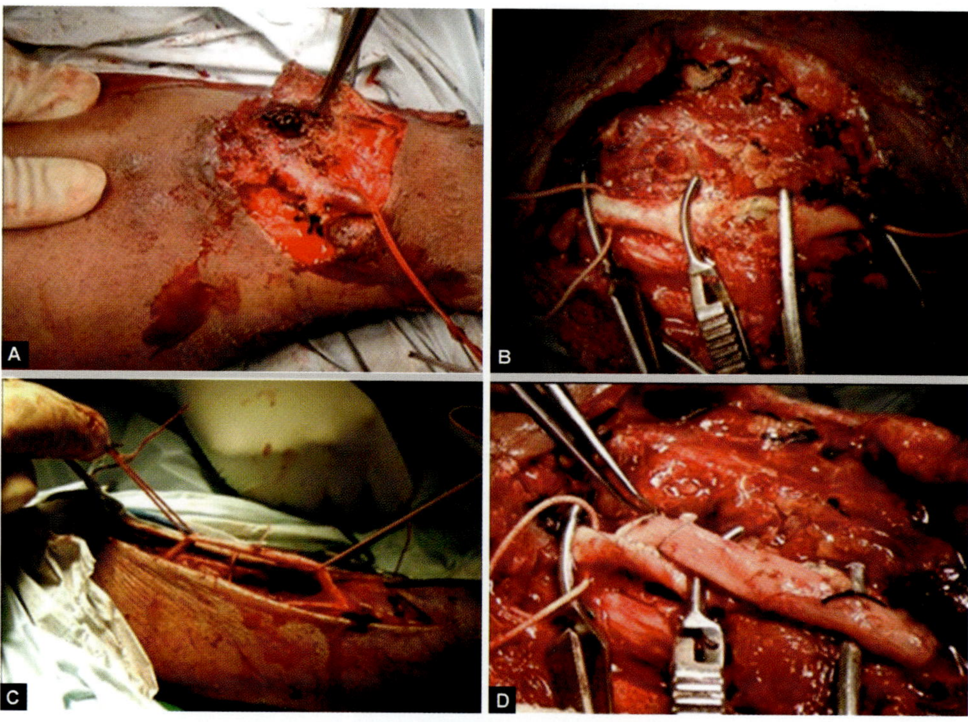

Figs 24.10A to D: (A) Ruptured fistula on exploration; (B) Unhealthy edges after excision of aneurysm; (C) Basilic vein graft being taken; (D) Interposition of basilic vein graft from above the AVF site to below it

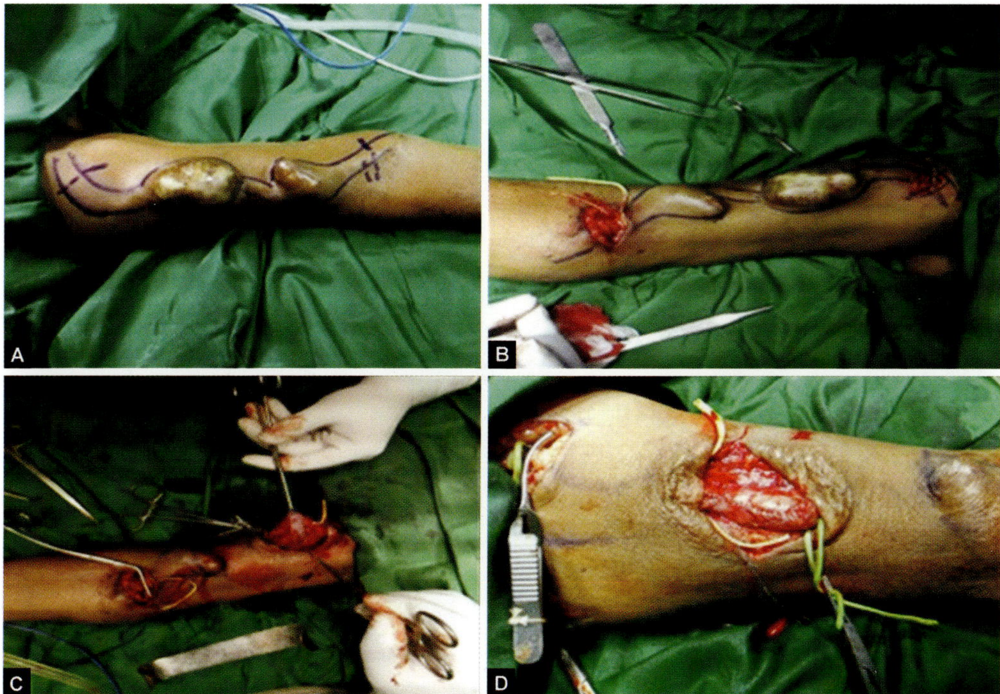

Figs 24.11A to D: (A) Marking of aneurysm of the venous limb; (B) Proximal and distal control of venous limb; (C) Excision of aneurysm; (D) Sutured venous wall of aneurysm

site and take control. This should be done by two separate incisions.

- Now the bleeding site should be explored.
- Aneurysm excised.
- Primary arterial repair, if possible.
- Autologous graft can be used, if required.

Aneurysmal Dilatation of Venous Limb (Figs 24.11A to D)

Recurrent point cannulation of the venous limb leads to weakening of the venous wall and aneurysmal dilatation. This can rupture and give rise to torrential bleeding. If central venous stenosis develops along with aneurysmal dilatation of the venous wall, there is bleeding from the cannulation site. Progressively skin over this area thins out and finally the aneurysm ruptures.

If patient presents with acute rupture, then bleeding should be compressed. A vascular clamp should be applied across the rent, include the surrounding skin in the clamp. This maneuver will arrest the bleeding, now the feeding artery should be controlled proximal and distal and fistula taken down.

If the patient presents with only sentinel bleed or thinning of the skin with aneurysmal dilatation. Partial excision of the aneurysm wall with plication can be done. To do this the venous limb should be controlled proximally and distally. Proximal clamp should be applied, then the aneurysm emptied completely and distal clamp applied. Elliptical incision is taken above the aneurysm and skin excised. Aneurysm is opened longitudinally and the thinned out wall is excised and the remaining wall is now closed transversely, if lot of redundancy is still present, it can be closed longitudinally. A rest of 3 weeks should be given to the fistula and re-cannulation should be done using rope ladder or button-hole technique.

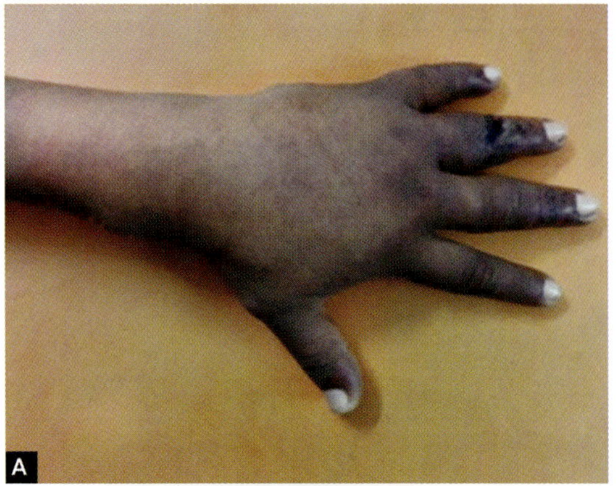

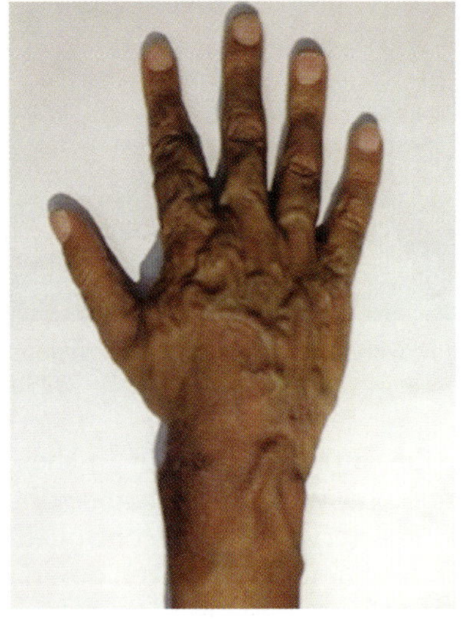

Figs 24.12A and B: Changes of venous hypertension

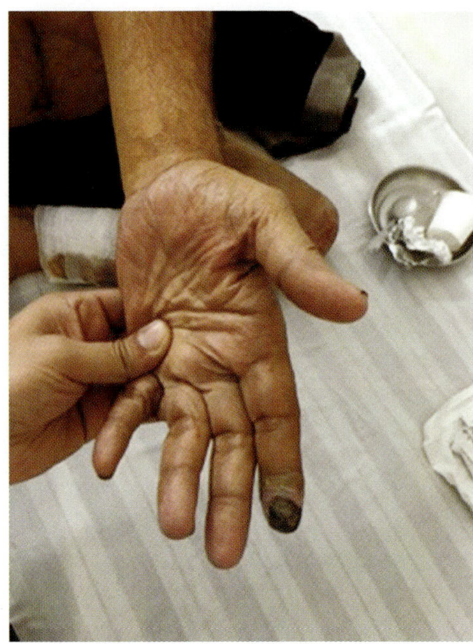

Fig. 24.13: Ischemic changes due to steal

Venous Hypertension (Figs 24.12A and B)

It is commonly seen in a side to side type of anastomosis done for AVF and more so in the radiocephalic AVF. The patient presents with pain, swelling, bluish discoloration of hand and dilated tortuous vessels can be seen on the dorsum of hand. It may cause a non-healing ulcer on hand. The treatment is ligation of the venous limb which feeds the blood to the hand.

The fistula is explored distal and proximal, arterial and venous control is taken and the limb of the vein feeding the hand is ligated, now all the blood from the fistula is diverted proximally reducing the venous hypertension. If this is not possible, the fistula has to be closed by ligation both the venous limbs.

Steal Syndrome (Fig. 24.13)

Steal syndrome occurs when the fistula steals away most of the blood from the limb and there is minimal or no blood flowing into the limb causing ischemic changes to the limb. It is not a very common occurrence as the compensatory mechanisms take care of the blood supply to the limb. In case of BC AVF, it is the anastomosis around elbow and in case of RC AVF, it is the ulnar artery.[2] In 1.6 to 8% patients develop unilateral ischemia.[3] Ischemic symptoms are more common in patients with comorbid illness like diabetes and in smokers.[2] Due to increasing age of the patients and increasing comorbidities number of patients with symptomatic steal syndrome are increasing. Prevention of steal syndrome can be done by meticulous surgical technique, making an arteriotomy of only 5–6 mm for brachial artery and 7–9 mm for radial artery. Vein should meet the artery at an angle of 90–120.

Ischemic polyneuropathy is a manifestation of decreased flow to the distal limb. It is seen in patients with diabetes in whom a BC AVF is created. It manifests as weakness in the arm, pain and paresthesia. On examination, there is weakness and sensory disturbance in the area supplied by median nerve. This syndrome may develop in a matter of hours after creation of AVF.

Management of Steal Syndrome

The outflow tract can be narrowed using various maneuvers, this decreases the amount of blood flow going into the venous limb as the resistance is increased and at the same time distal blood flow improves.[4] This can be achieved by:

- Excision of portion of the vein and suturing.
- Plication of the vein wall by mattress or continuous sutures.
- A polytetrafluoroethylene (PTFE) band can be placed across the venous limb to narrow the outflow tract.
- A small 4 mm PTFE graft can be interposed at the beginning of venous limb.

Distal revascularization and interval ligation procedure can be done. Here an autologous graft is placed between the artery proximal to AVF and artery distal to AVF and the artery immediately distal to AVF is ligated. If all of this does not work, then the fistula should be closed by ligating the venous limb. It is found that AVF increases the cardiac output by 15% and end diastolic pressure by 4%.[5]

AVF and Heart Failure

After creating AVF cardiac return increases, left ventricular hypertrophy may occur. All chronic kidney disease patient had some kind of ischemic heart disease (IHD) also they have left ventricular hypertrophy. It is very difficult to opine what causes cardiac morbidity AVF or IHD. Synthesis of natriuretic peptide by AVF increases intravascular volume. Incidence of left ventricular hypertrophy (LVH) after AVF creation is 12.2 to 17%.[6,7] Data suggest that ligation of the AVF does not decrease the LVH and may not provide the expected benefit.[5] In case congestive heart failure develops, fistula should be still ligated or outflow tract should be narrowed.

REFERENCES

1. Saxena AK, Panhotra BR, Al-Mulhim AS. Vascular access related infections in hemodialysis patients. Saudi J Kidney Dis Transpl. 2005;16: 46–51.
2. Scheltinga MR, van Hoek F, Bruijninckx CM. Time of onset in haemodialysis access-induced distal ischaemia (HAIDI) is related to the access type. Nephrol Dial Transplant. 2009;24:3198–204.
3. Leon C, Asif A. Arteriovenous access and hand pain: the distal hypoperfusion ischemic syndrome. Clin J Am Soc Nephrol. 2007;2:175–83.
4. Mickley V. Steal syndrome—strategies to preserve vascular access and extremity. Nephrol Dial Transplant. 2008;23:19–24.
5. London GM. Left ventricular alterations and endstage renal disease. Nephrol Dial Transplant. 2002;17:29–36.
6. Hiremath S, Doucette SP, Richardson R, Chan K, Burns K, Zimmerman D. Left ventricular growth after 1 year of haemodialysis does not correlate with arteriovenous access of low: a prospective cohort study. Nephrol Dial Transplant. 2010;25:2656–61.
7. Gallardo RM, Morong FV, Pino GG, Arias IC, Gallego RH, Magariños FG. Congestive heart failure in patients with advanced chronic kidney disease: association with pre-emptive vascular access placement. Nefrologia. 2012;32:206–12.

25
Quality Improvement Program

Abhishek Singh

All dialysis units must develop a quality improvement program. There should be good communication between dialysis technician, nephrologist and vascular surgeon. At risk fistula should be identified and closely followed. Unit must tract its AVF patency rate and strive to improve. All complications should be immediately reported and managed **(Fig. 25.1)**.

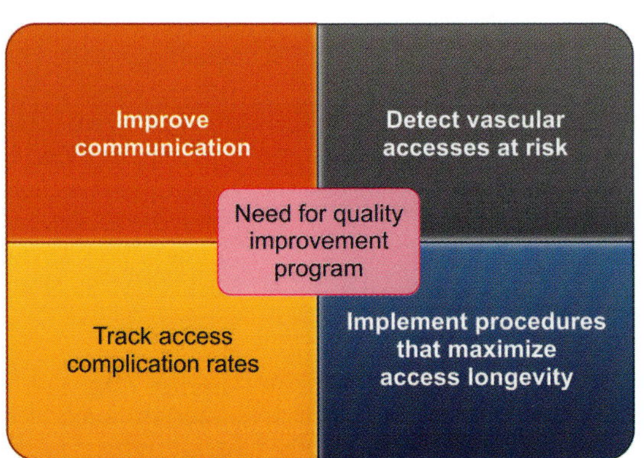

Fig. 25.1: AVF improvement program

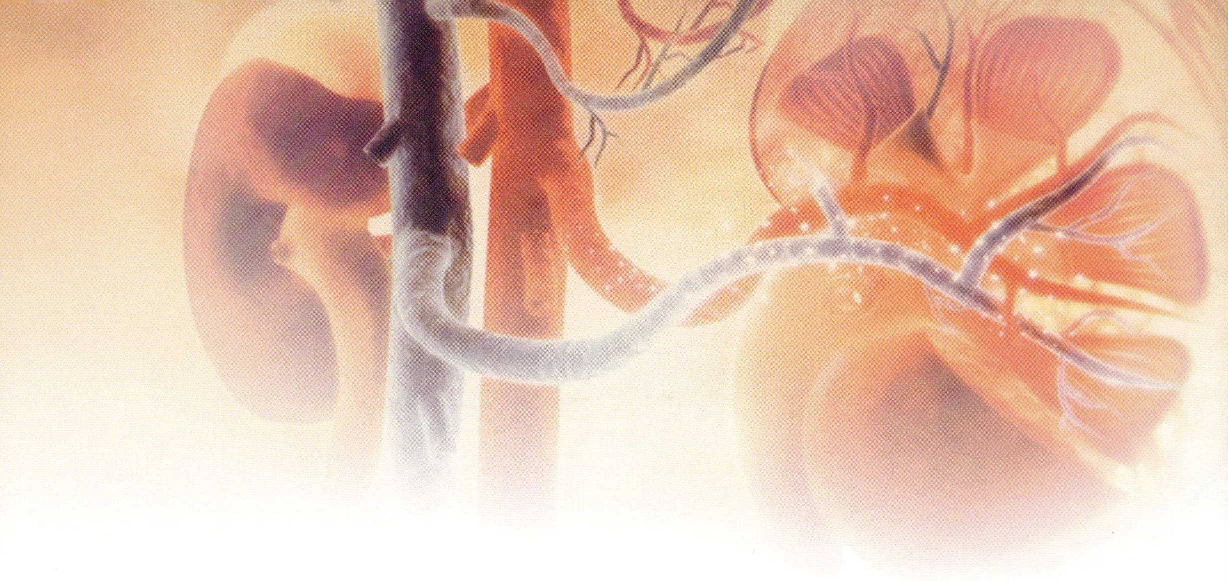

Part 2

Basics in Robotic Instrumentation, Docking and Port Placement

C H A P T E R S

26
Introduction

Ashwin Sunil Tamhankar, Surya Prakash Ojha, Puneet Ahluwalia, Gagan Gautam

A robot is defined as a computerized system with a motorized part, usually an arm that is capable of interacting with the environment.[1] The word robot comes from the word robota which means "drudgery" or "hard work" in Czech. The term was coined by Karel Capek in 1921. The famous Renaissance artist Leonardo da Vinci was said to have a mechanical lion that walked and roared.[2] As the necessity has always been the mother of invention, this field of robotic surgery has evolved over the last two decades gradually. It evolved in the form of different models, e.g. ROBODOC, AESOP, PROBOT, PAKY to the current advanced model of da Vinci Xi. Computer Motion Inc. founded in 1989 had the ZEUS™ robotic surgical system. Intuitive Surgicals Inc. founded in 1995 devised da Vinci surgical system. da Vinci™ surgical system got FDA approval for laparoscopic use in 2000 and for thoracoscopic use in 2001.[2] Robots are classified in various ways based upon the level of function.[3]

- *Passive robots:* These are static mechanical fixed devices which do not have power. These are first generation passive robots which were used majority for retraction, etc.
  Examples: Omni-Lapo Tract (Omnitract), Iron Intern (Automated Medical Products), Surg assistant (solos-endoscopy), Trocar Sleeve Stabilizer (Richard Wolfe), Bookwalter retraction system (Codman), Robotrac system (Aesculap), First Assistant (Leonard Medical), Endex laparoscopic holder (Andronic Medical).
- *Semi-active synergistic robots:* These models have some degree of autonomous motion with total four degrees of freedom. They are used in orthopedic use or stereotactic neurosurgery.
  Examples: LARS[4] (Laparoscopic Assistant Robotic System) (Johns Hopkins and IBM), Acrobot[5] (active constraint robot) (Imperial College, London), Steady-Hand robot (Johns Hopkins) NeuroMate[6] (Integrated Surgical Systems).
- *Active robots:* These have high degree of independent powered motion. These are used for camera holding with three degrees of freedom or head mounted navigation systems or cyberknife.
  Examples: AESOP3000,[7] EndoAssist, ROBODOC,[8] ORTHODOC,[8] CyberKnife,[9] PROBOT,[10] PAKY-RCM.
- Master-slave robotic systems
  Examples: ZEUS (Computer Motion), ARTEMIS (Advanced Robotics and Telemanipulator System for MIS), da Vinci system.

REFERENCES

1. Kumar R, Hemal AK. Emerging role of robotics in urology. J Minim Access Surg. 2005 Oct;1(4): 202–10.
2. Malone, Robert. "Robot". Collier's. 1996 ed. 115.
3. Singh I. Robotics in urological surgery: Review of current status and maneuverability, and comparison of robot-assisted and traditional laparoscopy. Computer Aided Surgery, January 2011;16(1):38–45.
4. Yang C, Taylor RH, Talamini MA. Human vs robotic organ traction during laparoscopic Nissen fundoplication. Surg Endosc. 1999;13(5):461–65.
5. Barrett AR, Davies BL, Gomes MP, Harris SJ, Henckel J, Jakopec M, Kannan V, Rodriguez y Baena FM, Cobb JP. Computer-assisted hip resurfacing surgery using the Acrobot navigation system. Proc Inst Mech Eng H. 2007;221(7): 773–85.
6. Li QH, Zamorano L, Pandya A, Perez R, Gong J, Diaz F. The application accuracy of the Neuro-Mate robot—a quantitative comparison with frameless and frame-based surgical localization systems. Comput Aided Surg. 2002;7:90–98.
7. Yavuz Y, Ystgaard B, Skogvoll E. A comparative experimental study evaluating the performance of surgical robots AESOP and EndoAssist. Surg Laparosc Endosc Percutan Tech. 2000;10:163–67.
8. Federspil PA, Geisthoff UW, Henrich D. Development of the first force-controlled robot for otoneurosurgery. Laryngoscope. 2003;113: 465–71.
9. Adler JR Jr, Chang SD, Murphy MJ. The Cyber-Knife: A frameless robotic system for radiosurgery. Stereotact Funct Neurosurg. 1997;69:124–28.
10. Arambula Cosio F, Davies BL. Automated prostate recognition: A key process for clinically effective robotic prostatectomy. Med Biol Eng Comput. 1999;37:236–43.

27
Overview of Instrumentation

Ashwin Sunil Tamhankar, Surya Prakash Ojha, Puneet Ahluwalia, Gagan Gautam

Starting from initial da Vinci model, this technology is evolved over past years to the current state of art da Vinci Xi system and SP system **(Fig. 27.1)**.

The basic model and principle of 'master slave' concept remains the same in all models. Basic model consists of surgeon console, patient cart, vision cart.

Operating Room Layout (Fig. 27.2)

The operating room (OR) layout will depend on the type of procedures being performed, and the location of booms, lights, anesthesia connections, operating table and other items.

Vision Cart Positioning

- Place outside the sterile field where it can be easily accessed by the circulating nurse, close enough to the patient cart to allow unrestricted camera cable and electro-cautery cord movement during surgery (~10 feet/3 meters).
- Position the monitor so it can be accessed by the circulating nurse and easily viewed by the patient side assistant.
- Cables between the vision cart and patient (e.g. insufflator, electrocautery, grounding pad, etc.) should be routed away from pathways.
- Maximize use of vision cart shelves with ancillary equipment (e.g. insufflators, video-recorders, etc.) to minimize OR footprint. Note: The vision cart requires a dedicated circuit and cannot be shared with ancillary equipment.

Surgeon Console Positioning

- Place outside the sterile field away from traffic flow or without impeding direct access to the patient (e.g. after scrubbing in).
- Rotate the console so there is a clear line of communication from the surgeon to the patient-side assistant that is within visibility of the patient.
- Fiberoptic cable should be routed away from doorways and heavy traffic.

Patient Cart Positioning

- Place cart in an open space in the operating room to prepare for the start-up sequence.
- Provide adequate room for full extension of the arms during draping.
- The area between the draping location and the operating table should be clear so the patient cart can be moved into the sterile field without obstruction.
- During surgery, the sterile draped cart will be positioned patient-side within the sterile operating field in a location where no one is expected to stand or require access the patient.

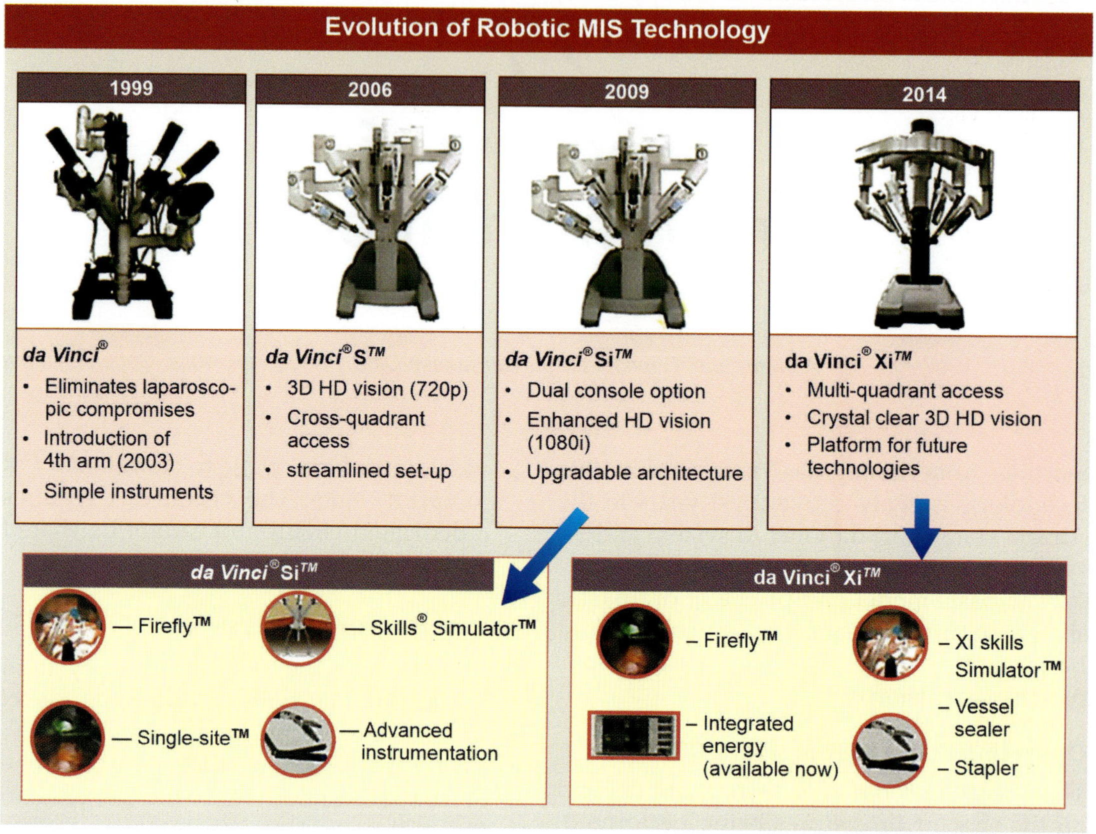

Evolution of Robotic MIS Technology
1999
2006
2009
2014
da Vinci®
Eliminates laparoscopic compromises
Introduction of 4th arm (2003)
Simple instruments
da Vinci® S™
3D HD vision (720p)
Cross-quadrant access
streamlined set-up
da Vinci® Si™
Dual console option
Enhanced HD vision (1080i)
Upgradable architecture
da Vinci® Xi™
Multi-quadrant access
Crystal clear 3D HD vision
Platform for future technologies
da Vinci® Si™
— Firefly™
— Skills® Simulator™
— Single-site™
— Advanced instrumentation
da Vinci® Xi™
– Firefly™
– XI skills Simulator™
– Integrated energy (available now)
– Vessel sealer
– Stapler

Fig. 27.1: Evolution of da Vinci system

Surgeon console
Patient cart
Vision cart

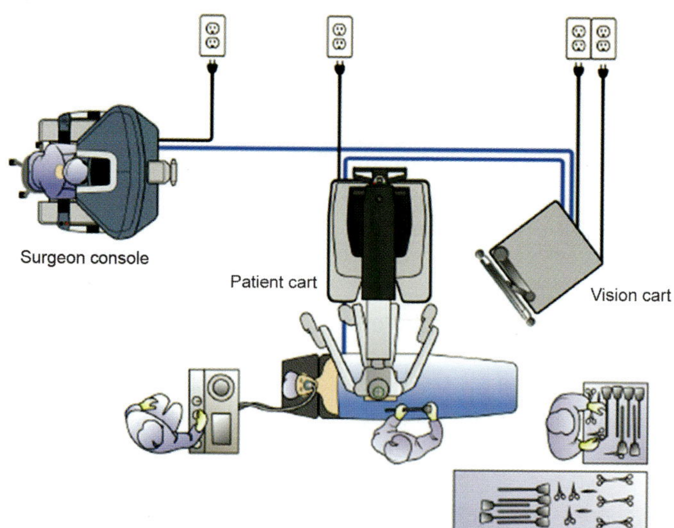

Fig. 27.2: Operating room layout

da VINCI X AND SI MODEL OVERVIEW

Surgeon Console Overview (Fig. 27.3)

- Stereo viewer
  - Infrared sensor
  - Speakers and microphone
- Right-side pod
  - *Power button:* Turns the da Vinci system on and off
  - *Emergency stop button:* Creates a recoverable fault and halts communication between the master controllers and the camera and instrument arms
- *Left-side pod:* Ergonomic controls
- *Touchpad:* Main control interface of the surgeon console
- *Master controllers:* Movements of the master controllers are precisely translated to the surgical arms in real time
- Footswitch panel
  - Arm swap pedal
  - Master clutch
  - Camera control
  - Activation pedals

Master Controllers (Fig. 27.4)

The master controllers (masters) enable the surgeon console operator to control the patient cart instruments and endoscope. The masters have two main parts, an orientation platform and a positioning arm.

- The orientation platform moves the instrument in the surgical environment. Positioning movements can be scaled to a 3:1 (fine), 2:1 (normal), or 1.5:1 (quick) ratio.
- The positioning arm rotates the instrument tips and opens and closes the grips of the instruments.

Finger Clutch (Fig. 27.5)

Finger clutch decouples the master from control of its instrument. While you hold the finger clutch, you can move the master and the instrument will not move. Unlike the master clutch pedal, the finger clutch applies only to its own master controller. So, when you apply one finger clutch, the other master's instrument remains in following. Applying the finger clutch enables you to reposition the master for comfort, and to reclaim space to maneuver when the master reaches its limits.

Stereo Viewer (Fig. 27.6)

The stereo viewer provides the intraoperative image to the console surgeon.

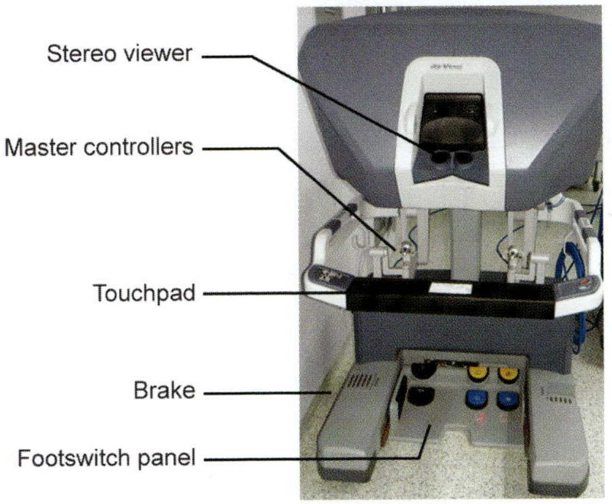

Fig. 27.3: Surgeon console overview

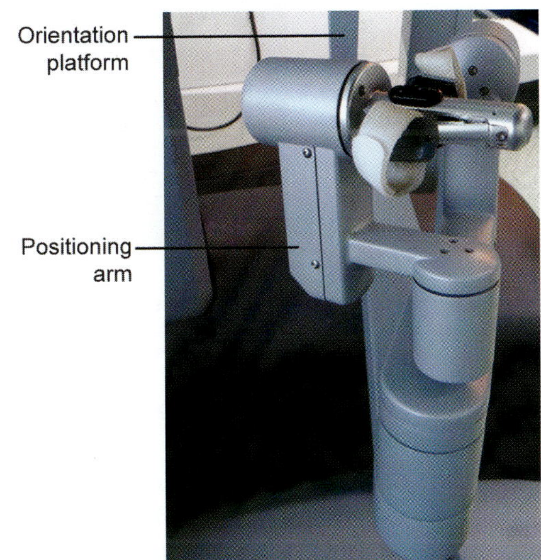

Fig. 27.4: Master controllers

Note: Intuitive surgical is likely to phase out Si model by 2024 and X model will become the workhorse. X is essentially an extension of Si with fourth generation lens and camera system. The arms of the X system are slender as compared to Si but are mounted on the similar cart.

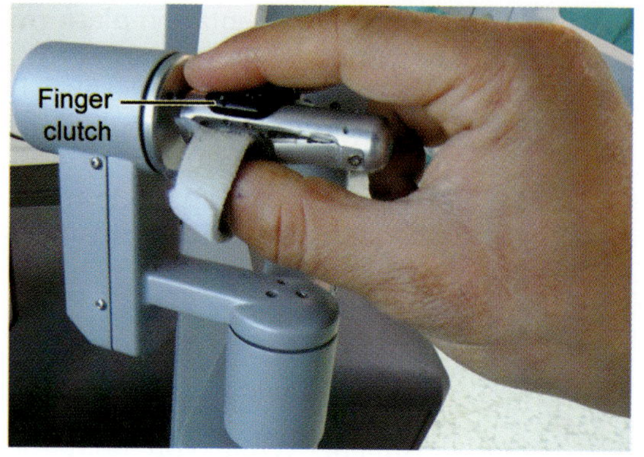

Fig. 27.5: Finger clutch

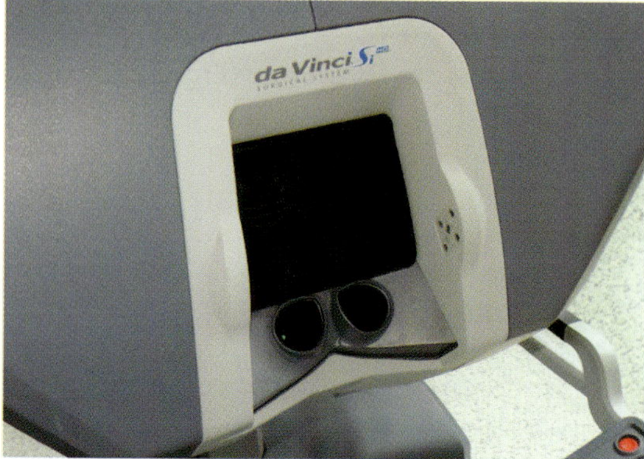

Fig. 27.6: Stereo viewer

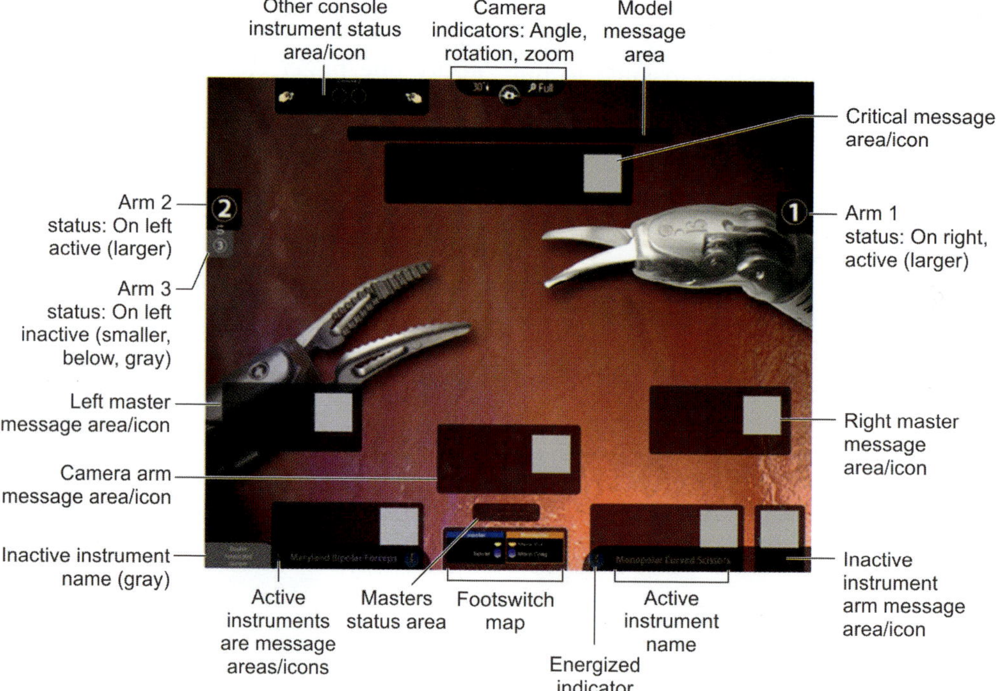

Fig. 27.7: Messages and icons on screen

With his or her head in the viewer, the surgeon can view the 3D image in full-screen mode or can choose to swap to TilePro™ mode.

Icons and text messages are overlaid on the video to provide extended information to the surgeon **(Fig. 27.7)**.

The system provides two-way audio-communications with the patient cart operator.

Left-side Pod Ergonomic Controls (Fig. 27.8)

The left-side pod provides the ergonomic adjustment controls for the surgeon console.

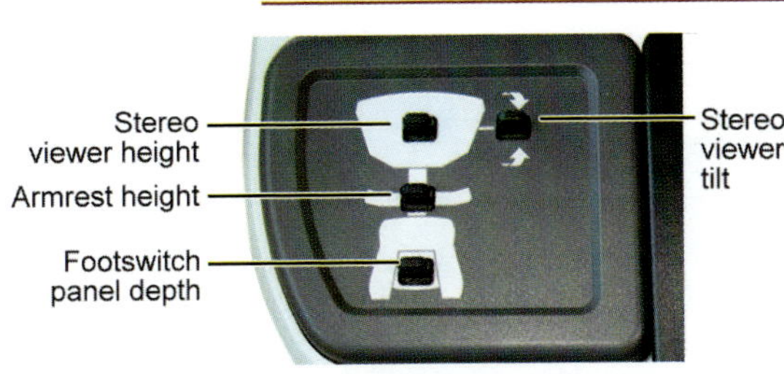

Fig. 27.8: Left-side pod ergonomic controls

Ergonomic Set up

To adjust the surgeon console ergonomics to your preference, perform the following steps:

- Adjust the chair height so your thighs are at a slightly downward angle relative to the floor. This ensures easy movement of the legs to activate the footswitches.
- Adjust the armrest height so your forearms rest comfortably on the armrest with your shoulders relaxed.
- Adjust the stereo viewer height to your preference.
- Adjust the stereo viewer tilt according to your preference. Tilting up allows for a more comfortable neck angle. Tilting down allows for more alignment of your hands and the instruments in the stereo viewer.
- Adjust the footswitch panel depth to your preference.

Right-side Pod Power and Emergency Stop (Fig. 27.9)

The right-side pod provides power and emergency stop buttons.

In case the machine needs to stopped in a exingent manner, the red button needs to be pressed.

The system classifies emergency stop as a recoverable fault, which one can override by pressing recover on the touchpad.

Footswitch Panel (Fig. 27.10)

Camera control and focus (X system camera has auto focus): Press the camera pedal to switch the masters from instrument control to camera (endoscope) control.

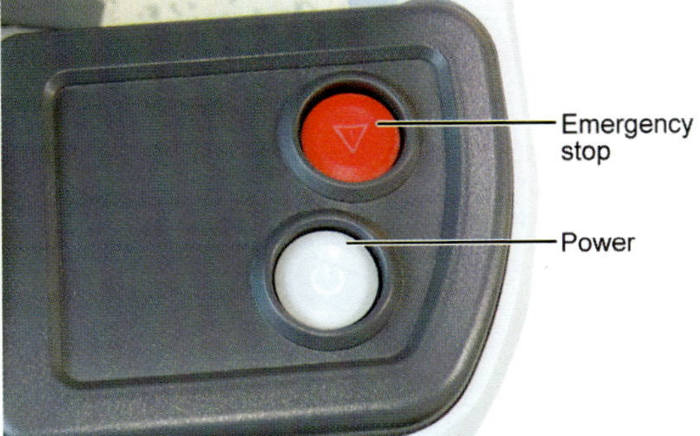

Fig. 27.9: Right-side pod power and emergency stop

Master clutch: Pressing the master clutch pedal decouples both masters from control of their instruments and enables you to move the masters easily while all instruments remain immobile.

Arm swap (left kick-plate): Swaps control between two instrument arms associated with the same master.

Energy Control Pedals (Table 27.1)

Right pair controls: The right pair of pedals controls energy activation for monopolar or secondary energy/bipolar energy instruments.

Left pair controls: The left pair of pedals controls energy activation for bipolar energy instruments, either standard or plasma kinetics.

Touchpad (Fig. 27.11)

The touchpad home screen displays the system status and controls instrument arms, camera arm, and energy controls.

*Vision Cart Overview (**Fig. 27.12**)*

Touchscreen monitor
- Single or dual console masters and instruments status area indicate association, masters status, finger clutch, associated arm number and instrument name/status. Message area
  - System status displayed
  - Critical messages are displayed

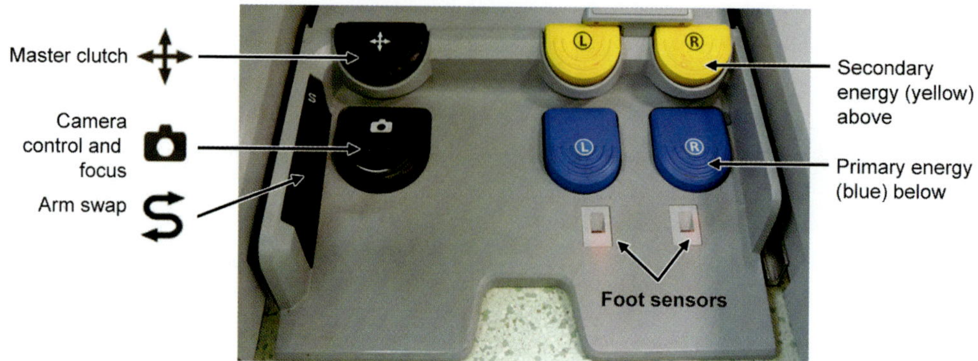

Fig. 27.10: Foot switch panel

TABLE 27.1: Energy types and associated pedal modes

Energy pedal	Bipolar (left pair)	PK (left pair)	Monopolar (right pair)	Harmonic (right pair)
Secondary energy (yellow)	<empty>	<empty>	Mono cut	Min
Primary energy (blue)	Bipolar	PK	Mono coag	Max

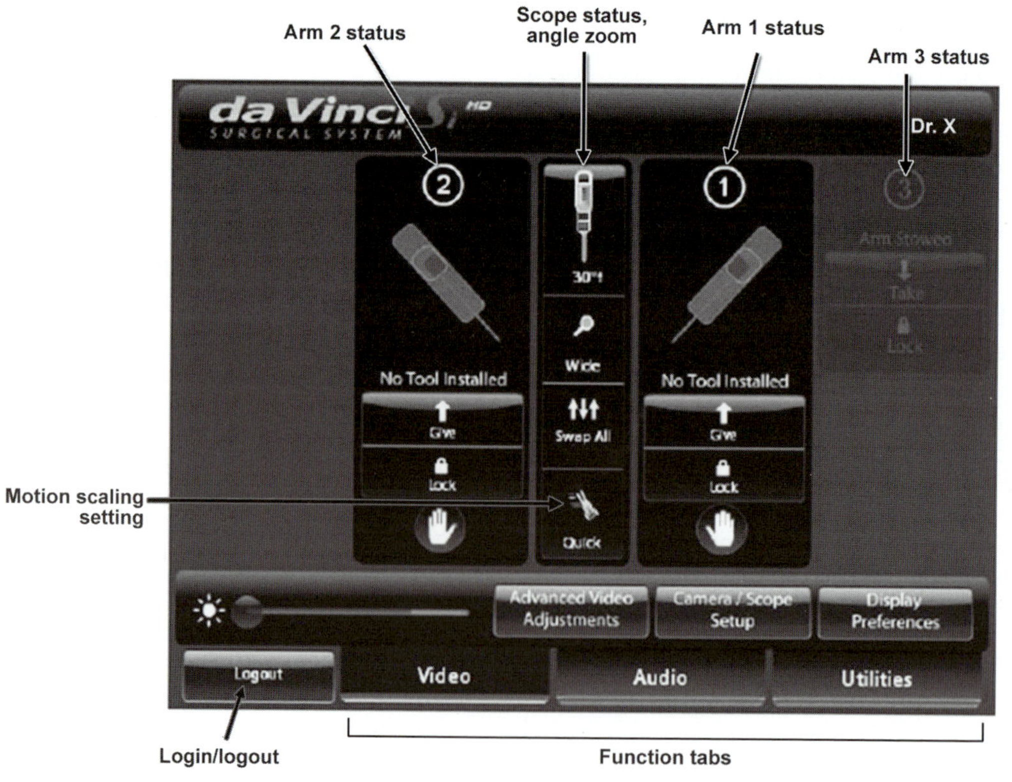

Fig. 27.11: Touchpad

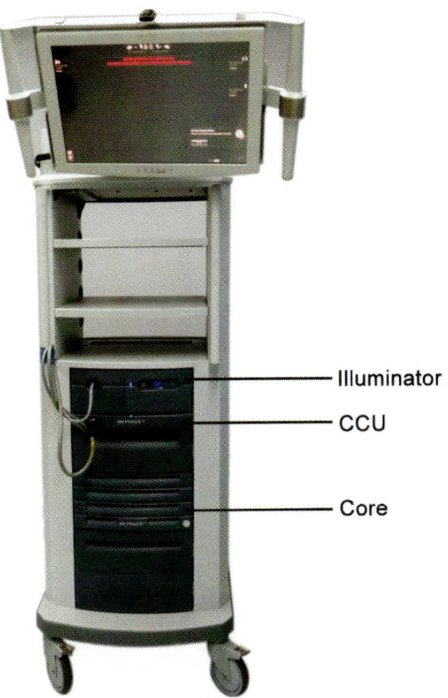

Fig. 27.12: Vision cart overview

- Instrument arm data
  - Surgeon name or console control
  - Instrument installed
  - Instrument arm message area
  - Instrument energized
- *da Vinci OnSite™:* Provides faster resolution through automated log retrieval, remote system status, remote diagnostics and servicing.
- Camera message area icon, camera angle, zoom and rotation indicator.
- *Telestration:* Drag your finger on the monitor, pressing slightly, to draw a colored line on video image.
- *Erase button:* Touch to erase all telestration marks from the touchscreen and surgeon console.

Illuminator

- *Lamp on/off:* Press and hold the lamp on/off button to turn illuminator on or off

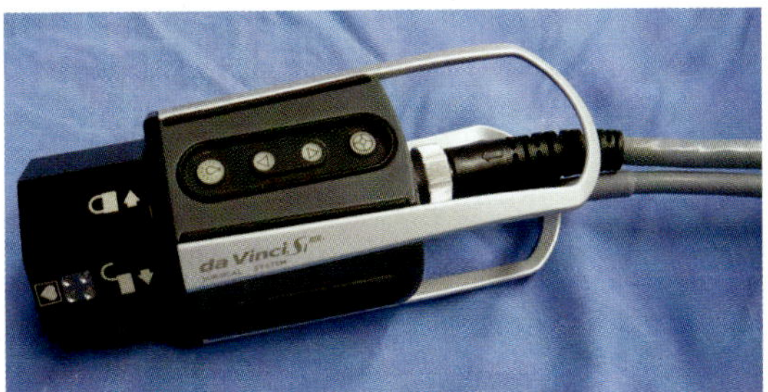

Fig. 27.13: High definition camera

- *Intensity control (–/+):* Press – and + buttons to adjust the brightness in 10% increments. Intensity control should always remain at 100%.
- ~1000 hours of service on each bulb

  Press and hold the – and + buttons at the same time to display the number of lamp hours accumulated (display counts up from 0000 to 1000).

  The system does not allow the use of third party lamps.

Camera control units (CCUs): Control acquisition and processing of camera image.

3D (HD) high definition camera (Fig. 27.13)

- *Wide-angle:* 60 field of view
- *Views:* Wide (16:9), full (5:4) and 2 levels of digital zoom (allowing for 2X and 4X magnification)
- *Vision control from camera head:* Vision set up button, focus control buttons, and illuminator lamp button.
- Store the camera head in its custom cutout in the vision cart drawer below the camera control unit. Coil the camera cables and loosely hang on the hook on the side of the vision cart.
- *Camera head:* The 3D camera head contains two HD video cameras. One camera is used for the right optical path and another for the left optical path.
- Camera top control buttons **(Fig. 27.14)**

Prerequisites before starting the procedure:
- White balance and caliberation not required for X system camera
- 3D calibration—manual calibration can be done by aligning the green and magenta crosshairs **(Figs 27.15 and 27.16)**.

Endoscopes (Figs 27.17 and 27.18)
- 12 mm or 8.5 mm: 0°, 30° up, 30° down

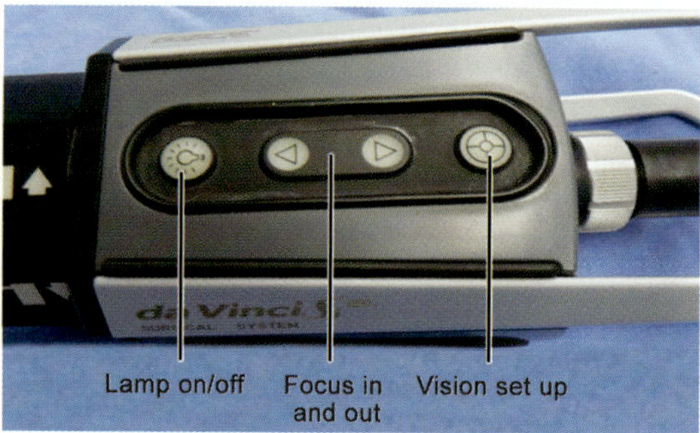

Fig. 27.14: Camera top control buttons

- When the endoscope is attached to the camera head, the system will automatically read and register the endoscope type using radiofrequency identification (RFID).

Core: The system's central connection point where system cables and auxiliary equipment are routed.

Patient Cart Overview (Fig. 27.19)

Camera Arm

- Camera arm set up joints
- Camera arm clutch button (press and hold vs quick click) moves the arm around the remote center but the remote center does not move.
- Camera arm port clutch button (press and hold) moves the patient cart set up joints manually and changes the position of the remote center (port position).

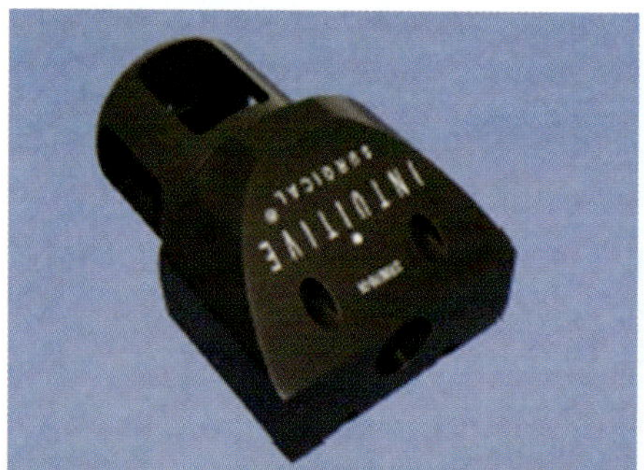

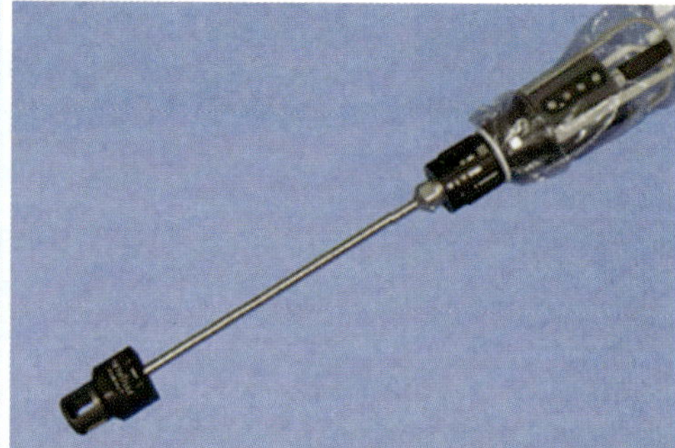

Fig. 27.15: 3D calibration

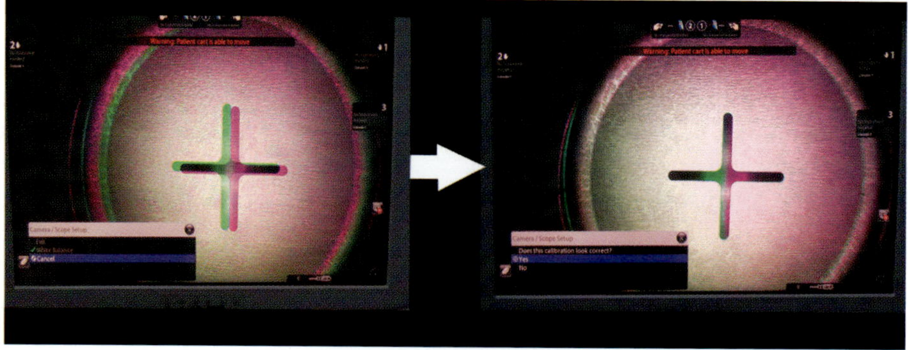

Fig. 27.16: 3D calibration

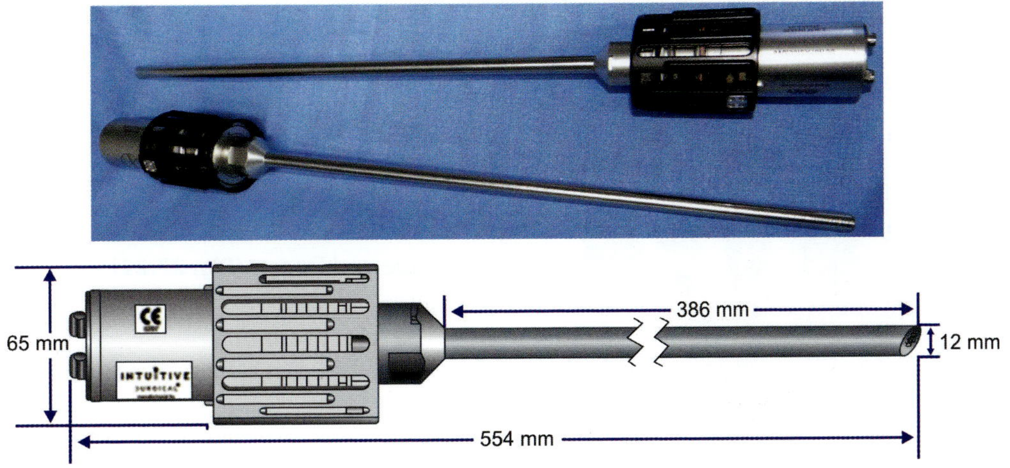

12 mm endoscope with dimensions

Fig. 27.17: Endoscope

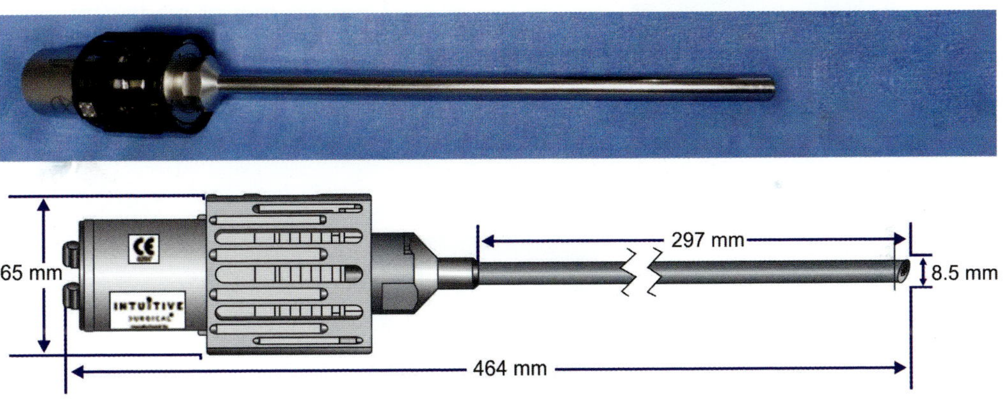

8.5 mm endoscope with dimensions

Fig. 27.18: Endoscope

- "Sweet spot" helps maintain the arm's optimal range of motion.
- Camera arm quick click cannula mount.

Instrument Arms

- Instrument arm set up joints
- Instrument arm numbers (1, 2 and 3)
- Instrument arm sterile adapter carriage and telescoping axis
- Instrument arm clutch button (press and hold vs quick click)

- Instrument arm port clutch button (press and hold)
- Instrument arm quick click cannula mount
- Movement of arm around remote center.

3rd Instrument Arm

Center column

Motor drive **(Fig. 27.20)**: Designed to provide faster/easier docking and operating room configuration.

- Power button

- Throttle enable switch
- Throttle

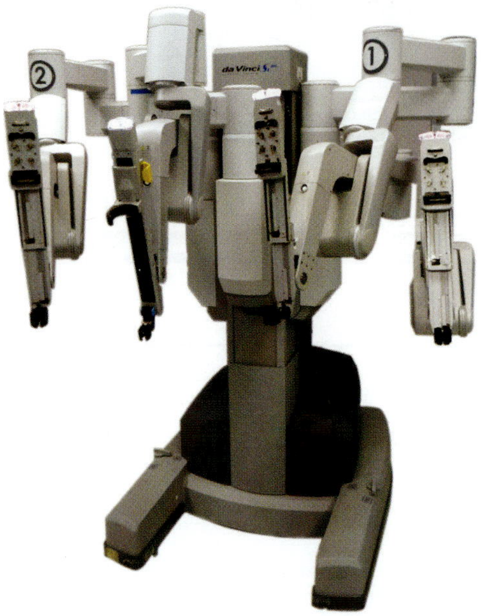

Fig. 27.19: Patient cart overview

- Cannula installed LED
- Battery status indicators show the amount of battery power

Flashing: Charge battery

Red: Insufficient charge for surgery
Base and shift switches (N and D)

Cannulae and Trocars *(Fig. 27.21)*

- *Instrument arm*
  - da Vinci cannula
    - *8 mm:* Reusable, 11 cm and 16 cm lengths
    - *8 mm with outlet:* Reusable, 11 cm and 16 cm lengths
    - *5 mm:* 11 cm cannula length
    - *8 to 5 mm reducer:* Reusable
    - Remote center markings
    - Cannula mount reads cannula type
  - Obturator
    - *8 mm blunt:* Reusable
    - *8 mm bladeless:* Disposable
    - *5 mm blunt:* Reusable

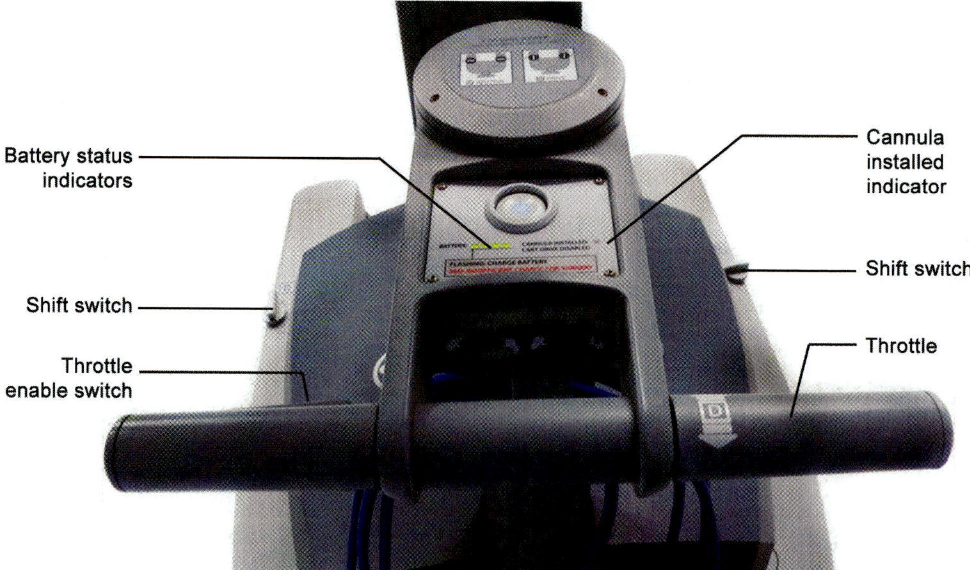

Fig. 27.20: Motor drive

- Cannula seal
  - *Green cannula seal:* Disposable, for 8 mm cannula
  - *White cannula seal:* Disposable, for 5 mm cannula

- *Camera arm*
  - 3rd party 12 mm and 8.5 mm trocars
  - Intuitive reusable 8.5 mm camera cannula
- *Assistant ports:* 3rd party cannula selected by the surgeon.

da VINCI Xi MODEL OVERVIEW

Surgeon Console Overview (Fig. 27.22)

- *3D viewer:* The high-resolution stereo viewer consists of two independent LCDs.
- *Hand controls (masters):* The two hand controls are positioned below the magnified, three-dimensional image of the surgical site. The surgeon grasps the masters while viewing the surgical site. The instrument tips, as seen in the 3D viewer, appear aligned with the surgeon's hands at the masters.

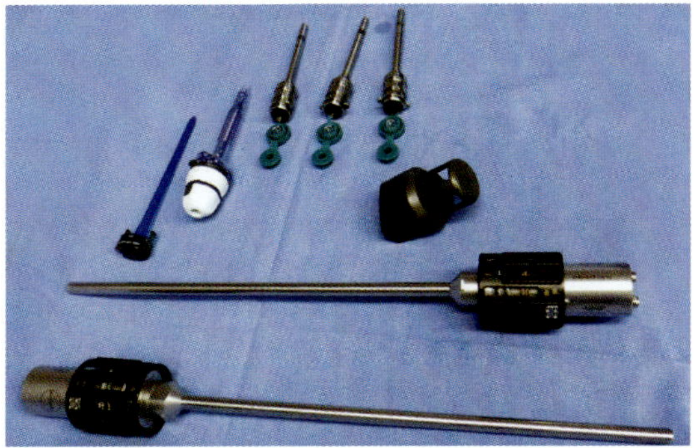

Fig. 27.21: Cannulae and trocars

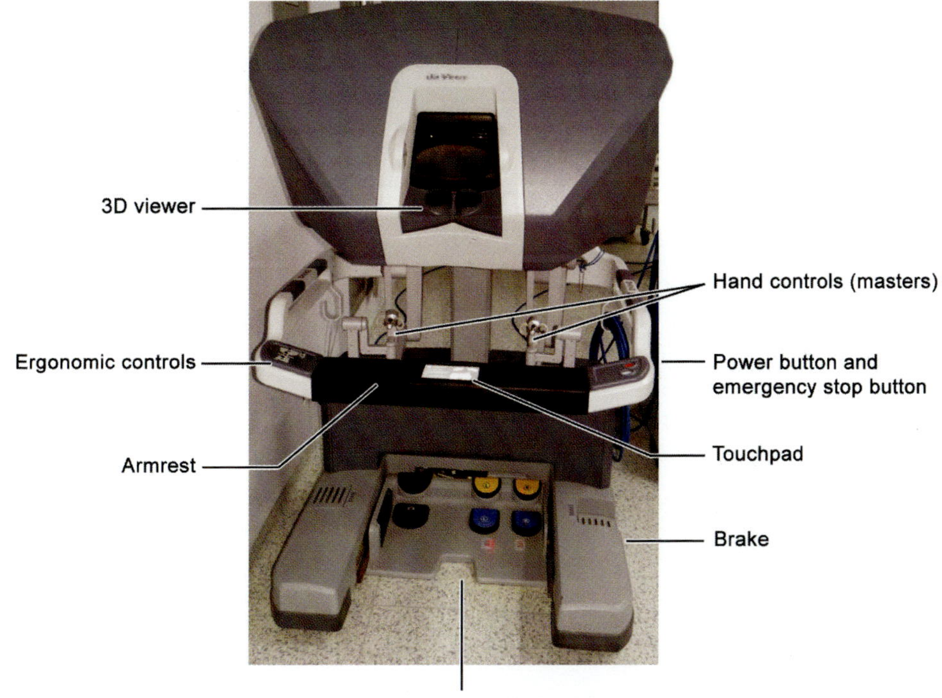

Fig. 27.22: Surgeon console overview

- *Armrest:* Contains a touchpad user interface, ergonomic controls for adjusting the ergonomics of the surgeon console, and power and emergency stop buttons.
- *Footswitch panel:* Houses foot pedals used to activate various system modes, such as endoscope control, as well as activate various instrument functions, such as monopolar and bipolar cautery.
- *Brakes:* There are two brakes located on the surgeon console base.

Patient Cart Overview (Fig. 27.23)

- *Boom:* The boom is an adjustable, rotating support structure for the arms.
  - *Boom pivot:* Alignment and extension of the boom along the column.
  - *Boom rotation:* Rotation of the boom cluster of arms.
- *Flex joint:* A joint that allows for the arm spacing to be adjusted.
- *Arm height joint:* A joint that allows for the arm height to be individually adjusted.
- *Patient clearance joint:* A joint that allows for adjustment of the arm to increase patient clearance.
- *Column:* The column moves the boom up or down.
- *Base:* The base includes a motorized cart drive for positioning and transportation, the patient cart electronics, and a connector panel.
- *Helm* **(Fig. 27.24):** The helm includes the handlebars with cart drive enable switches,

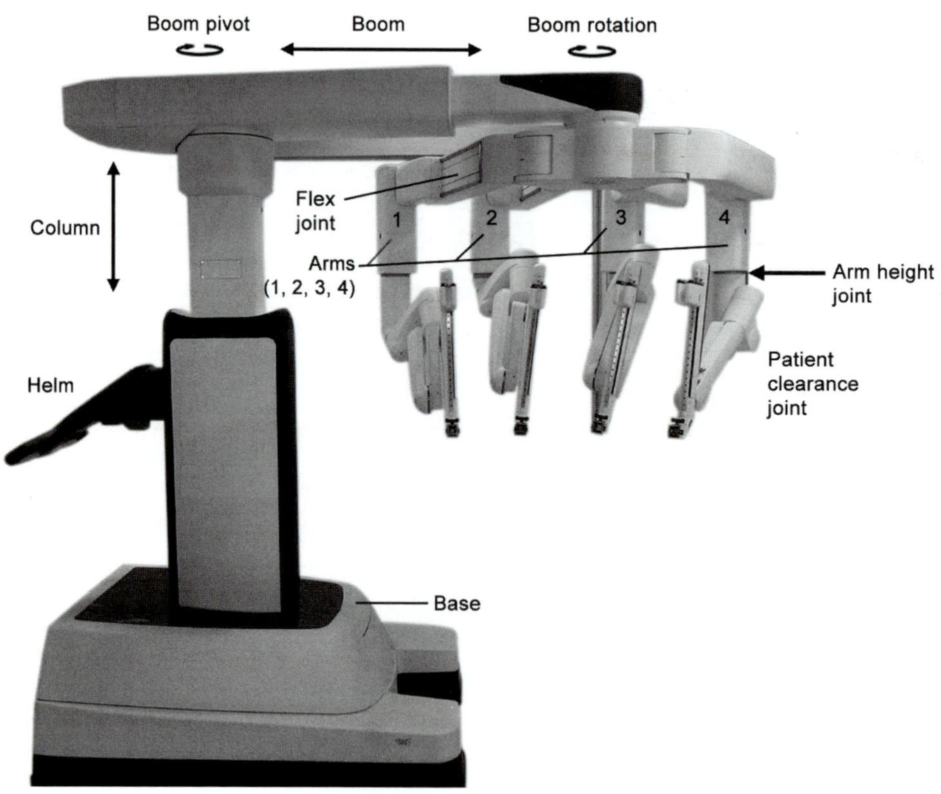

Fig. 27.23: Patient cart overview

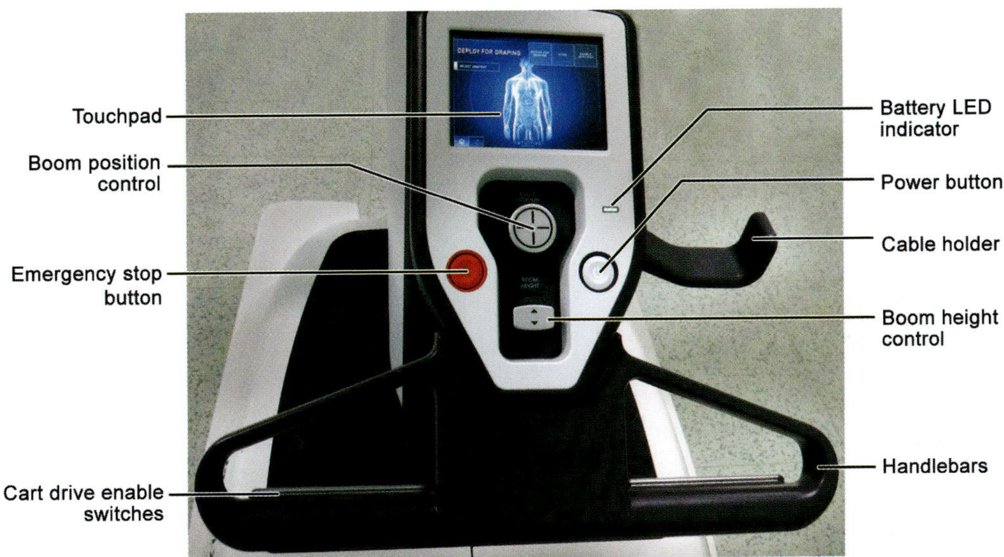

Fig. 27.24: The helm

a touchpad, two joysticks, power and emergency stop buttons, a cable holder, and a battery indicator. The handlebars and cart drive enable switches are used to maneuver the patient cart around the OR.

The Helm includes a touchpad for system messages and guided menu options, while the joysticks include boom position control and boom height control to manually orient the arms, boom and column.

- *Arm (1, 2, 3, 4) (Fig. 27.25):* The four instrument arms (also referred to as arms) hold and move the endoscope and instruments. The distal end attaches to the instrument/ endoscope cannula. The arms include set up joints that allow the user to connect the arms to the cannulae during set up.

Arm controls include

- *Instrument clutch:* User initiated movements to advance or retract the endoscope or instrument tip within the surgical site. User initiated movements of the arm about the remote center.

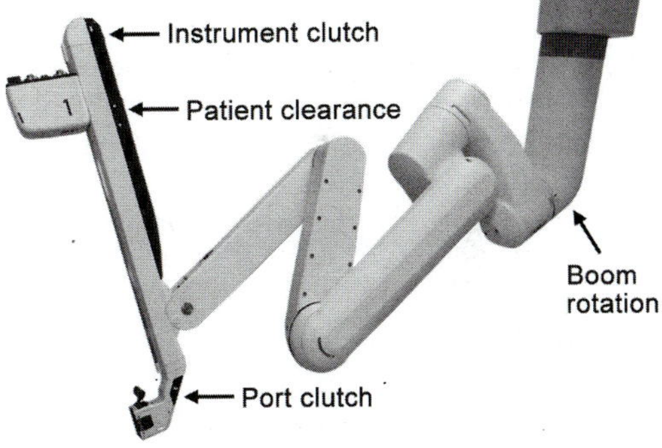

Fig. 27.25: The arm

- *Patient clearance:* Used to adjust the arm angle
- *Port clutch:* Used to reposition the arm to resolve and avoid potential arm collisions during the procedure. Also used to raise or lower the boom, space the arms together or apart (like a fan), or reduce tension at the port site. Examples include, bringing the arm to the cannula for docking, or stowing an arm for a 3-arm procedure.

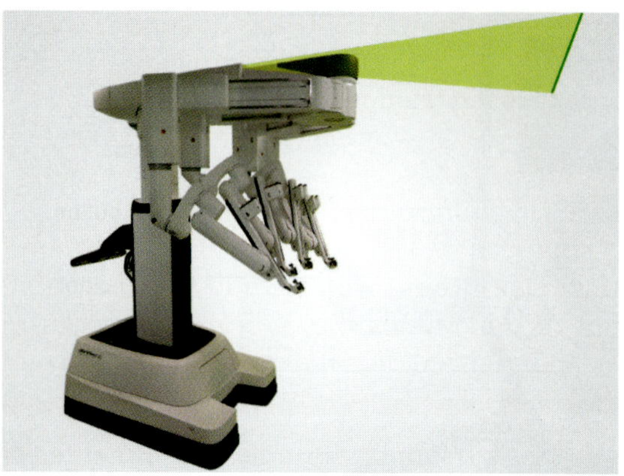

Fig. 27.26: Horizontal laser

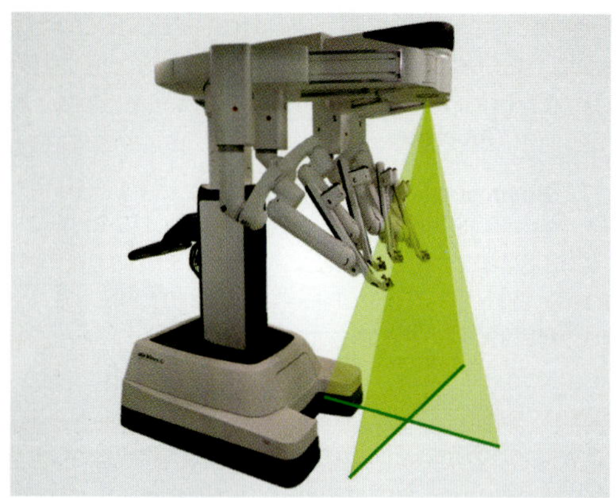

Fig. 27.27: Targetting laser

- *Boom rotation:* Used to rotate the boom cluster of arms.
- Patient cart lasers
  Horizontal laser (Fig. 27.26): The horizontal laser is mounted just below the highest point of the system and projects a horizontal line to the front of the system. The horizontal laser projects a horizontal line in front of the patient cart, highlighting possible collisions during powered patient cart movement.
  Targeting laser (Fig. 27.27): The targeting laser is mounted at the center of the boom and projects downward to assist positioning the patient cart at the patient. Targeting maximizes the range of motion of each arm helps manage arm spacing, and maximizes patient access. Additionally, the targeting laser activates during draping, when it is helpful to have a reference line for adjusting arm position.

Vision Cart Overview (Fig. 27.28)

- *Touchscreen:* The touchscreen monitor provides a view of the surgical site from the patient-side and a set of controls for endoscope and video configurations.
- *Accessory shelves:* Shelving units for accessory equipment, such as insufflators.

- *VIO dV:* Integrated electrosurgical unit (ESU) for instrument activation that can be used with robotic and laparoscopic instruments.
- *Endoscope controller:* Contains a high-intensity light source to illuminate the surgical site and the electronics for processing the video images from the endoscope.
- *Video processor:* Receives and processes video input from the endoscope and sends it through the system electronics to the touchscreen and 3D viewer.
- *System electronics (core):* Contains the electronics for advanced processing of the video image, system control algorithms, and control of ESUs when the surgeon uses the instrument function foot pedals.
- *Tank holders:* Two tank holders support use of an insufflator. To accommodate various size tanks, the tank holders have adjustable straps above and the lower bracket slides in and out after you loosen one screw on each side with a screwdriver. The tank holders can support two tanks, each weighing up to 50 lb (22.32 kg).

ENDOSCOPE (FIG. 27.29)

The endoscope acquires **(Fig. 27.30)** three-dimensional (3D) video from the surgical

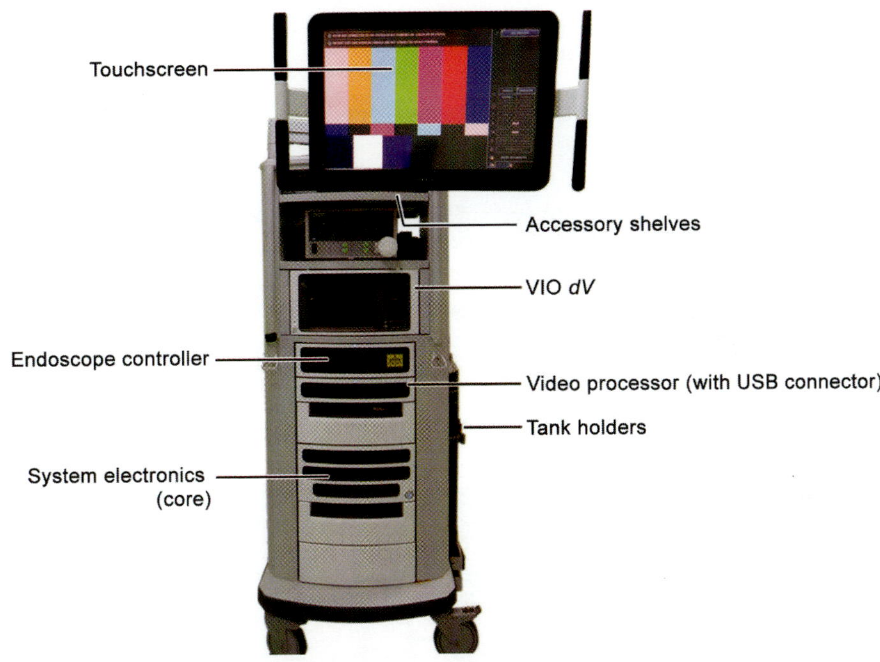

Fig. 27.28: Vision cart overview

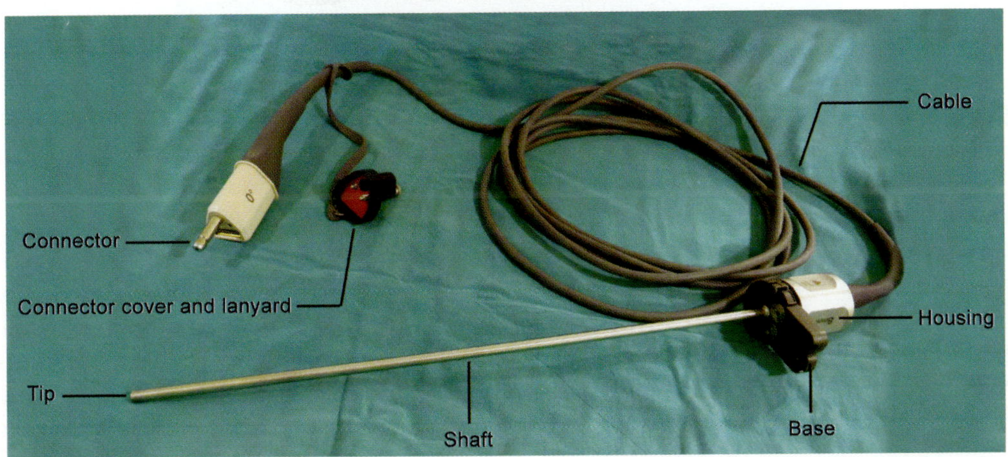

Fig. 27.29: Endoscope

site in high definition (HD). The HD video is processed by the system electronics in the vision cart and displayed on the surgeon console 3D viewer and vision cart touch screen.

8 mm endoscope is available in 0° and 30° (up or down) tip angles.

There are three light apertures (openings that emit light) in the vision system. The first aperture is on the endoscope controller.

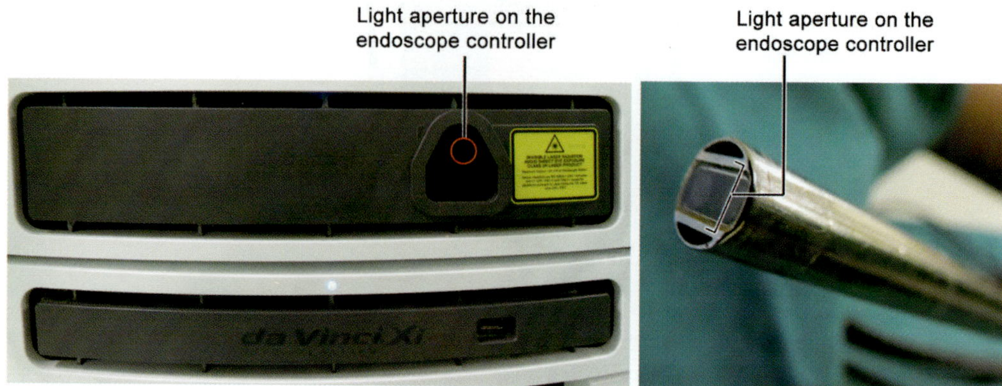

Fig. 27.30: Endoscope

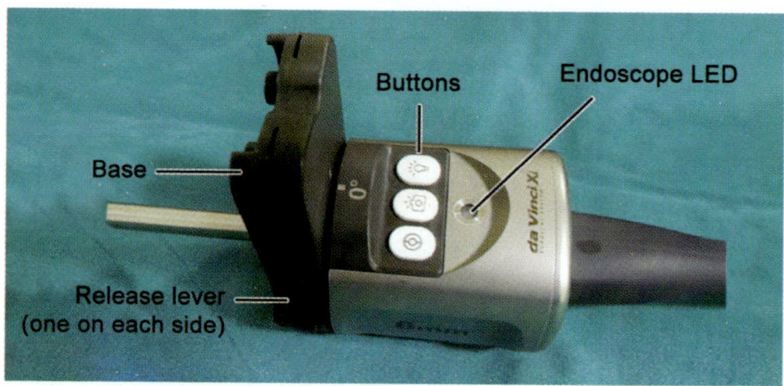

Fig. 27.31: Button controls of endoscope

Button controls of the endoscope **(Fig. 27.31 and Table 27.2)**.

The light guide and endoscope communication signals are integrated into a single cable, permanently attached to the endoscope. The endoscope cable connects directly to the endoscope controller on the vision cart to provide communication and illumination to the endoscope **(Fig. 27.32)**.

Audio System

The da Vinci Xi audio system consists of a set of microphones and speakers installed on both the patient cart and surgeon console, used for voice communication between the OR staff and the surgeon console operator. In addition, the audio system produces a variety of audible sounds (such as error tones), and voice annunciation messages.

EndoWrist Instruments Overview (Fig. 27.33)

The EndoWrist instruments have an articulating design at their distal tips that mimic the human wrist. Each instrument is used to perform a specific surgical task such as grasping, suturing, or tissue manipulation.

- *Instrument housing (A):* The instrument housing engages with the instrument sterile adapter and includes the:
  - *Release buttons (B):* The two release buttons, one on each side of the housing, are used to disengage the instrument from the instrument arm sterile adapter for removal.

TABLE 27.2: Button controls of the endoscope

Button	Adjustment	Description
	Left/right eye swap	Press to toggle the view on the vision cart touchscreen to the left or right endoscope image
	Targeting	Press and hold to activate the targeting features
	Take photo	Press to capture an image from the endoscope view. The system saves the image to a USB flash drive connected to the video processor on the vision case. The system records the left or right image based of which image is currently displayed on the touchscreen
	Illumination on/off	Press and hold to turn illumination on or off

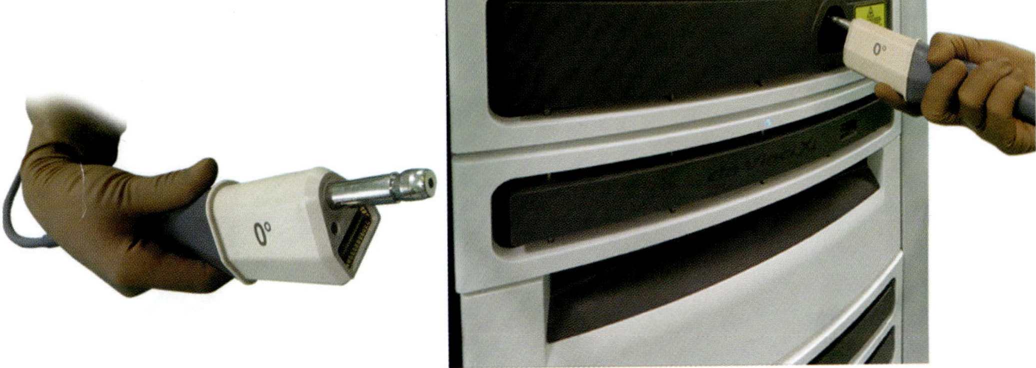

Fig. 27.32: Endoscope controller on vision cart

- *Flush ports (C):* Two flush ports are used for instrument reprocessing.
- *Discs (D):* The discs connect to the instrument wrist and translate the movements of the master hand controls from the surgeon console.
- *Shaft (E):* The shaft inserts through the cannula and rotates as controlled by the movements of the master hand controls.
- *Wrist (F):* The articulating wrist provides a wide range of movements.
- *Tip (G):* The instrument's end effector (for example, graspers, cautery hooks, blades)
- *Grip release socket (H):* Mechanism for manual grip release.
- *Maximum use indicator (I):* Indicates when the instrument has reached its maximum uses.

Different types of Forceps Available in da Vinci System (Si and Xi) **(Fig. 27.34)**

- Monopolar curved scissors (hot shears)
- Fenestrated bipolar forceps
- Cadiere forceps
- Maryland bipolar forceps
- Large needle driver
- Prograsp forceps

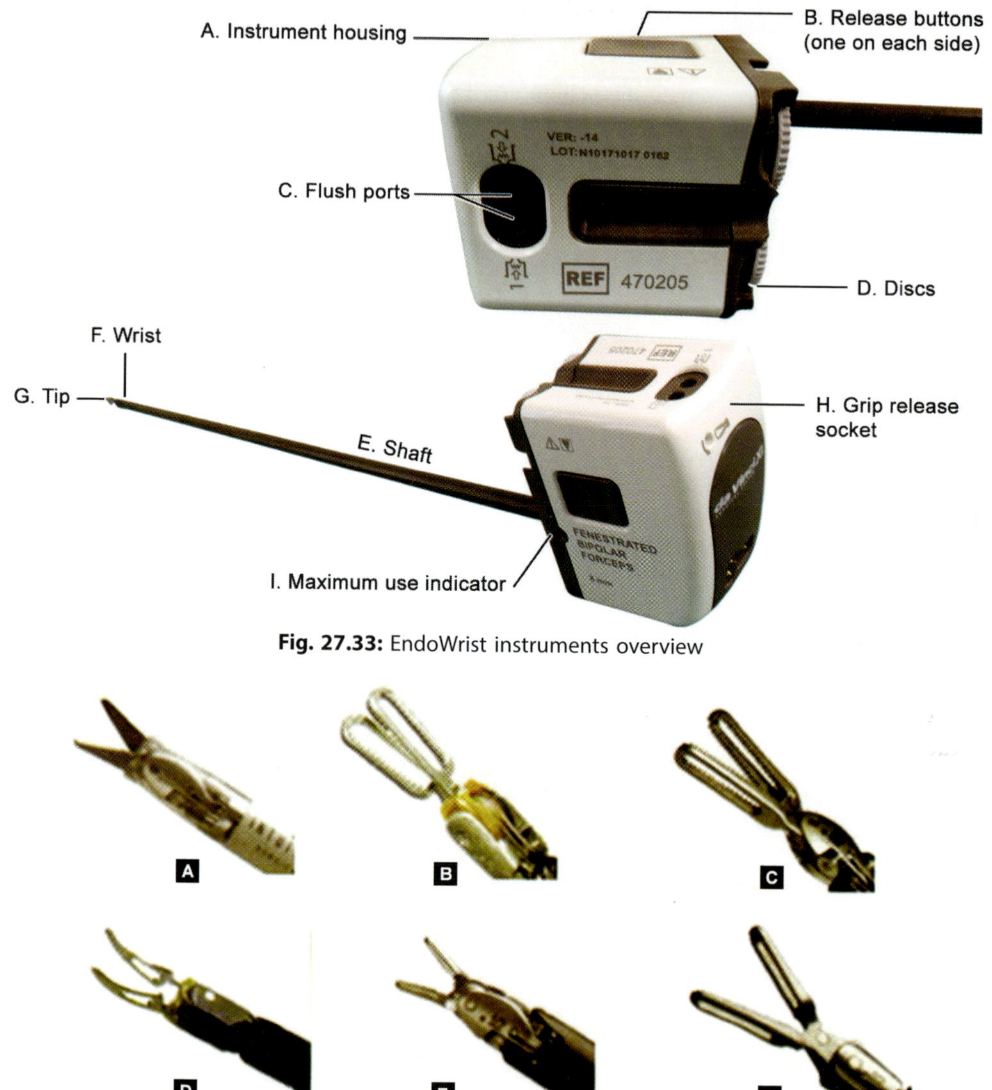

Fig. 27.33: EndoWrist instruments overview

Fig. 27.34A to F: Forceps type in da Vinci Si and Xi

Vessel Sealer and Stapler *(Fig. 27.35)*

Anti-fogging measures during use

- Use of zoom feature of the lens during use of cautery
- Avoid insufflation tube connection to camera port
- Use of warm saline for cleaning the lens

- The Clearify™ system is used to defog, clean, protect and white-balance the scope and clean the trocar.

Advantage of this system is that it avoids
Scope and lens damage, procedural delays, fire, burn, and hot water hazards.

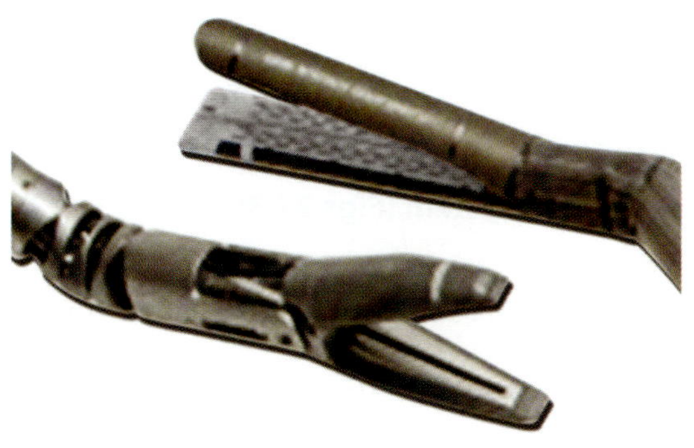

Fig. 27.35: Vessel sealer and stapler

Table 27.3: Sterilization and cleaning of instruments and accessories

Parameter	Value for Central and Eastern Europe, Middle East and Africa (EMEIA) and Asia
Sterilization type	Pre-vacuum
Preconditioning pulses	3
Minimum temperature	273°F (134°C)
Full cycle exposure time	3 minutes
Minimum dry time	50 minutes
Configuration	Place in sterilization tray and double wrap

- *AirSeal system:* Tri-lumen filtered tube set which optimizes gas flow, facilitates constant smoke evacuation, provides access port.

Sterilization and Cleaning of Instruments and Accessories (Table 27.3)

- Sterilization and cleaning of endoscopes
- Sterrad system with or without 100 NX express cycle

Advances in da Vinci Si Model

- *Visual resolution:* 1080i HD resolution provides visual clarity for precise visualization of target anatomy.
- *Ergonomic settings:* The console includes multiple ergonomic adjustments for surgeon comfort.
- *Surgeon touchpad:* An integrated surgeon control interface gives comprehensive information on control of video, audio and system settings.
- *Fingertip controls:* Master controllers allow exact control of the EndoWrist instruments. Motion scaling helps to coordinate the adjustments of hand-to-instrument movement ratios as per surgeon comfort to minimize errors.
- *Footswitch panel:* The footswitch panel enables the surgeon to perform different tasks such as swapping between different types of energy instruments.
- *Continual safety self-checks:* The system performs over one million safety checks per second, helping enhance safety and reliability.
- *Guided instrument exchange:* Allows for an efficient exchange of instruments during surgery.
- *Wide touchscreen:* Telestration capability facilitates team communication through touchscreen.
- *Audiovisual feedback:* Auditory and visual alerts mean the surgeon and OR team are constantly aware of system status and functions.
- *3D HD camera head:* A 3D HD camera with integrated controls assist in quick and convenient vision setup.
- *Motorized patient cart:* Docking becomes easier with the motor-driven patient cart.
- *Streamlined draping:* One-piece sterile draping with instrument adapters allows easy set up.
- *Firefly™ Fluorescence imaging:* Real-time endoscopic visual and near-infrared fluorescence imaging which enables vessel identification and solid organ perfusion (liver, kidney).
- *Single-Site®:* Trans umbilical entry enables a virtually scarless surgery. To avoid cannula collisions and arm interferences;

instruments and camera cross within the Single-Site port and use remote center technology.

- Skills Simulator™
- Advanced instrumentation
- Enables mechanical function of advanced instruments including EndoWrist One Vessel Sealer and EndoWrist Stapler 45.
- *5 mm instruments available:* Useful in head and neck surgery and pediatric surgery.
- The TilePro™ multi-input stereo viewer (Intuitive Surgical, Inc.) enables simultaneous display of multiple video inputs on the surgeon's console, integrating display of the patient's ultrasound, CT, MRI and intraoperative ultrasound images. This may be particularly beneficial in procedures like robot-assisted partial nephrectomy, partial cystectomy.[1]

Advances in da Vinci Xi Model

- Highly magnified 3D vision
- Enhanced ergonomics
- Targeting with laser beam
- Multi-quadrant improved access—camera can be mounted on any arm and instrument orientation can be flipped.
- Optics mounted at the tip of the scope allows better quality and color visualization to OR assistant.
- Integrated camera, scope, cable in handheld design
- Image capture available at endoscope head
- Integrated energy—ERBE VIO dV generator as an integrated energy source for instruments.
- Integrated table motion—wireless communication with integrated table which allows table motion while the surgeon operates.
- Firefly™ Fluorescence Imaging, EndoWrist Vessel Sealer and EndoWrist Stapler
- Single port upgrade possible for NOTES surgery.

Disadvantage

No 5 mm instruments available.

DRAPING

da Vinci Si System (Figs 27.36 to 27.43)

Procedure

- Circulating nurse delivers the instrument arm drape to the scrub nurse in sterile fashion, with the instrument arm sterile adapter facing above.
- Scrub nurse unfolds the drape on a sterile table after that.
- Tent the opening of the drape and grip the outside with your finger and thumb. Hold the top of the drape with the other hand. Lower the drape over the instrument arm insertion axis.
- Once the system recognizes the sterile adapter; wheels on the sterile adapter will spin, and you will hear beeps.
- Attach the molding over the cannula mount.

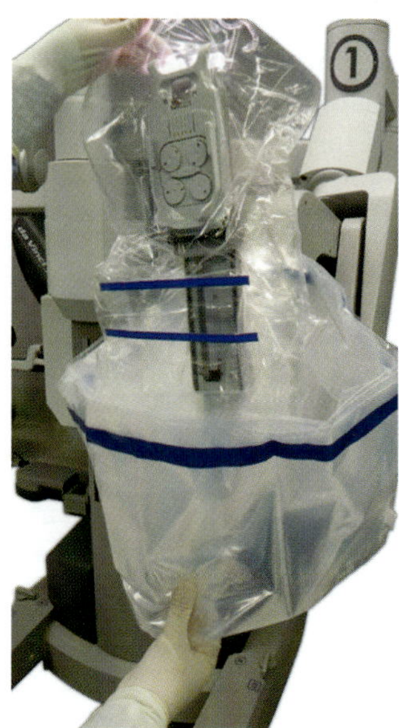

Fig. 27.36: Lowering the drape over the insertion axis

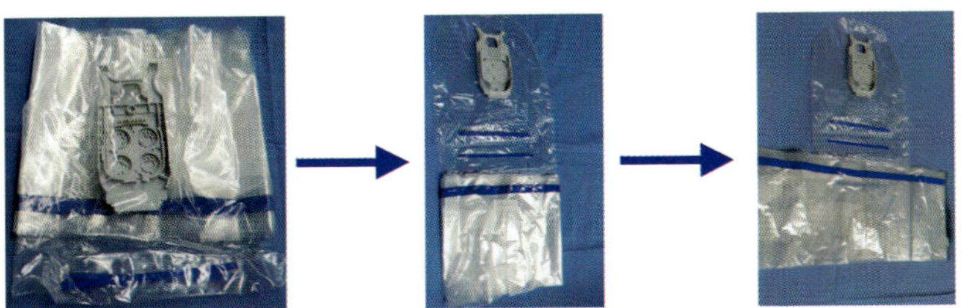

Fig. 27.37: Unfolding instrument arm drape

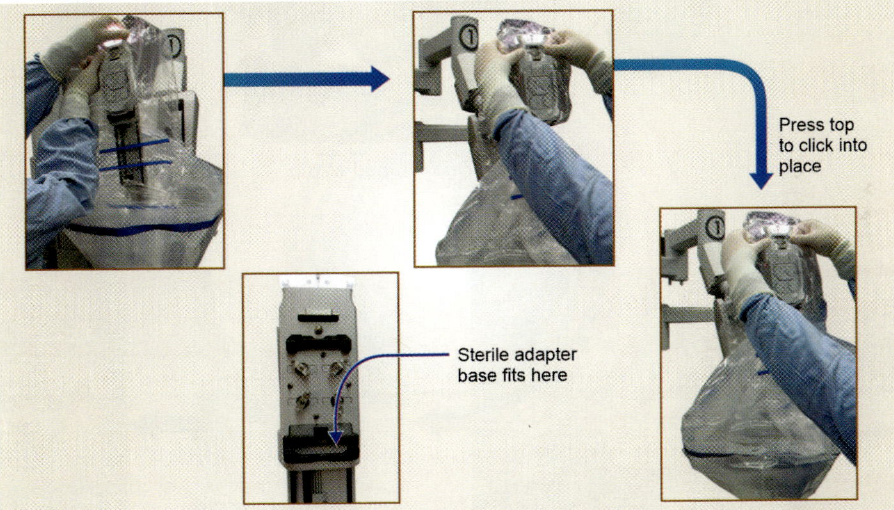

Fig. 27.38: Installation of sterile adapter

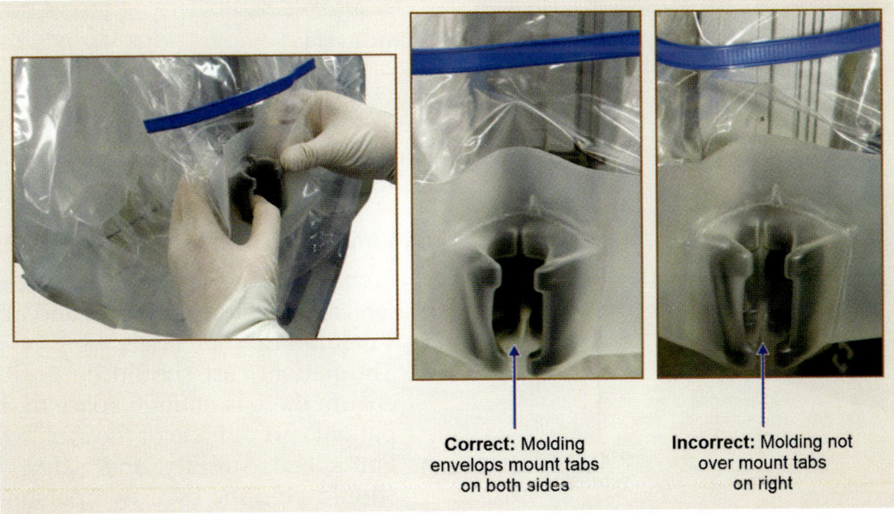

Fig. 27.39: Cannula mount molding

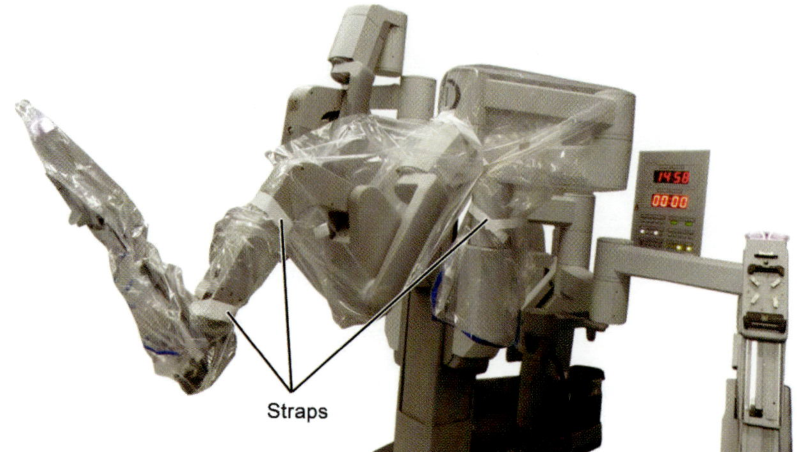

Fig. 27.40: Final draped arm

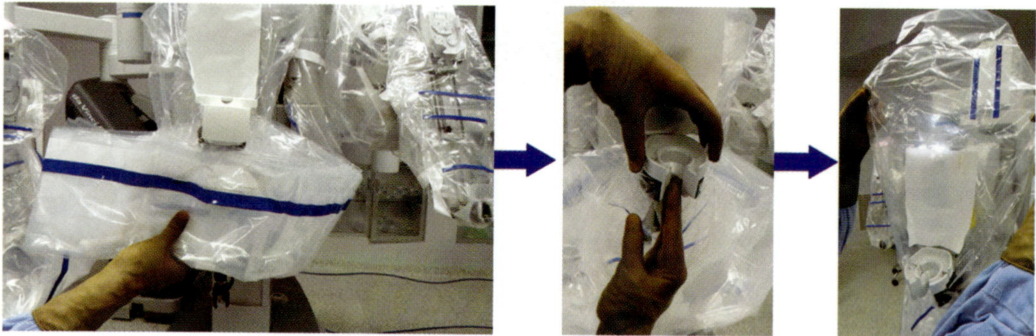

Fig. 27.41: Camera arm draping

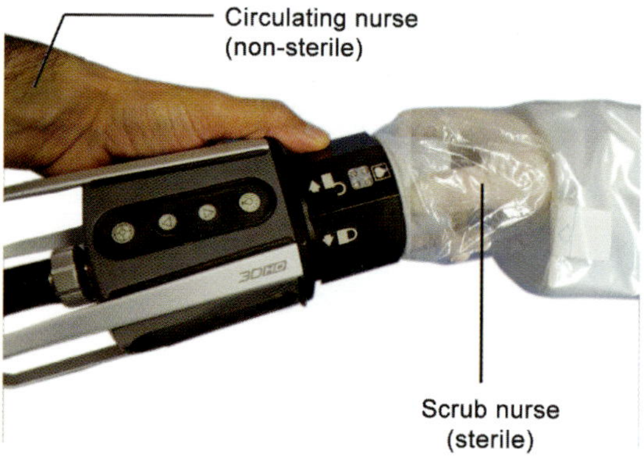

Fig. 27.42: Camera head draping

- Wrap all white drape straps snugly around the instrument arm, and attach each strap to itself.

da Vinci Xi System (Figs 27.44 to 27.56)

- *4 arm drapes:* Includes instrument sterile adapter, cannula sterile adapter and arm clip.
- 1 column drape.
- The patient cart should be positioned to ensure there is enough space to drape the patient cart outside of the sterile field.
- For speed, sterility and safety, draping should be done by a two-person team: A sterile user (scrub nurse or surgical assistant)

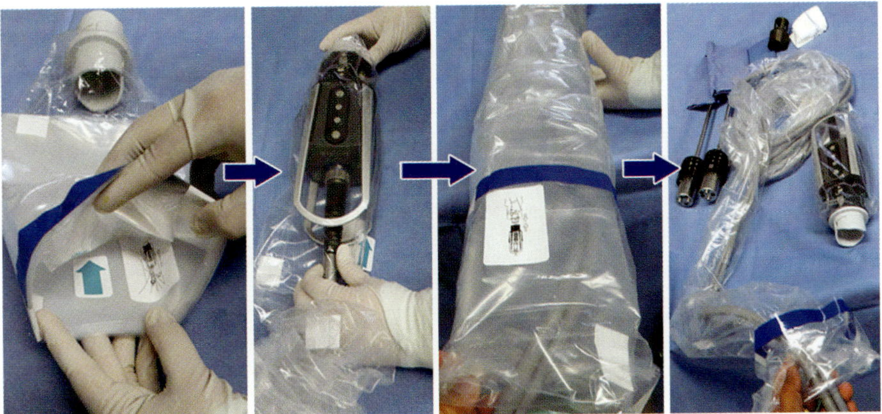

Fig. 27.43: Camera head drape

Instrument sterile adapter   Cannula sterile adapter   Arm clip

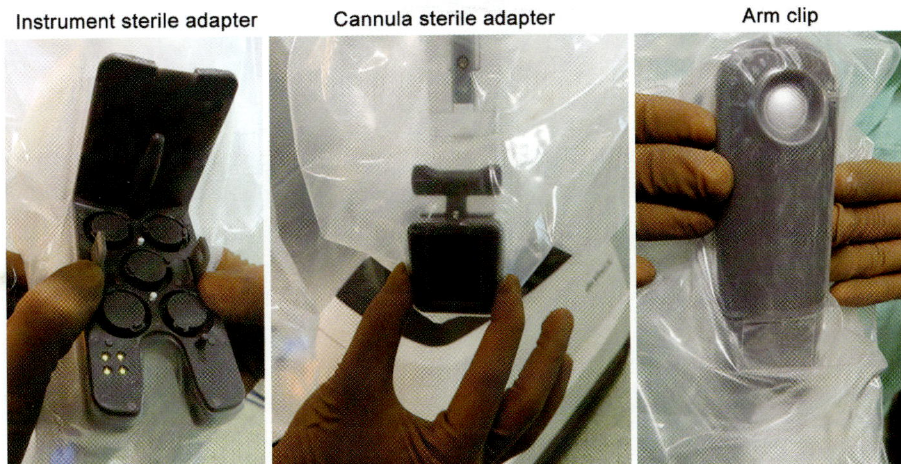

Fig. 27.44: Adapter for arms

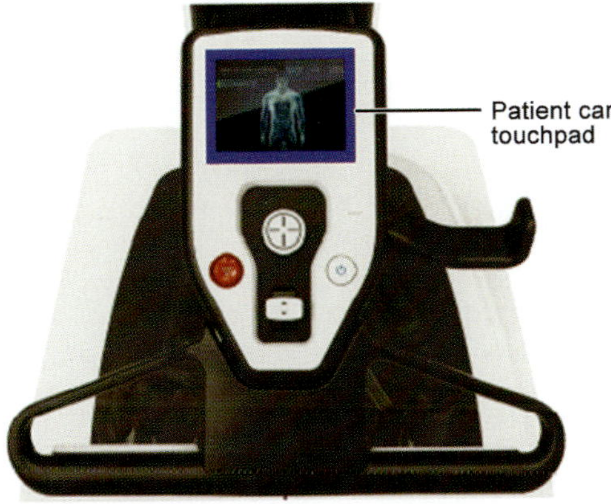

Fig. 27.45: Patient cart touchpad

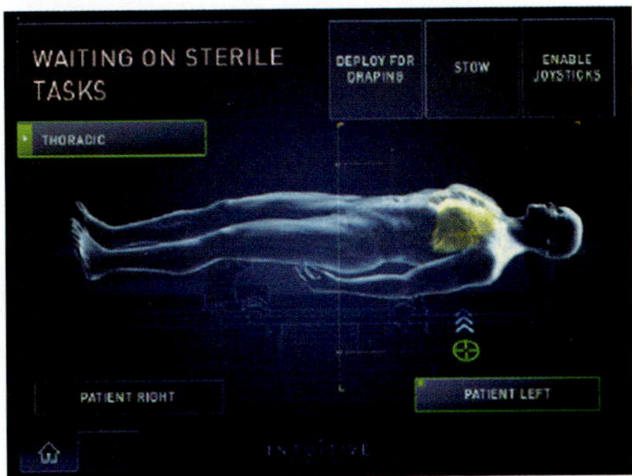

Fig. 27.46: Monitor

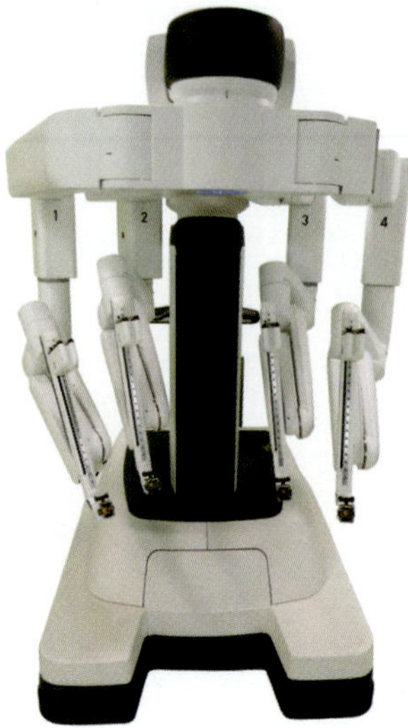

Fig. 27.47: Deployment for draping

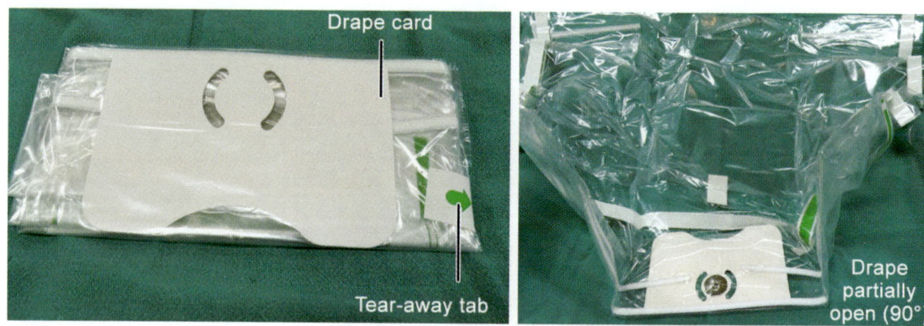

Fig. 27.48: Drape overview

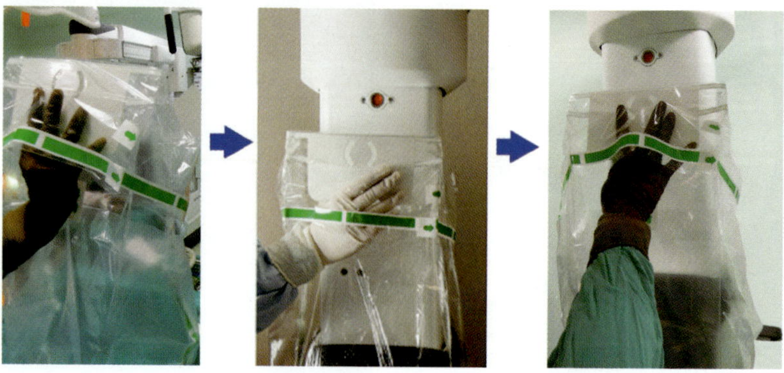

Fig. 27.49: Central column sterile draping

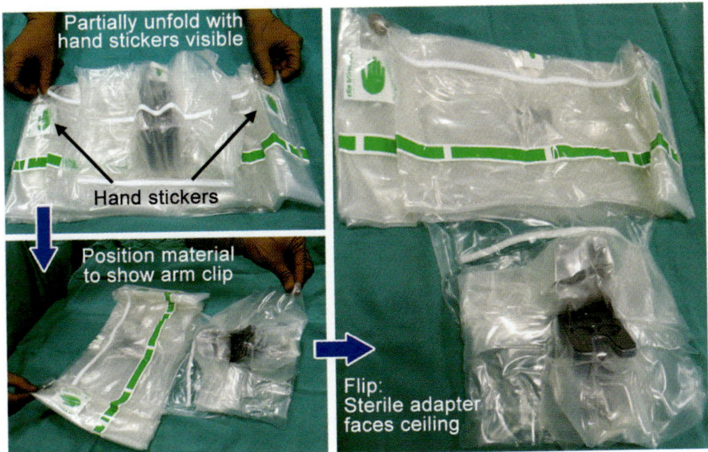

Fig. 27.50: Unfolding of arm drape

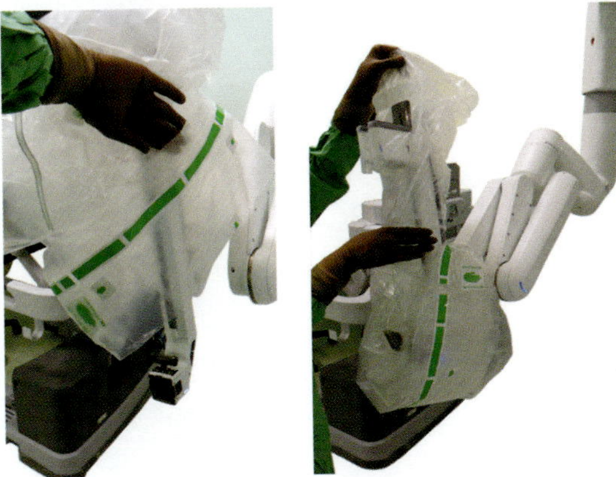

Fig. 27.51: Arm draping

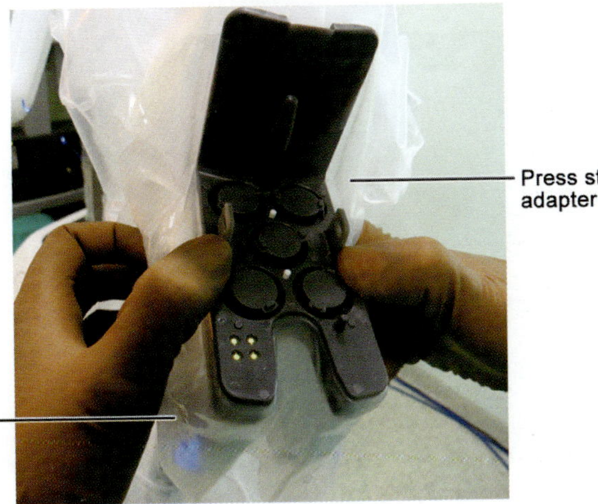

Fig. 27.52: Aligning adapter with the arm

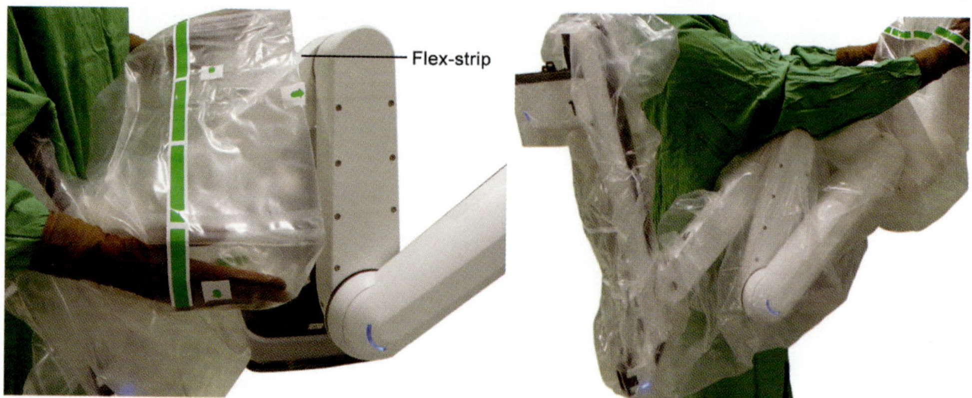

Fig. 27.53: Draping the arm

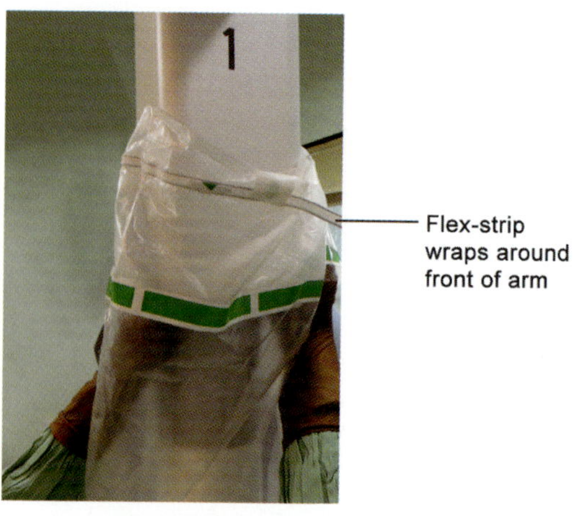

Fig. 27.54: Alignment of drape

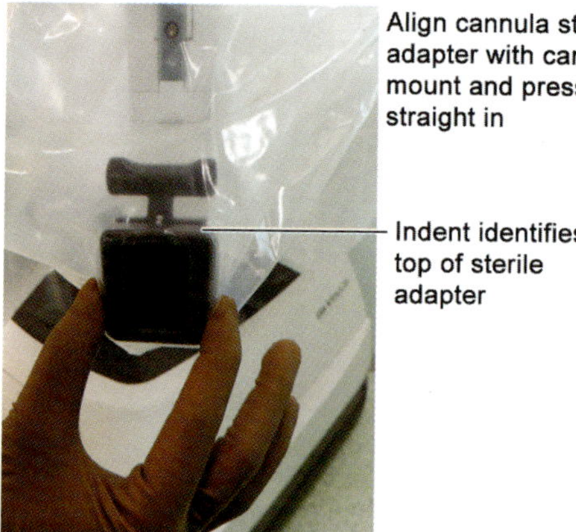

Fig. 27.55: Alignment of adapter

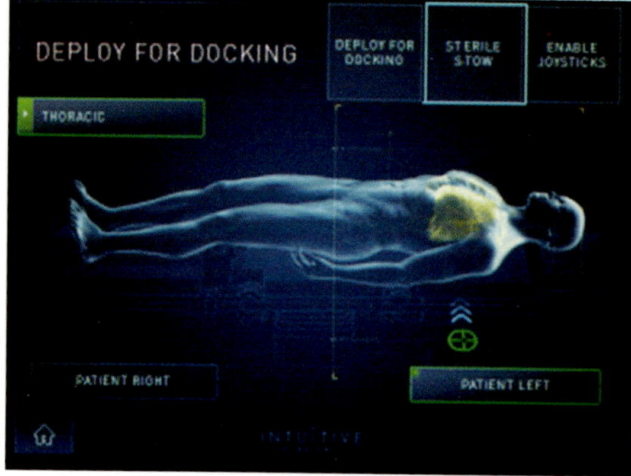

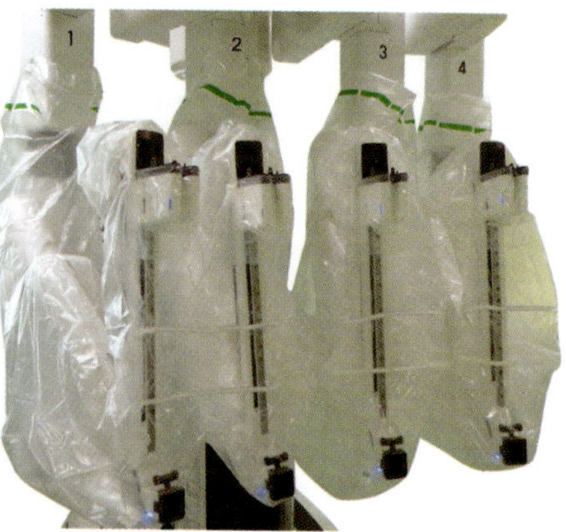

Fig. 27.56: Sterile stow (system is ready for use)

and a non-sterile user (circulating nurse) who can handle non-sterile components.

- The patient cart touchpad provides instructions to deploy the boom and arms for draping, install the drapes, and sterile stow the arms until the procedure.

REFERENCE

1. Singh I. Robotics in urological surgery: Review of current status and maneuverability, and comparison of robot-assisted and traditional laparoscopy. Computer Aided Surgery January 2011;16(1):38–45.

28
Patient Positioning and Port Placement

Ashwin Sunil Tamhankar, Surya Prakash Ojha, Puneet Ahluwalia, Gagan Gautam

PATIENT POSITIONING

Upper Tract Surgery (Fig. 28.1)

Lateral decubitus position with pressure padding with pneumatic cuffs on calf.

Lower Tract Surgery

da Vinci Si System *(Fig. 282)*

Trendelenburg position with lithotomy position with pressure padding and chest

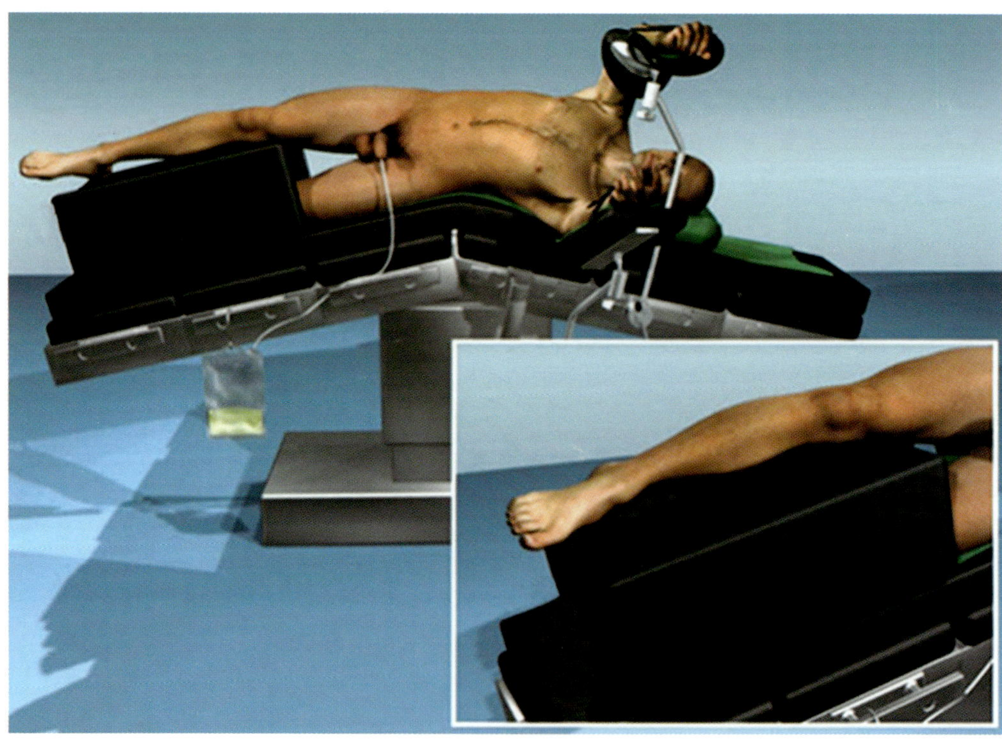

Fig. 28.1: Lateral decubitus position

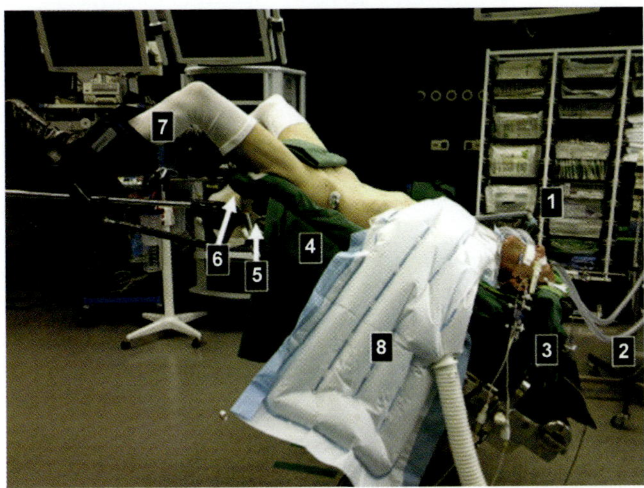

Fig. 28.2: Trendelenburg position with lithotomy. (1) Head end of patient; (2) Anesthesia trolley; (3) Head rest; (4) Arm tucked under drape; (5 and 6) Thigh support; (7) Lithotomy; (8) Patient warmer

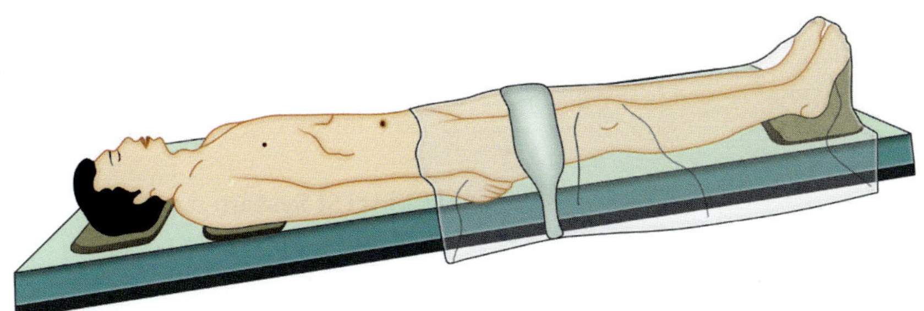

Fig. 28.3: Supine Trendelenburg position

Note: For X system patient positioning is same as Si. For a pelvic procedure the robot is positioned between the legs of the patient which are placed in the lithotomy/split leg position

strapping is required as the docking is done from the foot end with patient cart placed between the legs of the patient.

Pneumatic cuffs are placed around the calf of both legs to minimize the risk of deep venous thrombosis.

da Vinci Xi System (*Fig. 28.3*)

Supine Trendelenburg position with pressure padding and chest strapping is required as the docking is done from the side of table.

Pneumatic cuffs are placed around the calf of both legs to minimize the risk of deep venous thrombosis.

Problems Associated with Steep Head Low Position

- Mean arterial pressure changes by 2 mm Hg every inch change in vertical height.
- Raised pressures in the circle of Willis.
- Respiratory compromise—reduced vital capacity, compliance, functional reserve capacity.
- Raised intracranial pressure—effect of raised arterial and venous pressure along with cerebral vasodilatation because of hypercapnia.
- Raised intraocular pressure

- Calf ischemia and compartment syndrome can be precipitated because of head low position along with increased pressures because of pneumatic compression.

PORT PLACEMENT

General Principles

- All basic principles of laparoscopy for port placement remains the same in cases of robotic surgery. Triangulation for complete optimization in a lesser working space is applicable in robotics surgery as it is the advanced form of minimal access surgery (MIS) **(Fig. 28.4)**.
- *Remote center technology (**Fig. 28.5**):* The instrument arms and the camera arm on da Vinci surgical systems use remote centre technology. The remote center is the fulcrum point around which the da Vinci system moves the instrument. When the remote center of cannula is placed correctly in the patient's body wall, moving the patient cart arms around the remote center exerts minimal pull and tug at the port site, which lends itself to reduced pain and faster healing of the incision.
- *Insufflation:* Initial access can be by Veress needle or open method (Hassan) as in laparoscopy.
- *Burping:* This encompasses holding the trocar and pressing the set joint button while lifting the robot arm and trocar above so as to create more working space between the target organ and the instrument.

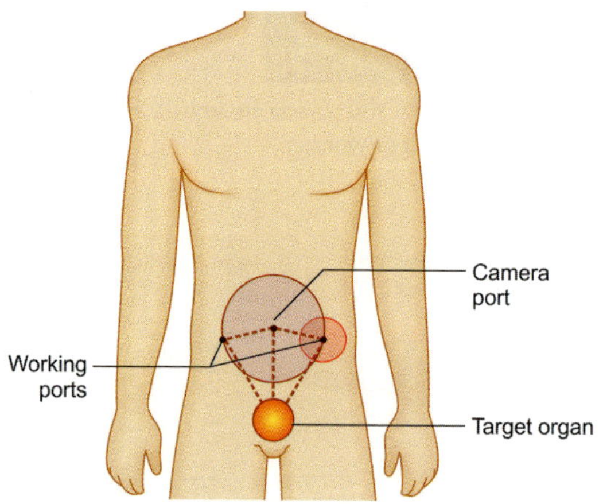

Fig. 28.4: Triangulation in port placement

da Vinci Si System

The goals of port placement are to avoid patient cart arm collisions and to maximize instrument and endoscope range of motion.

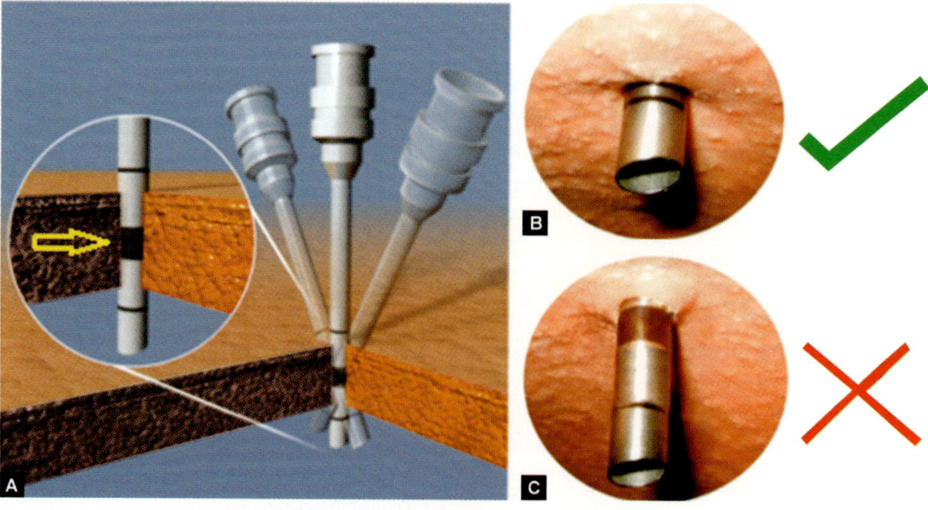

Figs 28.5A to C: Remote center technology

Some generic guidelines of the port placement in Si system are:

- Insufflate prior to marking out port placement.
- Camera port
  - Place the camera port so it aligns with the patient cart tower and target anatomy in a straight line.
  - Place the camera port 10–20 cm away from the target anatomy when possible (closer to 20 cm when possible)
- *Instrument arm placement:*
  - For arms 1 and 2, measure 8–10 cm from the camera port, perpendicular to the axis between the target anatomy and camera port.
  - For arm 3, measure an additional 8–10 cm from the closest da Vinci port
  - Triangulate as needed
  - Instrument arms should be at least 10 cm from target anatomy
- Instrument arm 3 considerations:
  - Location of internal anatomy to be retracted
  - Place on the same side as scissors
  - Place on the opposite side from assistant
- Non-robotic accessory ports should be at least 5 cm away from other ports, should be on opposite side of arm 3 with clear approach to target.

- Maintain at least 8–10 cm spacing between da Vinci Si ports.

da Vinci Xi System

- Straight line port placement allows da Vinci Xi instrument arms to work in parallel, maximizing surgical workspace and minimizing arm interference **(Fig. 28.6)**.
- This is important if instrument reach behind the ports and/or in line with the ports is required.
- Triangulated port placement may also be used.
- Insufflate the abdomen before measuring port placement.
- Following insufflation, mark the locations of instrument and accessory ports.
- Identify the surgical workspace:
  - If two quadrants or less, place the target in center of the surgical workspace boundary.
  - If greater than two quadrants, consider dual docking
- Place the initial endoscope port 10–20 cm from the target anatomy
- Place the initial endoscope port at the edge, or beyond the edge of the surgical workspace. This avoids losing perspective over the surgical workspace.
- If more than 20 cm from the target anatomy, consider dual docking.

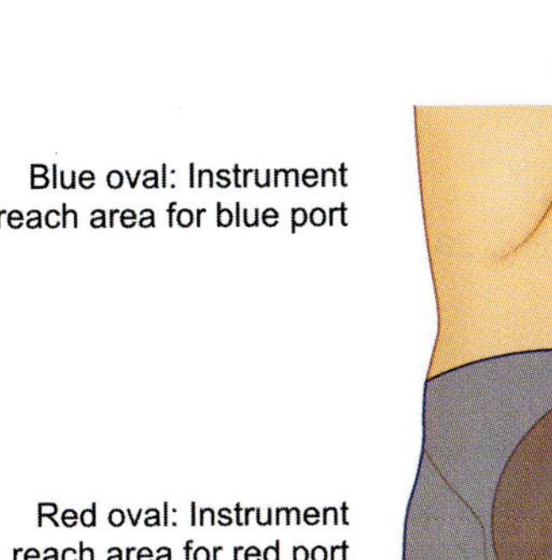
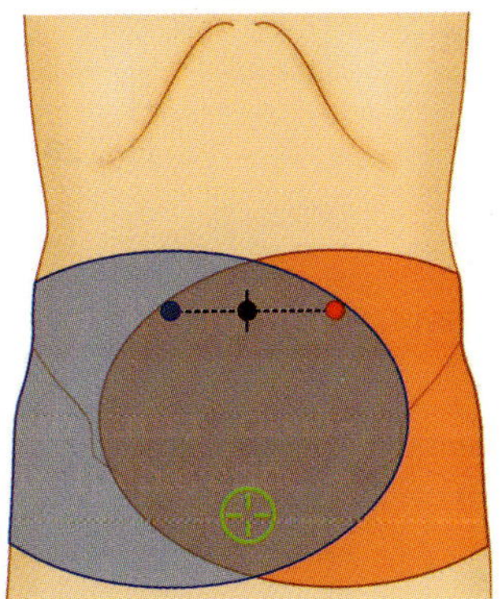
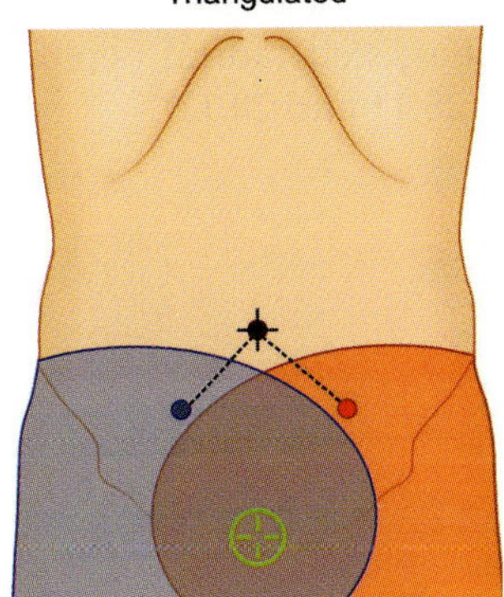

Fig. 28.6: Port placement in da Vinci Xi system

- Place remaining ports 6–10 cm apart (8 cm recommended) in a perpendicular line relative to the target anatomy.
- If space is limited, minimize distance between ports to 6 cm.
- Assistant port placement
  - Place assistant ports as needed, as far away as possible (at least 7 cm) from robotic ports.
  - Place in line with or triangulated between robotic ports to maximize access and minimize instrument arm interference.
  - Do not place an assistant port between a robotic port and the target anatomy.
  - Consider what the assistant needs to do or access.
  - Consider which side of the patient the assistant will be on.
  - Ensure the assistant is facing the target anatomy and can access the arms for instrument exchanges and intraoperative endoscope cleaning.
  - Consider using longer length laparoscopic instruments to add distance between the assistant and the da Vinci Xi instrument arms.

Schematic Representative of Port Placement of Surgeries

- Robot-assisted radical nephrectomy **(Figs 28.7 and 28.8)**
- Robot-assisted partial nephrectomy **(Figs 28.9 and 28.10)**
- Robot-assisted radical nephroureterectomy **(Figs 28.11 and 28.12)**

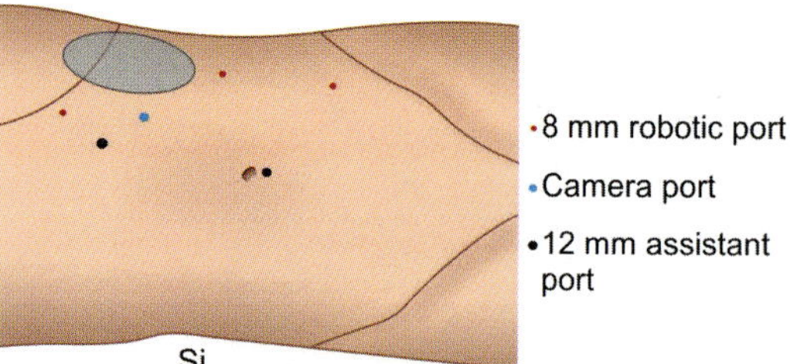

Fig. 28.7: da Vinci Si system

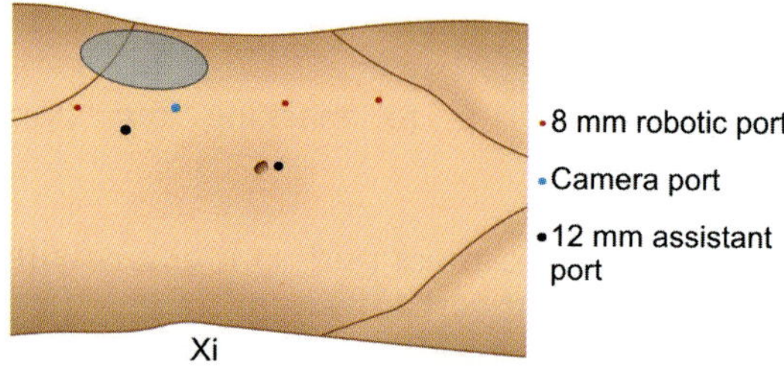

Fig. 28.8: da Vinci Xi system

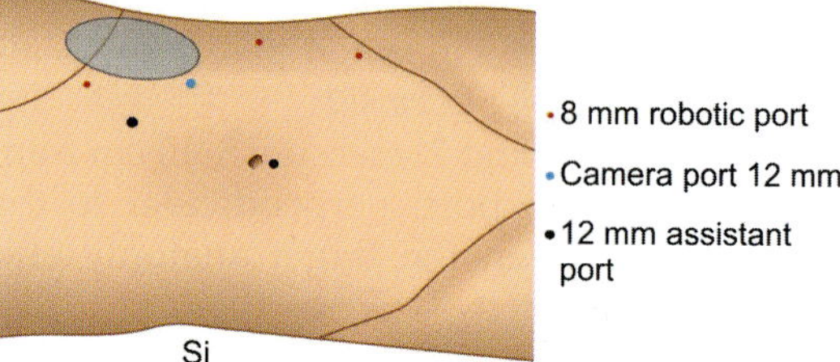

Fig. 28.9: da Vinci Si system

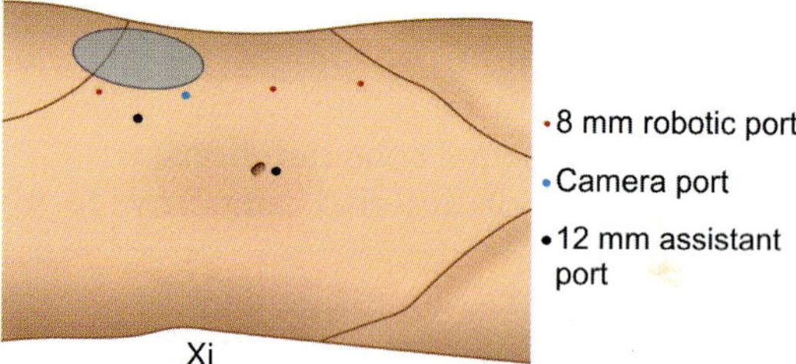

Fig. 28.10: da Vinci Xi system

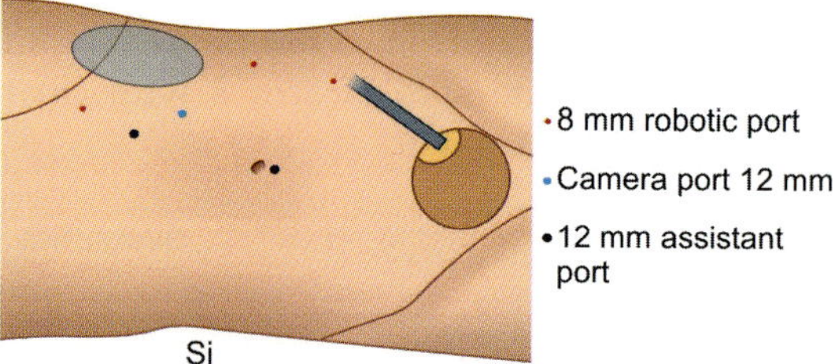

Fig. 28.11: da Vinci Si system

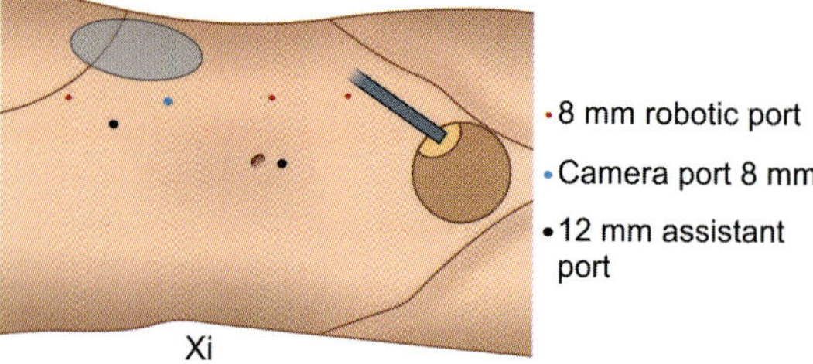

Fig. 28.12: da Vinci Xi system

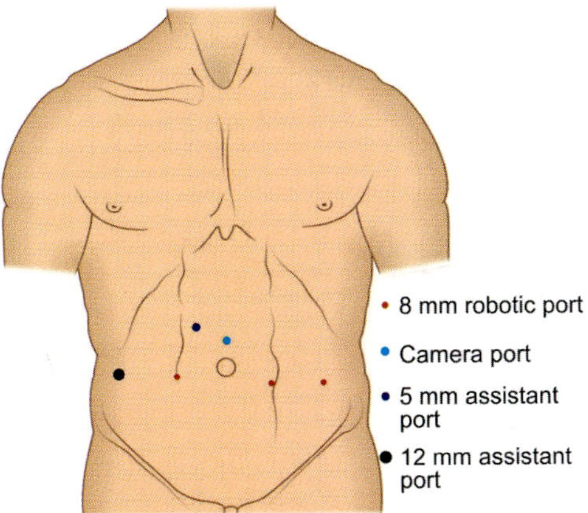

Fig. 28.13: da Vinci Si system

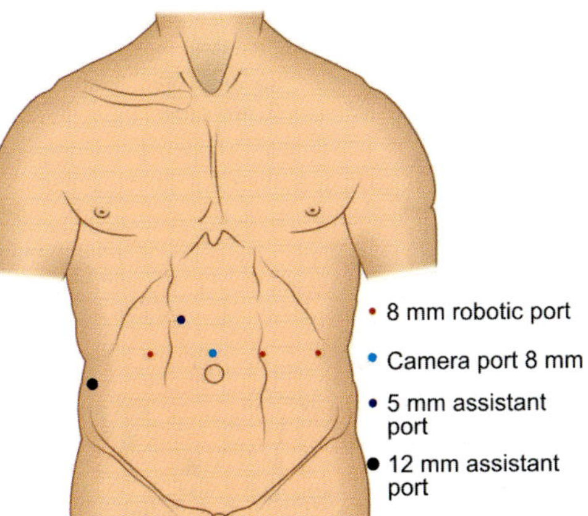

Fig. 28.14: da Vinci Xi system

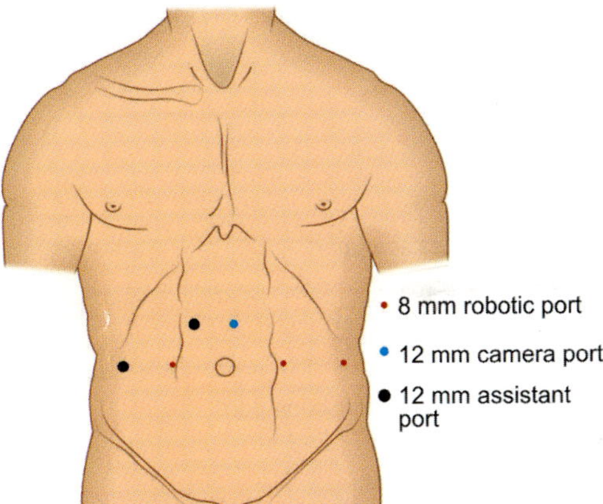

Fig. 28.15: da Vinci Si system

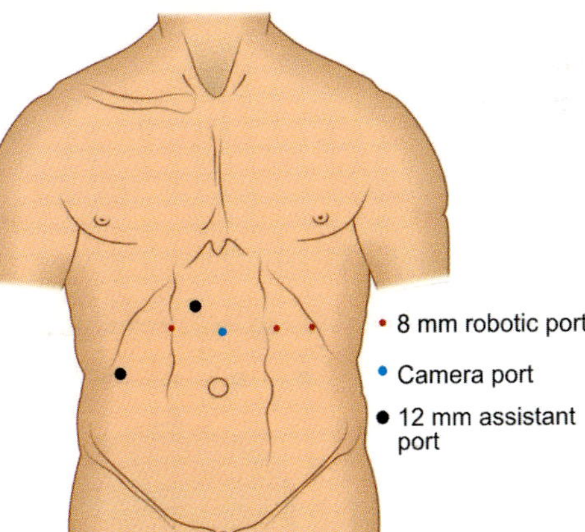

Fig. 28.16: da Vinci Xi system

- Robot-assisted radical prostatectomy **(Figs 28.13 and 28.14)**
- Robot-assisted radical cystectomy **(Figs 28.15 and 28.16)**
- Robot-assisted retroperitoneal lymph node dissection **(Figs 28.17 and 28.18)**

TARGETING (FIG. 28.19)

It is applicable for da Vinci Xi system only.

Once the patient cart is deployed and the initial endoscope arm is docked, targeting is performed.

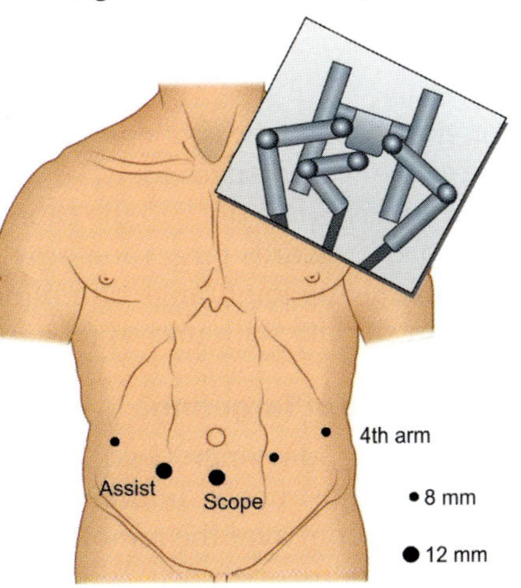

Fig. 28.17: da Vinci Si

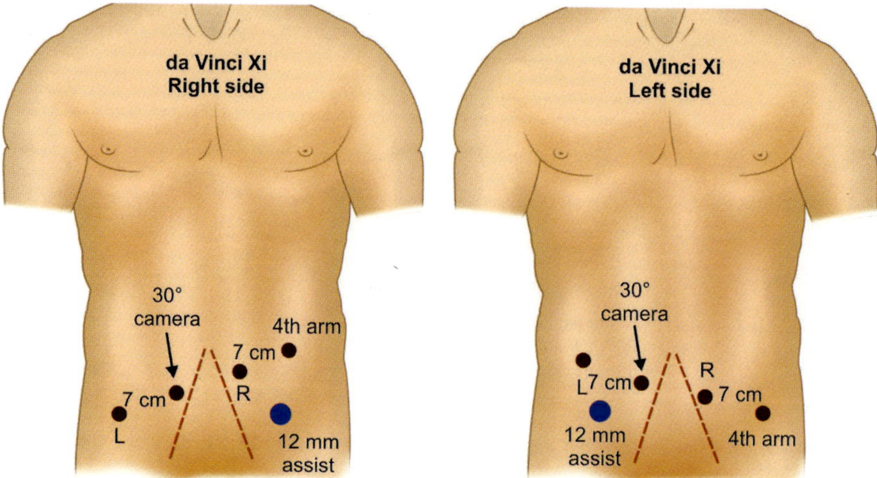

Fig. 28.18: da Vinci Xi

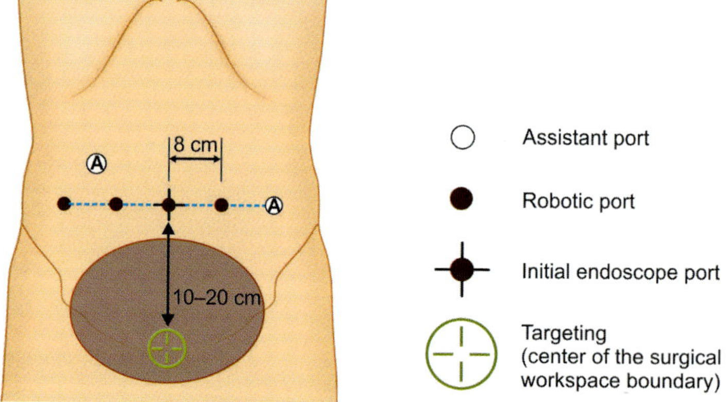

Fig. 28.19: Role of targeting

Targeting aligns the patient cart boom over the surgical workspace to:

- Ensure all arms can dock to the cannulae
- Orient arms towards target anatomy
- Maximize set up joint range of motion
- Maintain sterility with undraped boom.

What is the Role of Targeting?

During targeting, da Vinci Xi system makes the following adjustments simultaneously:

- Center the boom over the remote center of the initial endoscope port (occurs only if arms 2 and 3 are docked).
- Rotate the boom to point toward the target anatomy **(Fig. 28.20)**.
- Adjust the system height to maximize sterility between the boom and instrument arms, while ensuring reach to low, lateral ports (i.e. there is enough space between the docked arm remote center and the underside of the boom to maintain sterility).

DOCKING

Once the targeting is complete, docking of the other arms and instrument is performed.

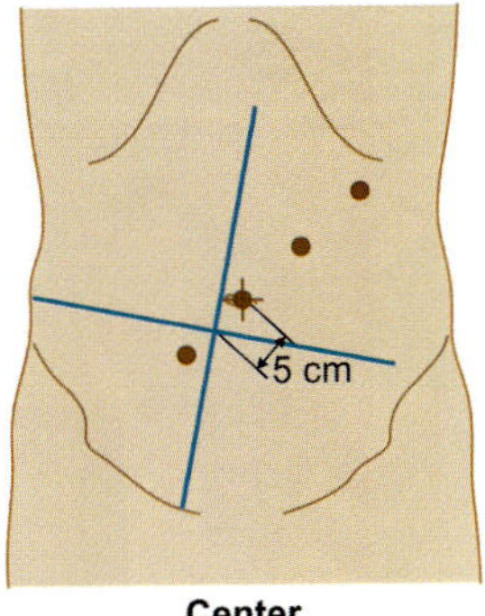
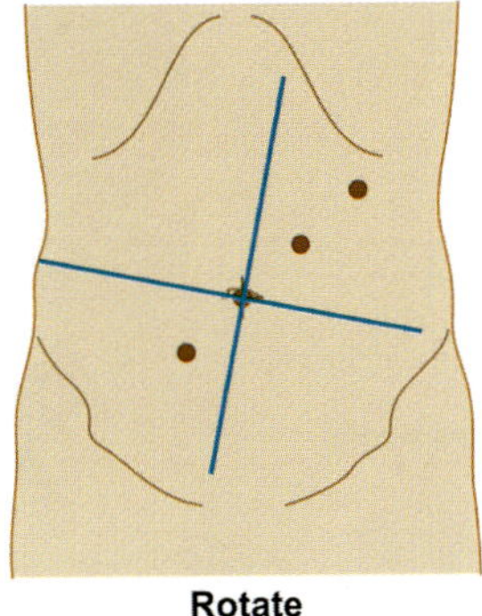
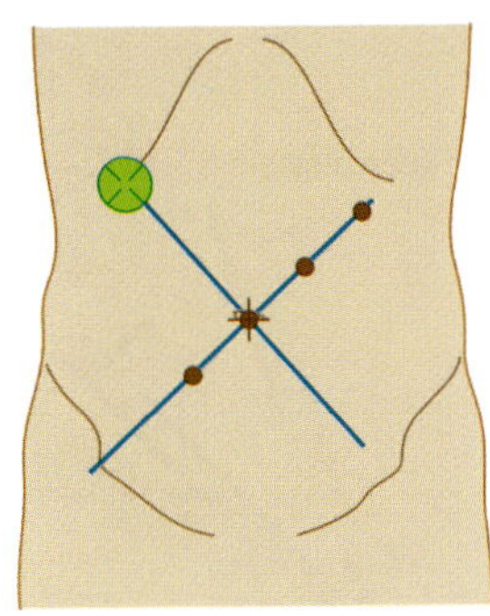

Fig. 28.20: Role of targeting

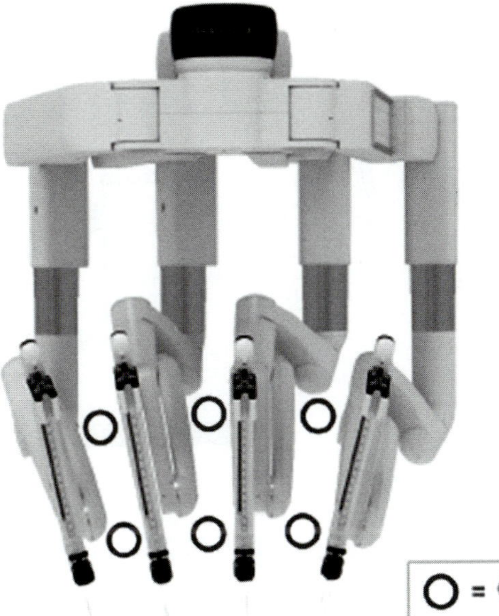

Fig. 28.21: Docking of the robotic arms: Importance of the boom

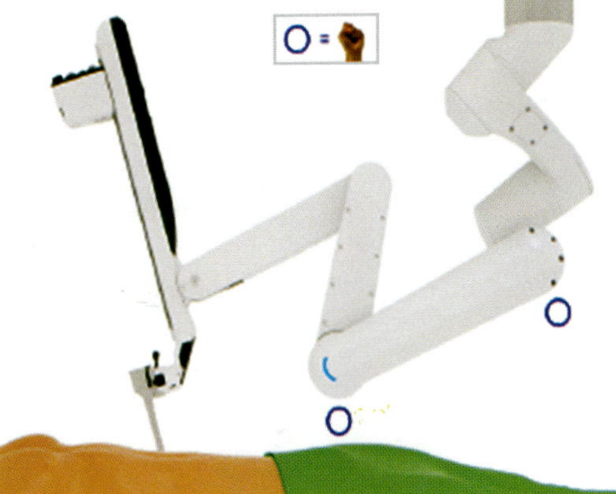

Fig. 28.22: Docking of the robotic arms: Importance of the joints

- If needed, use the port clutch button to space the arms (about a fist's spacing) **(Fig. 28.21)**. This helps resolve and avoid potential arm collisions during a procedure. It is recommended to position the arms as close together as possible while still allowing each axis to move without interference.
- Starting with the arms closest to the initial endoscope arm, use the port clutch and flex joints to bring arms together, using one hand to measure about a fist's space between the arms. This ensures sufficient space for the arms to work in parallel and for patient clearance adjustment.
- If needed, use the patient clearance button on each arm to adjust the arm angle. Adjust the angle "up" for increased patient clearance, or "down" for increased instrument access.
- After the arms are spaced, lower the patient clearance joints with about a fist's space to the patient or other sterile obstacles. This ensures maximum instrument reach **(Fig. 28.22)**.

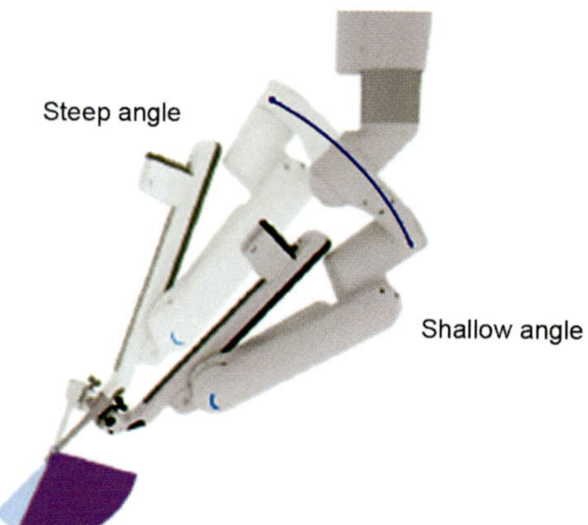

Fig. 28.23: Patient clearance

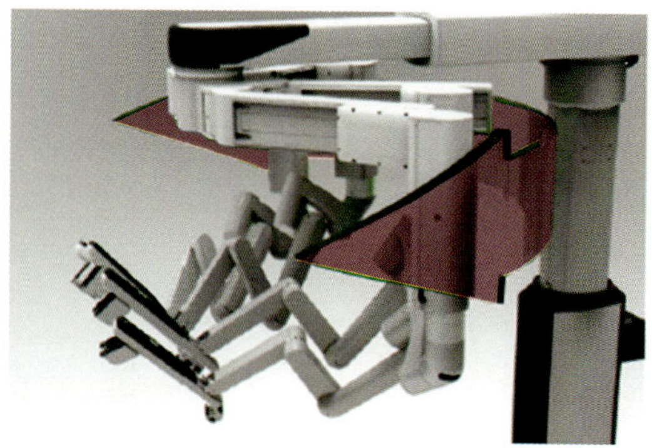

Fig. 28.24: Boom rotation

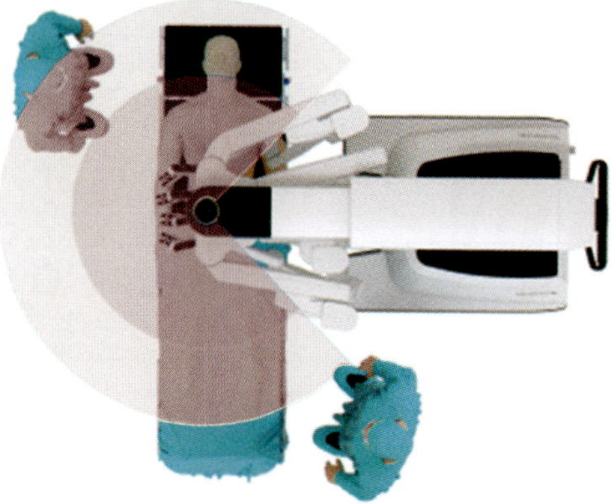

Fig. 28.25: Boom rotation

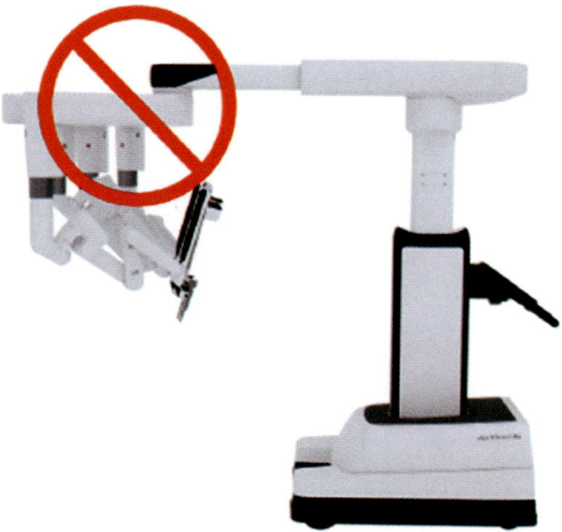

Fig. 28.26: Boom rotation

PATIENT CLEARANCE

Patient clearance **(Fig. 28.23)** is a pair of buttons that allows users to adjust the arm to a steep or shallow angle.

- Steep angles are used to make more room under the arm (patient clearance)
- Shallow angles are used to achieve the maximum working range of motion (instrument reach).

What Patient Clearance does?

- Adjust the arm angle
- The remote center does not move
- Cannot be initiated when the surgeon console is in control.

Boom Rotation (Figs 28.24 to 28.26)

What Boom Rotation does?

- Rotate the boom
- Located on arms 1 and 4 only
- The boom can only be rotated when there are no cannulae installed.

Total access of 2700 rotation on both sides is permissible in da Vinci Xi system.

Over-rotation of 1800 to opposite side should be avoided.

Guided Tool Change (Fig. 28.27)

To provide an efficient and safe method for instrument exchange or reinsertion, the system can assist the patient cart operator by guiding an instrument into the patient. Guided tool change helps guide the instrument tip to a location just short of the last position of the previously installed instrument tip.

- Intraoperative tips and tricks for improvement in movements of arms
    - Arm-to-arm interference **(Fig. 28.28)**
        - Near front end of the arm (near the instrument):
          Solution: Use the flex joints to bring the arm close to the adjacent arm. This allows the arms to work in parallel, minimizing interference.
        - Back end of the arm (near the patient clearance joint) **(Fig. 28.29)**

Solution: Use the patient clearance button to adjust the arms away from each other (up or down). This increases the space between the joints and minimizes interference.

Increasing Instrument Reach

- When desired surgical workspace to be increased is in-line with the ports:
  Use of flex joints: Starting with the arm closest to the desired area of reach (near the boundary of the surgical workspace),

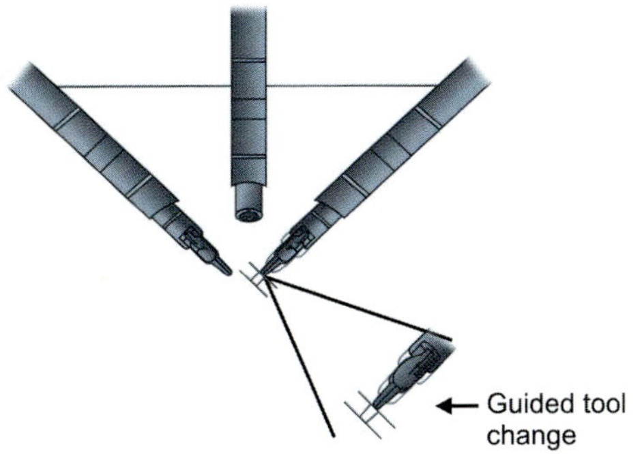

Fig. 28.27: Guided tool change

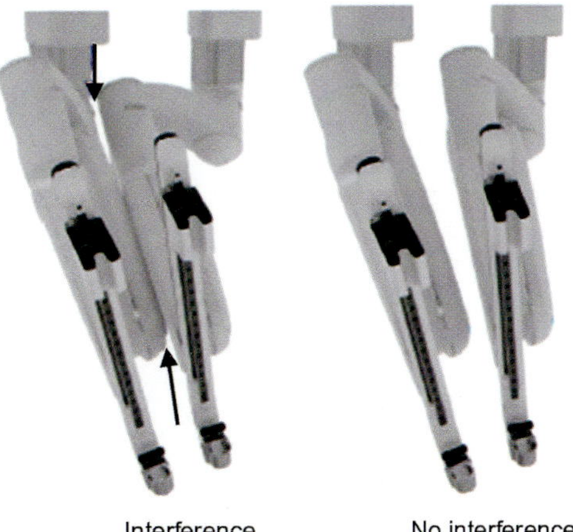

Fig. 28.29: Arm to arm interference

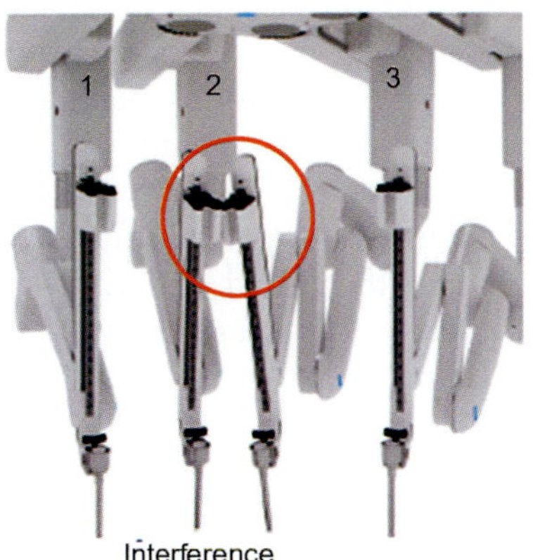

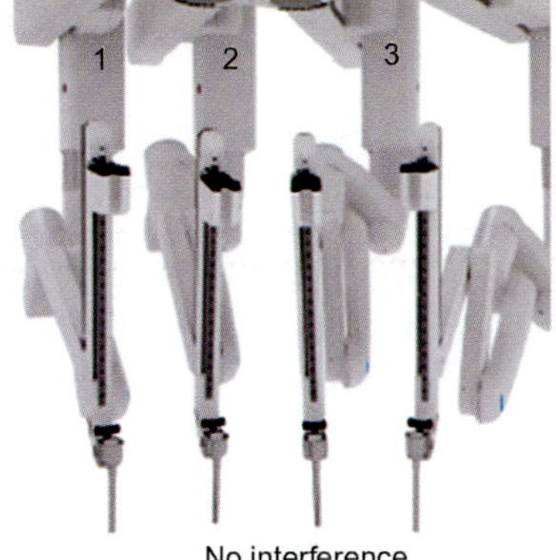

Fig. 28.28: Arm to arm interference

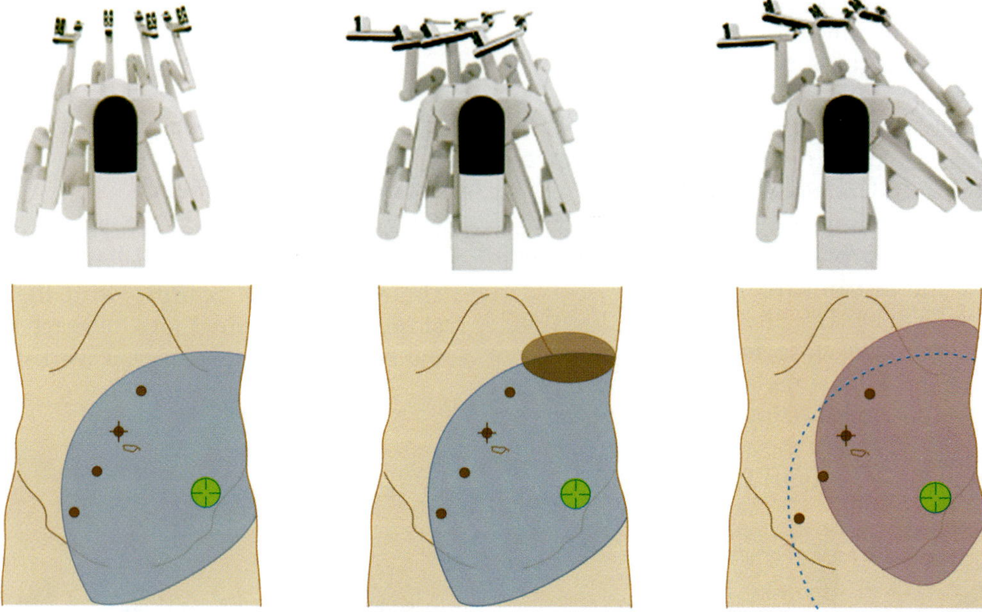

Fig. 28.30: Use of flex joints

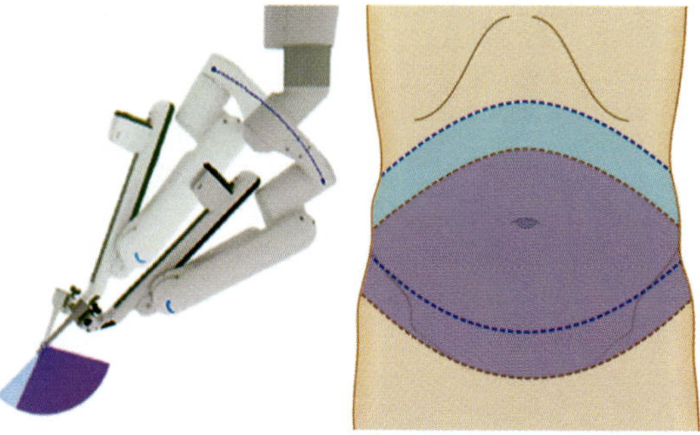

Fig. 28.31: Lowering of patient clearance joint

adjust all arms towards the direction where reach is desired **(Fig. 28.30)**.

- When desired workspace to be increased is beyond the level of the ports **(Fig. 28.31)**: Consider lowering the patient clearance joint where available so that the workspace is increased beyond the level of port.

Dual Docking (Fig. 28.32)

Dual docking can be used in procedures requiring a surgical workspace larger than two quadrants (for example, if the initial endoscope port cannot be placed 10–20 cm from the target anatomy, and two targets are necessary), and when working beyond the level of the ports does not provide enough instrument reach.

Steps of Dual Docking

- Identify the surgical workspace. If larger than two quadrants, or if the initial endoscope port cannot be placed 10–20 cm from the target anatomy, split the surgical workspace in half.
- Identify a target anatomy in each half.
- Place the initial endoscope port at equal distance between the two target anatomies (approximately 10–20 cm from each target).
- Place the remaining ports in a line between the two target anatomies.
  - Consider placing five ports in a line, allowing two right-hands or two left-hands in either set up. The lateral port

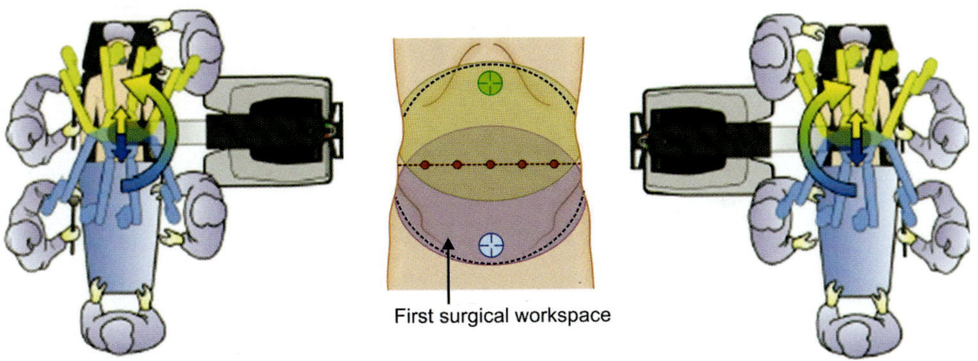

Fig. 28.32: Dual docking

(not docked to an instrument arm) can be used as an assistant port.

- The surgical workspace that is in-line with the ports is the most difficult to access. This may affect how the surgical workspace is divided and what target anatomies are identified.
- Set up the system for the first target anatomy.
- When ready to dual dock (for example, access the second target anatomy or additional workspace), remove all instruments and undock all arms.
- While the boom and instrument arms require readjustment, the patient cart location does not require readjustment.
- Position the boom to reach the target anatomy. Rotate the boom towards the column, this avoids a range of motion limit.
- Dock the initial endoscope port and perform targeting and docking.

Robot Malfunctions

Robot malfunctions may be classified as temporary (recoverable and capable of being electronically overridden) or critical (non-recoverable and thus necessitating a system shutdown or outage), resulting in the robotic assistance having to be aborted.

In a large-scale multi-institutional evaluation of robotic equipment malfunction, the authors found that the robotic components that most commonly experienced critical malfunctions were the optics (34%) and robotic arms (34%), followed by the masters (10%) and power supply (15%), and then unknown components (7%), with an overall critical malfunction rate of approximately 0.4%.

29
System Troubleshooting

Ashwin Sunil Tamhankar, Surya Prakash Ojha, Puneet Ahluwalia, Gagan Gautam

TECHNICAL SUPPORT

Support system is active for 24 hours for all seven days a week.

CONVERTING TO OPEN SURGERY OR OBTAINING IMMEDIATE ACCESS TO THE PATIENT

Following steps should be considered for immediate patient access
1. Remove the instruments from the patient
2. Remove the endoscope from the patient
3. Disconnect the cannulae from the arms
4. Move the arms away from the patient
5. If necessary, move the patient cart away from the patient.

TROUBLESHOOTING THE PATIENT CART DRIVE

In case of problem with automated drive mode, place the patient cart into manual drive. This manual drive feature lets you move the cart without using the powered motor drive.

UNEXPECTED MOTION

Unexpected motion occurs when the arm brakes are overpowered which can be because of excessive force on the patient and collisions of patient cart components (arms, nearby objects). If the system detects unexpected set up joint motion, the arm LED for the associated set up joint illuminates amber and a message appears on screen.

To clear the error, press the port clutch button for that arm. This also relieves any potential excessive force on the patient.

SYSTEM POWER ISSUES

When the da Vinci Xi system or an individual component (surgeon console, patient cart, and vision cart) fails to power on normally; or, fails to undergo an automatic, controlled power-down sequence the system might experience anomalous behavior.

If the entire system or either the surgeon console, patient cart, or vision cart fail to power on normally after pressing a component power button, check the AC power connections.

If all AC power connections are sound, follow the steps below:
1. Remove AC power from the vision cart and surgeon console by switching each AC power switch to off (indicated by "O" near each switch).
2. On the patient cart, press the EPO button to remove all power; it will remain partially pressed in.
3. Wait two seconds and then press the EPO button to reset it; it will rebound to its fully extended ready position.

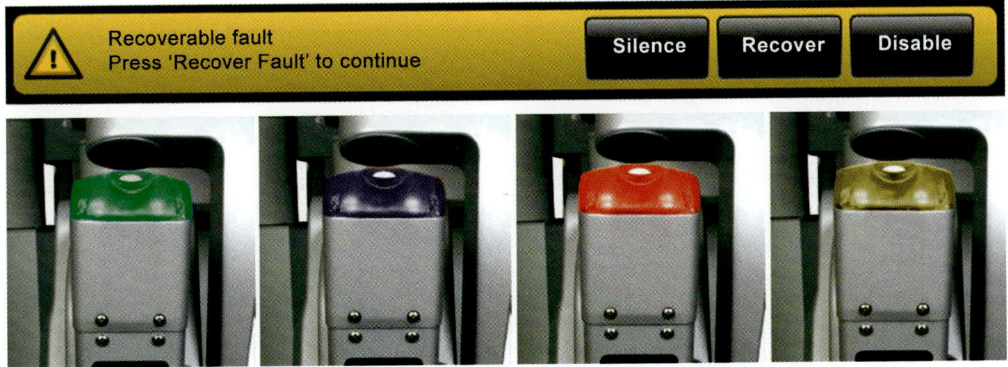

Fig. 29.1: da Vinci Si system arm LED colors

4. Switch on the vision cart and surgeon console AC power switches.
5. Verify that the patient cart AC power switch is in the on position (if not, switch it on). After 30 seconds, all three system components return to default standby mode. All three power buttons will be amber.
6. Power on the system normally, by pressing the power button on either the surgeon console, patient cart, or vision cart.

Restarting the System

Restart from Automatic High Temperature Power Down

This controlled power down prevents system damage. When the system detects overheating, it automatically initiates a 60-second power down sequence.

System Faults, Recoverable Faults and Non-recoverable Faults (Figs 29.1 and 29.2)

The system determines whether the fault is recoverable or non-recoverable.

If the fault is recoverable, you can override it by touching recover fault on the touchpads or touchscreen. The alarm silences and the system recovers after a few seconds.

If a fault is non-recoverable, the system has to be restarted.

Patient cart arm indicator of Xi system **(Table 29.1)**.

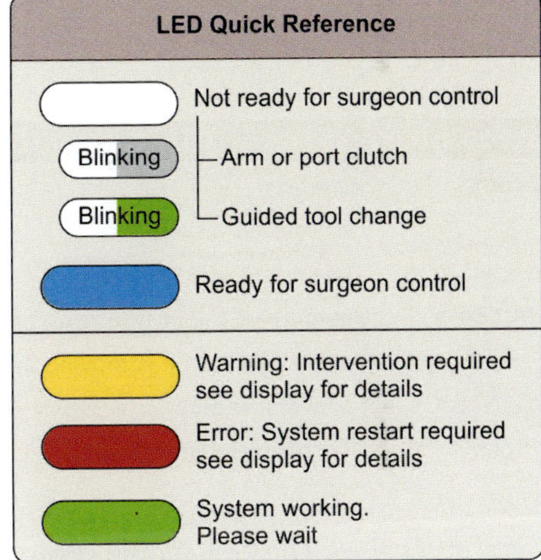

Fig. 29.2: da Vinci Si system arm LED colors

Patient cart boom LED indicator of Xi system **(Table 29.2)**.

STANDARD OF PRACTICE

Association of surgical technologies (AST) developed the following standard of practice (SOP) to support healthcare facilities (HCF) and reinforce best practices as related to the role and duties of the Certified Surgical Technologist (CST), the credential conferred by the National Board of Surgical Technology and Surgical Assisting (NBSTSA) during robotic surgical procedures.

TABLE 29.1: Patient cart arm indicator of Xi system

LED status	Meaning
Off	Unpowered/disabled/stowed
Blue/solid	The system is operating properly
Blue/blinking	• Instrument clutch or port dutch is in progress
	• Patient clearance should be considered to improve instrument reach
Blue/pulsing	• The arm is performing an activity which requires the user to wait for a brief period, for example, instrument engagement
	• The user is adjusting the patient clearance of the arm
Green/blinking	Guided tool change is in progress
Amber/solid	Recoverable fault
Amber/blinking	Arm-related issue that the user normally can resolve, including issues associated with instruments, for example, during a homing failed message
Red/solid	Non-recoverable fault

TABLE 29.2: Patient cart boom LED indicator of Xi system

LED status	Meaning
Off	Unpowered/disabled
Blue/solid	The system is operating properly
Blue/pulsing	Patient cart boom is moving and targeting laser is not active
Green/pulsing	Patient cart boom is moving and targeting laser is active
Amber/solid	Recoverable error
Red/solid	Non-recoverable error

Standard of practice I: The CST should complete training specific to the robotic device being used at the HCF.

Standard of practice II: It is recommended that the HCF designate an individual in the surgery department as the Robotics Team Leader.

Standard of practice III: The CST must have a thorough understanding of the two robotic components in order to be able to participate in setting up the components when scrubbed in or as an assistant circulator.

Standard of practice IV: The CST must have a thorough understanding of the specialty EndoWrist® instruments in order to properly handle and care for the instruments.

Standard of practice V: The CST should demonstrate the knowledge and skills with the preoperative preparation and set up of the system's components.

Standard of practice VI: The CST at the sterile field assists the surgeon in performing a safe robotic surgical procedure.

Standard of practice VII: The CST should work with troubleshooting system technical errors.

Standard of practice VIII: The CST must be prepared for conversion to an open procedure such as in the event of a patient emergency, e.g. unanticipated hemorrhage.

Standard of practice IX: The CST is responsible for break-down of the sterile back table including the initial decontamination of the robotic instrumentation and accessory items.

CONCLUSION

Robotic surgical platforms have a rapid and far reaching impact on the performance of minimally invasive surgical procedures in urologic surgery as well as other disciplines. The robot assistance in laparoscopic urological surgery tends to improve the level of dexterity and the degree of maneuverability. It leads to scaling of movements giving more precision for more intricate surgeries because of the intuitive nature of the working system.

ACKNOWLEDGMENTS

- da Vinci Si surgical system user manual P/N 550650-04 Rev. A 2011.09.
- da Vinci Xi surgical system user manual P/N 551400-08 Rev. A 2015.08.
- AST Standards of Practice on the Perioperative Role and Duties of the Surgical Technologist during Robotic Surgical Procedures. Approved October 11, 2013. Revised April 23, 2014.

30
Newer Robots on the Horizon

Aruj Shah, Arvind P Ganpule

Intuitive Surgical has commanded the market with sequential iterations of the da Vinci model (the S, Si and Xi). However, there are many issues that plague the platform. The lack of competition has hindered any control on costs and the initial high cost as well as recurring costs is a sore point for most hospitals. Insurance companies do not cover the additional cost associated with robotic platform over laparoscopy.[1] There is concern over the lack of haptic feedback. The setup is unwieldy and docking process takes a significant amount of time. The bulky operation cart occupies a large amount of space and limits access to the patient.

The expiration of patents has opened the market and several new contenders have become available or are currently in development. In this chapter, we look at the alternatives available in the market currently **(Fig. 30.1)**.

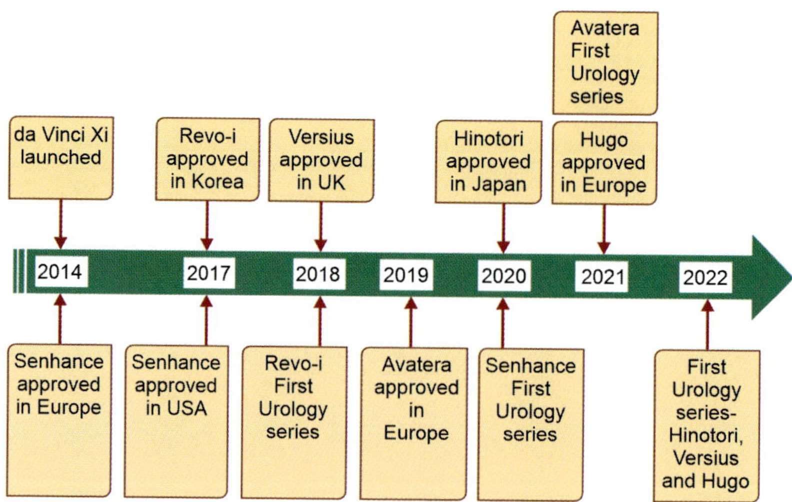

Fig. 30.1: Timeline of the various surgical robotic systems in urology

SENHANCE SURGICAL ROBOTIC SYSTEM (TRANSENTERIX, MORRISVILLE, NC)

Introduction

Originally known as ALF-X by the Sofar company, it was bought by US based Transenterix which later renamed it.[2] It was approved for use in Europe and USA in 2014 and 2017 respectively.

Components

It consists of a cockpit (remote control unit), a 3D high definition monitor, an infrared system for eye tracking, keyboard, touchpad, foot pedal, 4 independent arms and reusable laparoscopic instruments **(Fig. 30.2)**.[3]

The optics and needle holder require a 10 mm trocar for access. 5 mm ports are needed for all other instruments.

Unique Features[4]

- Any 3-D system of optics can be adapted for use with it
- The camera can be controlled simply by viewing various parts of the operative field (eye tracking)
- Haptic feedback helps in suturing and dissection.
- The same monitor can be viewed by the surgeon and the rest of the surgical team

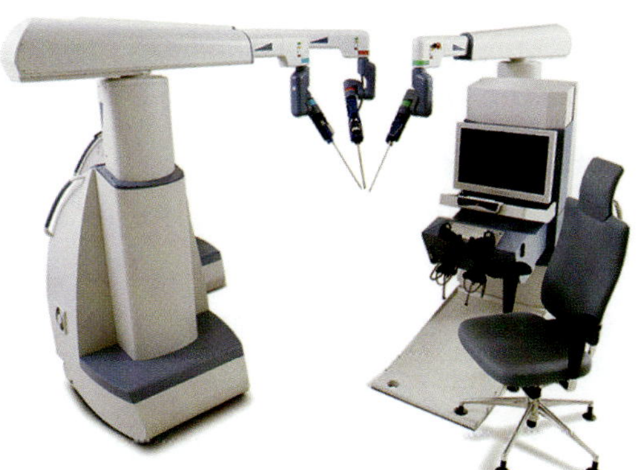

Fig. 30.2: Senhance surgical system

- Recurring cost is less as the laparoscopic instruments are reusable
- Surgeons trained in laparoscopy can easily migrate to this platform

Shortcomings

- The substantial size hinders access to the patient in case of an emergency.
- Urological publications are in porcine models. Marketed currently for use in gynecological or colorectal procedures. In Europe, it is CE marked for non-cardiac thoracic and abdominal applications.[5]
- The system uses non-wristed instruments that mimic laparoscopy.

REVO-I ROBOTIC SURGICAL SYSTEM (MEERE COMPANY, SOUTH KOREA)

Introduction

The Korean Ministry of Knowledge selected the Meere Company in 2010 to develop a surgical robot. The MSR-5000 REVO-I was launched in 2015 after several models and 20 odd animal studies.[6] It received Korean FDA approval in mid 2017.

Components

The systems include reusable instruments, four armed operation cart and a control console **(Fig. 30.3)**.

Unique Features[7]

- The 7.4 mm instruments allow seven degrees of freedom
- The instruments are reusable up to twenty times
- The latest version incorporates haptic feedback
- Availability of integrated online and off-line training courses including the Revo-Sim VR simulator
- *Multiple instruments can be used with this system including:* Forceps, needle holders, clip appliers and energy instruments that can be both monopolar or bipolar.

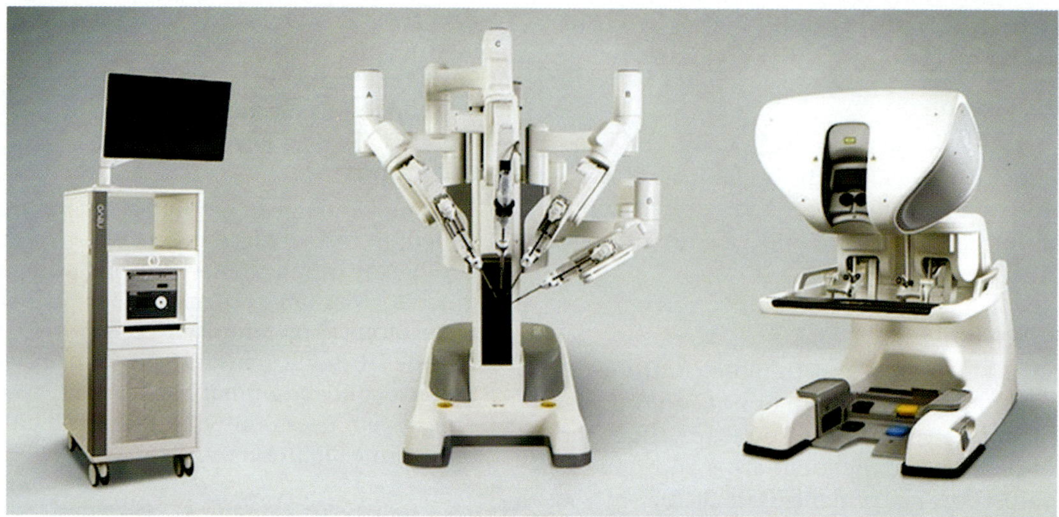

Fig. 30.3: REVO-I robotic surgical system

- *Newer energy sources:* Revo SONIC uses ultrasonic vibrations to simultaneous cut and seal the tissue.

Shortcomings

As compared to the da Vinci, there is lesser range of motion of the needle driver.[8]

VERSIUS SURGICAL SYSTEM (CMR LTD., CAMBRIDGE, UK)

Introduction

Launched by the Cambridge Medical Robotics (CMR), it received the European CE Mark in March, 2019.[5] It is a small, modular open console surgical robot designed for laparoscopic, gynaecological, upper GI, colorectal, thoracic, and urological surgeries.

Components[5]

It features an open console and five robotic arms called BSU (bedside unit) **(Fig. 30.4)**. To provide greater flexibility, each BSU has its own wheeled cart. In order to impersonate the human arm movement, the robotic arm has a shoulder, an elbow, and a wrist joint. The instruments measure 5 mm in diameter.

Unique Features[9]

- The surgeon can adopt either a standing or a sitting position.
- V-wrist technology allows 360° of wrist motion and 7 degrees of freedom
- The system provides haptic feedback
- The modular design permits greater flexibility of positioning
- The system is mobile and compact sized. Thus in case of an emergency, it is easier and faster to convert to open surgery, thereby facilitating hybrid manual—robotic procedures.
- *Versius trainer:* A small unit that plugs directly into a standard Versius console to deliver a variety of training exercises.

Shortcomings

As compared to the da Vinci, arm collisions were more frequently reported.[10]

THE HUGO RAS SYSTEM (MEDTRONIC, MINNEAPOLIS, MN, USA)

Introduction[11]

The first procedure was conducted in Chile (2021). It was approved for use in Europe for

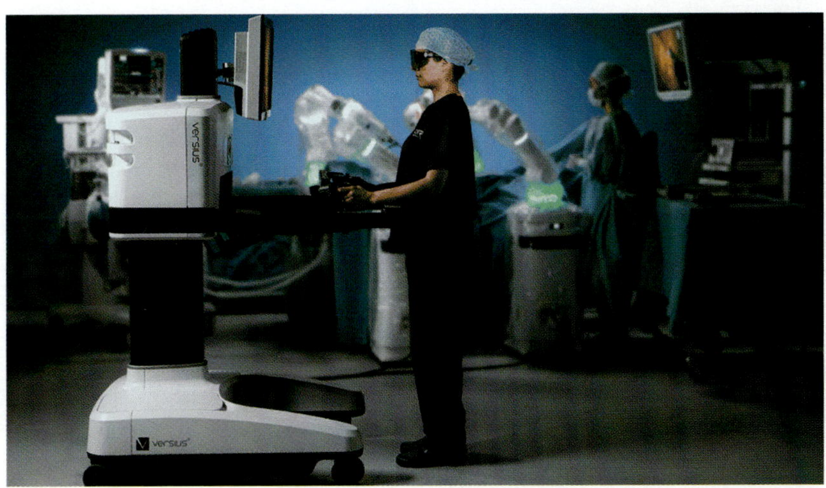

Fig. 30.4: Versius surgical system

TABLE 30.1: Overview of the robotic surgical systems available in India at the time of publication

	da Vinci	*Hugo RAS*	*SSI Mantra*	*Versius*
Console	Closed	Open	Open	Open
Optics	8 mm 3D HD	Karl Storz 3D Tipcam S (12 mm)	Information not available	10 mm 3D 0 degree
Energy sources	Monopolar/bipolar/ SynchroSeal/Vessel Sealer Extend	Monopolar/bipolar/ LigaSure	Monopolar/bipolar	Monopolar/bipolar
Instrument size	8 mm	8 mm	8 mm	5 mm
Haptic feedback	No	Information not available	Information not available	Yes
Reusability	Yes	Yes	Yes	Yes
Instrument and arm control	Manipulator mimics the end effectors via pinching or grasping motion	Manipulator is trigger operated	Information not available	Manipulator resembles a game controller
Arm switching	Feature provided by foot pedal	Information not available	Information not available	Feature provided by axillary controls on hand controller

urological and gynecological procedures in 2022. Pursuant to an investigational device exemption (IDE) from the US FDA, the Expand URO US trial is in progress.

Components[12]

It consists of four arm carts, a console and a system tower. It features an open console with a 32-inch 3D high definition display to be used with special glasses. The two arm controllers have pistol grip like handgrips and a foot pedal for controlling the reserve arm, energy sources and the camera. Endoscopic vision is provided by Karl Storz 3D Tipcam S **(Table 30.1)**.

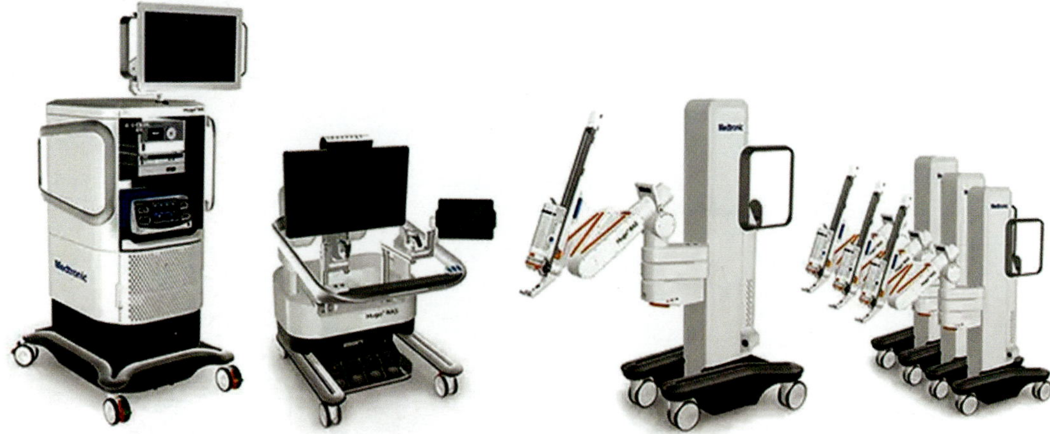

Fig. 30.5: The Hugo RAS system

Unique Features[13]

- Each robotic arm is independent and extendible which permits greater flexibility of positioning and reduces collision risk **(Fig. 30.5)**.
- Six different joints on each arm promises a greater manoeuvring range.
- The bedside assistant has more working space as the independent arms allow for better flexibility of positioning.

Shortcomings

- There is increased complexity of docking multiple robotic arms independently.
- In one study, the authors noted that the docking process was longer with the Hugo RAS.[14]

SSI MANTRA (SS INNOVATIONS PVT LTD)

Introduction[15]

SSI MANTRA stands for the company making it—SS Innovations and Multi Arm Novel Tele Robotic Assistance. The company is founded and named after a cardiothoracic surgeon of Indian origin, Dr. Sudhir Srivastava. The first installation was at the Rajiv Gandhi Cancer Institute and Research Centre in New Delhi in late 2022.

Components[16]

It is a modular multi-arm system with an open console **(Table 30.1)**, up to 5 robotic arms and a 32-inch three dimensional 4K monitor **(Fig. 30.6)**.

Unique Features[17]

- It is a more affordable robotic system—one-third the cost of its global competitors
- The modular robotic arm carts provide greater flexibility
- Digital user guide touch panel (23 inch) for patient related information
- Allows for superimposition of 3D holographically reconstructed DICOM images.

Shortcomings

- Individual cart arms occupy more space in the OT, reduce patient access, take longer to undock in case of emergency
- Intraoperative port hopping is not possible: Independent 4 surgical carts with dedicated camera arm

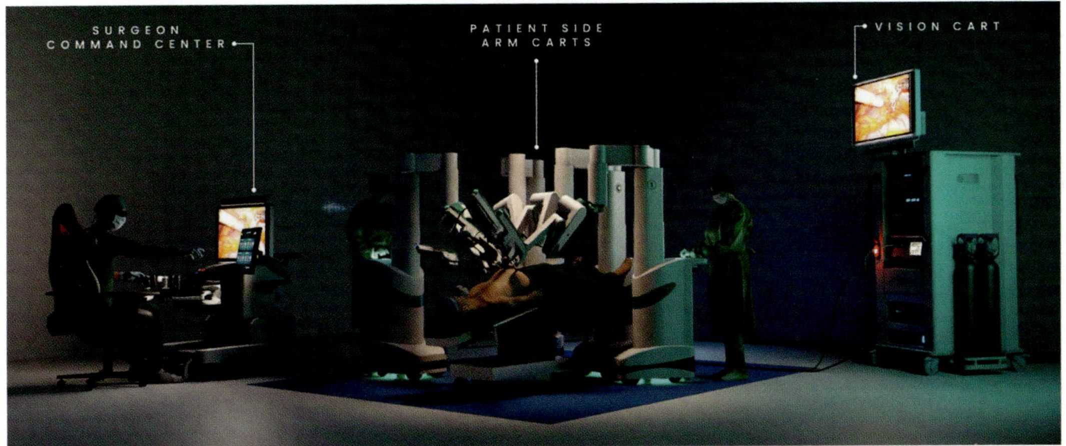

Fig. 30.6: SSI MANTRA

- Dual console not available, hence training residents takes a hit
- Unavailability of integrated energy source

DA VINCI SINGLE-PORT (SP) PLATFORM (INTUITIVE SURGICAL INC, SUNNYVALE CA)

Introduction[18]

In 2010, the da Vinci single-site platform was developed to integrate the utility of single-port surgery and robotic surgery. The FDA approved its use for urological procedures in 2018.

Components[19]

The only entry point is a 25 mm multichannel port **(Figs 30.7A and B)**. 12 × 10 mm 3D high definition camera provides 73 degree field of view. Intracorporeal triangulation is achieved with the help of three double jointed instruments which provide 7 degrees of freedom. A 'relocation' pedal helps to shift the entire robotic arm without moving the instruments. The instruments' relative position is tracked by the navigation interface, an image overlay.

Unique Features

- A dual surgeon console setup helps in training residents

- According to a meta-analysis, SP systems were related with shorter hospital stays while demonstrating equivalence in terms of operative time and blood loss.[20]
- Improved cosmetic outcomes as only a single incision is placed on the body.
- Two flexible joints allow for greater power and increased free access to the target anatomy.

Shortcomings

- Even surgeons with experience on multi-port systems will face a learning curve on transition to single port system
- The 'elbow' joint produces a right angle and thus requires a larger workspace in comparison to straight instruments.
- The cannula setting must be lifted from the GelPass port to ensure space for a secondary trocar to help with suctioning and irrigation.[21]

THE AVATERA (AVATERAMEDICAL, JENA, GERMANY)

Introduction[22]

For use in gynaecology and urology, it was approved in Europe in November 2019. The first clinical use was in 2022 at the University of Leipzig Medical Center, Germany.

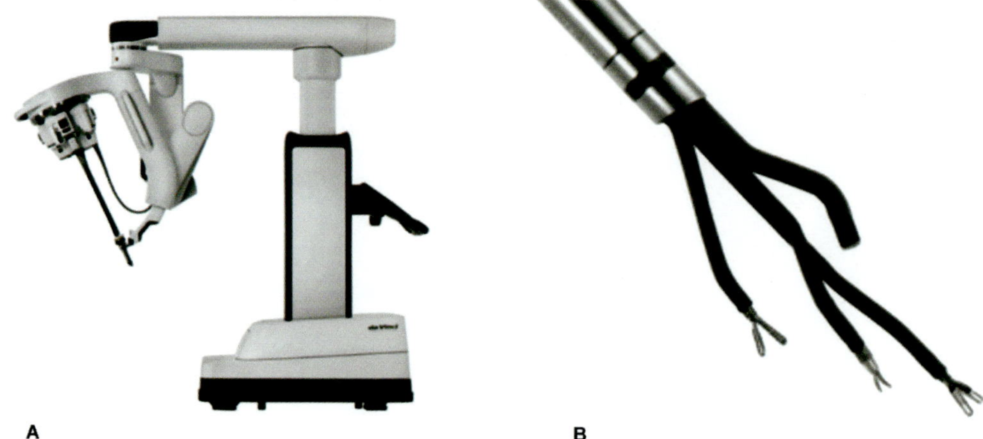

Figs 30.7A and B: (A) da Vinci single-port robotic system; (B) Single 25 mm port with endoscope and 3 instrument arms

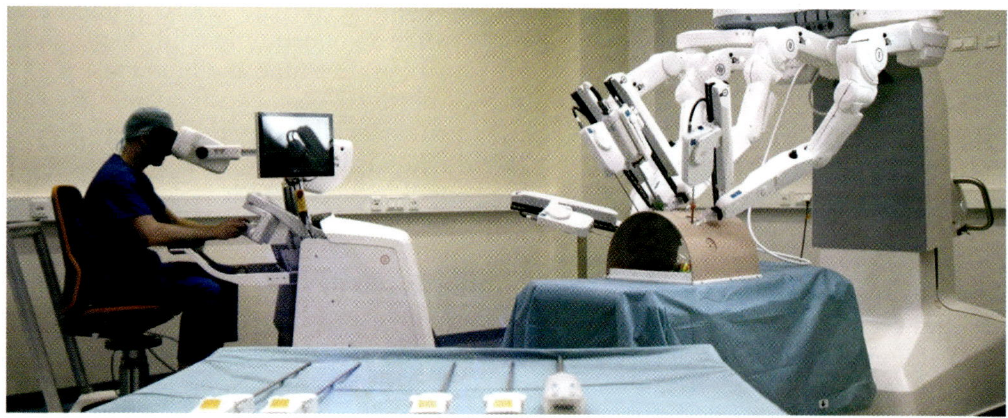

Fig. 30.8: The Avatera system

Components[23]

The Avatera consists of a robotic cart, 4 arms and a console unit **(Fig. 30.8)**. The surgeon wears an eyepiece which keeps his/her ears and mouth uncovered. Looplike handles are used to control the instruments. The system uses disposable 5 mm instruments which offer 7 degrees of freedom.

Unique Features[24]

- It saves space as it has only two main parts: Surgical robot and control unit.

- The slender eyepiece facilitates easy communication by keeping the surgeon's ears and mouth uncovered.
- Single use concept saves cost by eliminating the cumbersome and expensive sterilization processes.
- Availability of VR simulator for training.

Shortcomings

The feasibility of this new system for cystectomy and nephrectomy requires further studies.

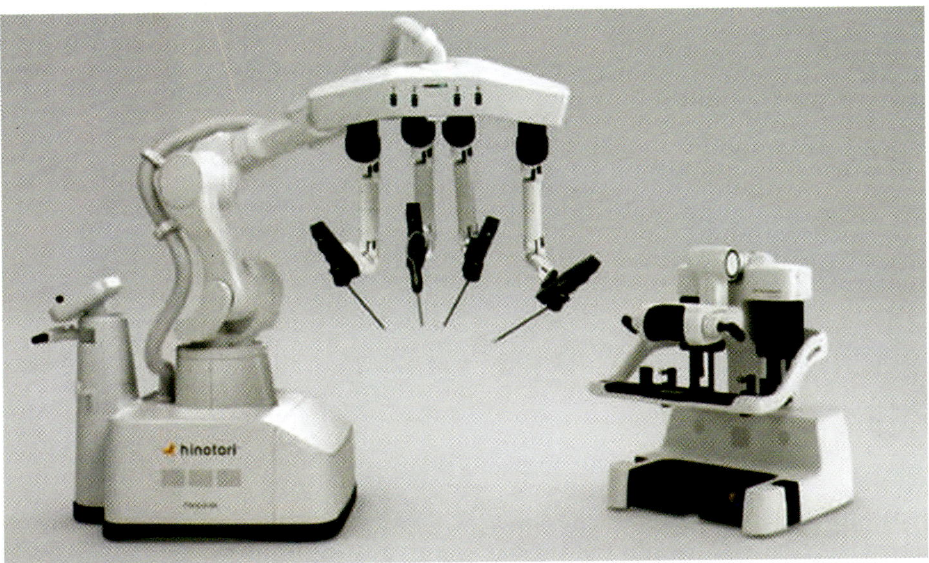

Fig. 30.9: Hinotori surgical robot system

THE HINOTORI ROBOTIC SYSTEM (MEDICAROID, KOBE, HYOGO, JAPAN)

Introduction[25]

Medicaroid Corporation is a joint venture by Kawasaki and Sysmex Corporation. Its initial surgery, radical prostatectomy was carried out at the International Clinical Cancer Research (ICCRC) at Kobe University Hospital. It is approved for use in Japan.

Components[26]

It is composed of the three units: Surgeon Cockpit, Operation Unit and Vision Unit **(Fig. 30.9)**. It consists of a patient cart with four 8-axis operation arms and a semi-closed surgeon console. Three dimensional view of the operative field is provided by a microscope-like eyepiece. Loop-like handles are used to control the wristed instruments.

Unique Features[26]

- It offers smoother movements by adding 8th degree of freedom in its 4 arm operational unit.

- Transitioning between the da Vinci and Hinotori should be straightforward as both the systems are quite similar to use.
- It boasts a 'docking-free' system, designed to reduce interference between arms and with the bedside assistant.
- Availability of training simulation system.

THE DEXTER ROBOT (DISTALMOTION SA)

Introduction[27]

The Dexter surgical robot is European CE-marked for use in gynecology, general surgery and urology. It integrates the affordability of laparoscopy with the perks of robotic surgery **(Fig. 30.10)**. A simple and a radical prostatectomy were the first urological procedures carried out with the Dexter robot in June, 2022 at Bern.

Components[27]

The open console is mobile and can be adapted to either a standing or a seated position. The two arms can be realigned to change trocar sites intraoperatively. It uses disposable 8 mm

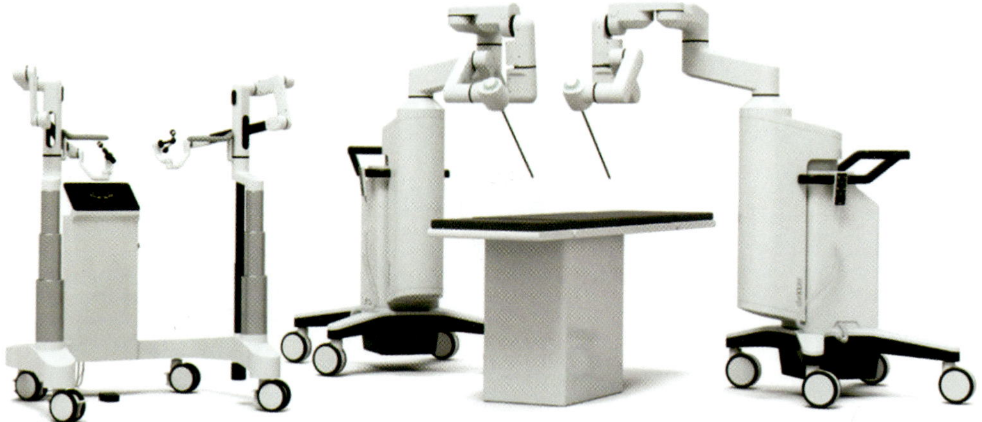

Fig. 30.10: The Dexter robot

articulated instruments for dissection and suturing using monopolar and bipolar intruments **(Fig. 30.10)**.

Unique Features[28]

- The surgeon can easily switch between robotic surgery and laparoscopy as he remains sterile while operating at the console.
- It can be used with any commercial laparoscopic tower and is engineered to work with all laparoscopic instruments.
- Integrates seamlessly into any operating room and can be easily transported between operating rooms
- Single use instruments ensure consistently reliable performance
- It provides haptic feedback to the surgeon
- Availability of simulator based training

REFERENCES

1. Assessment of Out-of-Pocket Costs for Robotic Cancer Surgery in US Adults - PMC [Internet]. [cited 2023 Jul 20]. Available from: https://www.ncbi.nlm.nih.gov/pmc/articles/PMC6991257/

2. The Future of Robotic Surgery in Pediatric Urology: Upcoming Technology and Evolution Within the Field - PMC [Internet]. [cited 2023 Jul 20]. Available from: https://www.ncbi.nlm.nih.gov/pmc/articles/PMC6614201/

3. First experience in colorectal surgery with a new robotic platform with haptic feedback | Request PDF [Internet]. [cited 2023 Jul 20]. Available from: https://www.researchgate.net/publication/319758179_First_experience_in_colorectal_surgery_with_a_new_robotic_platform_with_haptic_feedback

4. What's New | Senhance Surgical System [Internet]. [cited 2023 Jul 20]. Available from: https://www.senhance.com/us/home

5. Robotic surgical systems in urology: What is currently available? - PMC [Internet]. [cited 2023 Jul 20]. Available from: https://www.ncbi.nlm.nih.gov/pmc/articles/PMC7801159/

6. (PDF) Retzius-sparing Robot-assisted Radical Prostatectomy using Revo-i robotic surgical system: Surgical Technique and Results of the First Human Trial [Internet]. [cited 2023 Jul 20]. Available from: https://www.researchgate.net/publication/324479396_Retzius-sparing_Robot-assisted_Radical_Prostatectomy_using_Revo-i_robotic_surgical_system_Surgical_Technique_and_Results_of_the_First_Human_Trial

7. Revo | Robotic Surgical Solution [Internet]. [cited 2023 Jul 20]. Available from: http://revo-surgical.com/render/view/index/

8. Robotic surgery: new robots and finally some real competition! - PubMed [Internet]. [cited 2023 Jul 20]. Available from: https://pubmed.ncbi.nlm.nih.gov/29427003/

9. Versius - CMR Surgical [Internet]. [cited 2023 Jul 20]. Available from: https://cmrsurgical.com/versius.

10. Transition from da Vinci to Versius robotic surgical system: initial experience and outcomes

of over 100 consecutive procedures - PubMed [Internet]. [cited 2023 Jul 20]. Available from: https://pubmed.ncbi.nlm.nih.gov/35752748/

11. New multiport robotic surgical systems: a comprehensive literature review of clinical outcomes in urology - PMC [Internet]. [cited 2023 Jul 20]. Available from: https://www.ncbi.nlm.nih.gov/pmc/articles/PMC10265325/

12. The new robotic platform HugoTM RAS for lateral transabdominal adrenalectomy: a first world report of a series of five cases - PMC [Internet]. [cited 2023 Jul 20]. Available from: https://www.ncbi.nlm.nih.gov/pmc/articles/PMC9834370/

13. HugoTM RAS System | Medtronic [Internet]. [cited 2023 Jul 20]. Available from: https://www.medtronic.com/covidien/en-us/robotic-assisted-surgery/hugo-ras-system.html

14. Robot-Assisted Laparoscopic Radical Prostatectomy Utilizing Hugo RAS Platform: Initial Experience - PubMed [Internet]. [cited 2023 Jul 20]. Available from: https://pubmed.ncbi.nlm.nih.gov/36205571/

15. SSI MANTRA: How This 'Made-In-India' Robotic Surgery System Is Setting A Shining Example [Internet]. [cited 2023 Jul 20]. Available from: https://swarajyamag.com/science/ssi-mantra-how-this-made-in-india-robotic-surgery-system-is-setting-a-shining-example

16. India's first indigenously developed surgical Robot – SSI Mantra – Flawlessly Executes Robotic Lung Surgery at Nitrd, a First by a Central Govt Hospital - Modern Medi Health | Medical, Healthcare And Wellness Magazine [Internet]. [Cited 2023 Jul 20]. Available From: Http://Modernmedihealth.com/Indias-First-Indigenously-Developed-Surgical-Robot-Ssi-Mantra-Flawlessly-Executes-Robotic-Lung-Surgery-At-Nitrd-A-First-By-A-Central-Govt-Hospital/

17. SSI Mantra - SS Innovations International Inc. [Internet]. [cited 2023 Jul 20]. Available from: https://ssinnovations.com/ssi-mantra/

18. Robotic Single-Port Donor Nephrectomy with the da Vinci SP® Surgical System - PMC [Internet]. [cited 2023 Jul 21]. Available from: https://www.ncbi.nlm.nih.gov/pmc/articles/PMC8692076/

19. Robotic perineal radical prostatectomy and pelvic lymph node dissection using a purpose-built single-port robotic platform | Request PDF [Internet]. [cited 2023 Jul 21]. Available from: https://www.researchgate.net/publication/305312923_Robotic_perineal_radical_prostatectomy_and_pelvic_lymph_node_dissection_using_a_purpose-built_single-port_robotic_platform

20. Single-port versus multiport robotic-assisted radical prostatectomy: A systematic review and meta-analysis on the da Vinci SP platform - PubMed [Internet]. [cited 2023 Jul 21]. Available from: https://pubmed.ncbi.nlm.nih.gov/34985775/

21. Robotic single-port surgery using the da Vinci SP® surgical system for benign gynecologic disease: A preliminary report - ScienceDirect [Internet]. [cited 2023 Jul 21]. Available from: https://www.sciencedirect.com/science/article/pii/S1028455920300127

22. Avateramedical robot-assisted surgery system progresses to [Internet]. [cited 2023 Jul 21]. Available from: https://www. globenewswire.com/en/news-release/2022/05/10/2439328/0/en/avateramedical-robot-assisted-surgery-system-progresses-to-clinical-use.html

23. (PDF) The Availability, Cost, Limitations, Learning Curve and Future of Robotic Systems in Urology and Prostate Cancer Surgery [Internet]. [cited 2023 Jul 21]. Available from: https://www.researchgate.net/publication/369275915_The_Availability_Cost_Limitations_Learning_Curve_and_Future_of_Robotic_Systems_in_Urology_and_Prostate_Cancer_Surgery

24. Avatera system - avateramedical [Internet]. [cited 2023 Jul 21]. Available from: https://www.avatera.eu/en/avatera-system

25. Japan: Surgical support robot succeeds in first surgery: Removal of prostate cancer | Tokio X'press [Internet]. [cited 2023 Jul 22]. Available from: http://tokiox.com/wp/japan-surgical-support-robot-succeeds-in-surgery-removal-of-cancer/?lang=en

26. System Hinotori Robotic Assisted Surgery System Product Medicaroid [Internet]. [cited 2023 Jul 22]. Available from: https://www.medicaroid.com/en/product/hinotori/

27. Distalmotion Dexter surgical robot receives European CE Mark [Internet]. [cited 2023 Jul 22]. Available from: https://www.therobotreport.com/distalmotion-dexter-surgical-robot-receives-european-ce-mark/

28. Distalmotion | Dexter [Internet]. [cited 2023 Jul 22]. Available from: https://www.distalmotion.com/dexter

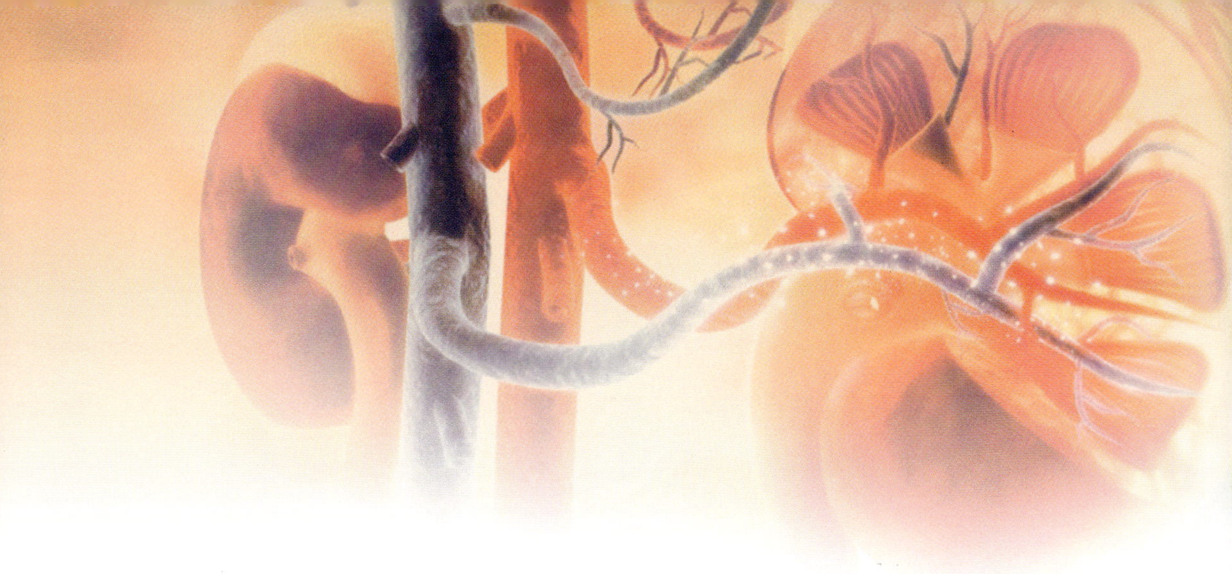

Part 3

Partial Penectomy and VEIL

CHAPTERS

31
Introduction

Srivatsa N, Raghunath S Krishnappa, Nagaraja VH, Tejus C

Treatment of the primary penile cancer lesion aims to remove the tumor completely, while preserving as much of the penis as possible without compromising radicality. Local recurrence has a little effect on long-term survival so that organ preservation strategies can be used wherever possible.

Close to 80% of penile carcinomas occur distally, involving the glans and/or prepuce, which are potentially amenable to organ-preserving surgery.

The overall quality of the available research evidence is low for organ preserving procedures as the overall burden of penile cancers is low. There are no randomized controlled trials or observational studies for surgical management of localized penile cancer nor studies comparing surgical and non-surgical modalities. Penile preservation appears to be superior in functional and cosmetic outcomes. It is the primary treatment method for men with localized penile cancer. However, there are no randomized studies comparing organ-preserving and ablative treatment strategies, only retrospective studies with a poor level of evidence or less exist as of date.

While many minimally invasive and less disfiguring therapeutic options exist for management of early penile cancers. Glansectomy and partial penectomy remain by far the most commonly performed procedures. Li J et al, in 2011 published their series of cases undergoing partial penectomy and illustrated the complications and outcomes over a 4-year period. All cases which are T2/T3 present in the distal shaft of the penis qualify for partial penectomy and is the current standard of care.

A traditional 2 cm excision margin has been challenged as unnecessary for patients undergoing partial penectomy for squamous cell carcinoma. Conservative techniques involving surgical margins of even less than 10 mm appear to offer excellent long-term oncological control.

Lesions which after a negative surgical margin on frozen section analysis cannot be of functional utility for voiding are disqualified from the choice of partial penectomy.

Tumor location especially with reference to the meatus, size, histology, stage as well as patient factors play an important role in the choice of surgical treatment.

A true concern of penile preserving surgery is the potential risk of recurrence, both local as well as distant.

For all surgical treatment options, the intraoperative assessment of surgical margins by frozen section is recommended as tumor-positive margins lead to local recurrence. Total removal of the glans (glansectomy) and prepuce has the lowest recurrence rate for the treatment of small penile lesions (2%). Negative surgical margins are imperative when using penile-conserving treatments and a margin of 5 mm is considered oncologically safe.

32
Surgical Technique

Srivatsa N, Raghunath S Krishnappa, Nagaraja VH, Tejus C

STANDARD TECHNIQUE (Figs 32.1A TO D)

The surgery is usually carried out with regional anesthesia with the patient in supine position. The genitalia is prepared and draped in a sterile manner. A tourniquet is positioned around the base of the phallus and the incision is outlined circumferentially using a marker pen. This step is vital to avoid skewing of incision and loss of excess skin which is vital for a good reconstruction subsequently. The penile lesion itself can be covered with a condom or sterile surgical glove. The circumferential incision is carried down through the skin and subcutaneous tissue. The neurovascular bundle is identified, mobilized and divided. At this stage, attention is paid to the isolation of urethra. The corpus spongiosum is then divided to gain access to the urethra. Maximum length of

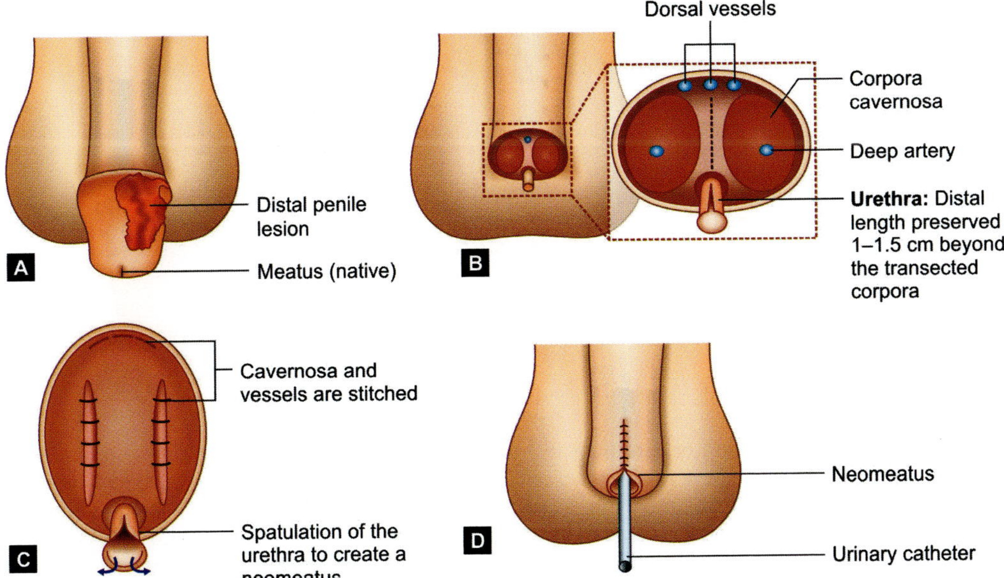

Figs 32.1A to D: Schematic diagram of standard technique of partial penectomy

healthy urethra is isolated which facilitates preservation of maximum penile length subsequently. The corpora cavernosa are then divided sharply in a manner which provides a further distal length of the urethra of 1.5 to 2 cm. The corporal vessels are bipolarized and the tunica of corpora approximated with running sutures of 3–0 PDS. The polydioxanone serves to remain in the repaired tissue for a longer time till occurrence of complete healing but subsequently get absorbed leaving no risks of long-term retention like suture granulomas or sinus formation. The penile skin is then brought over as a hood on the distal penis and a small opening is made in the reapproximated penile skin to accommodate the urethra. The urethral neomeatus is then matured similar to a stoma creation. The dorsal aspect of the distal urethra is incised and is folded back and sewn to the penile skin. When this neomeatus is complete, a Foley catheter is left indwelling for 48–72 hours and a pressure dressing applied to prevent any hematoma formation **(Figs 32.1A to D)**.

PARACHUTE TECHNIQUE (Figs 32.2A TO F)

Parachute technique was described in 2010 by the Brazilian group of Korkes and Machado et al with better cosmetic results and better

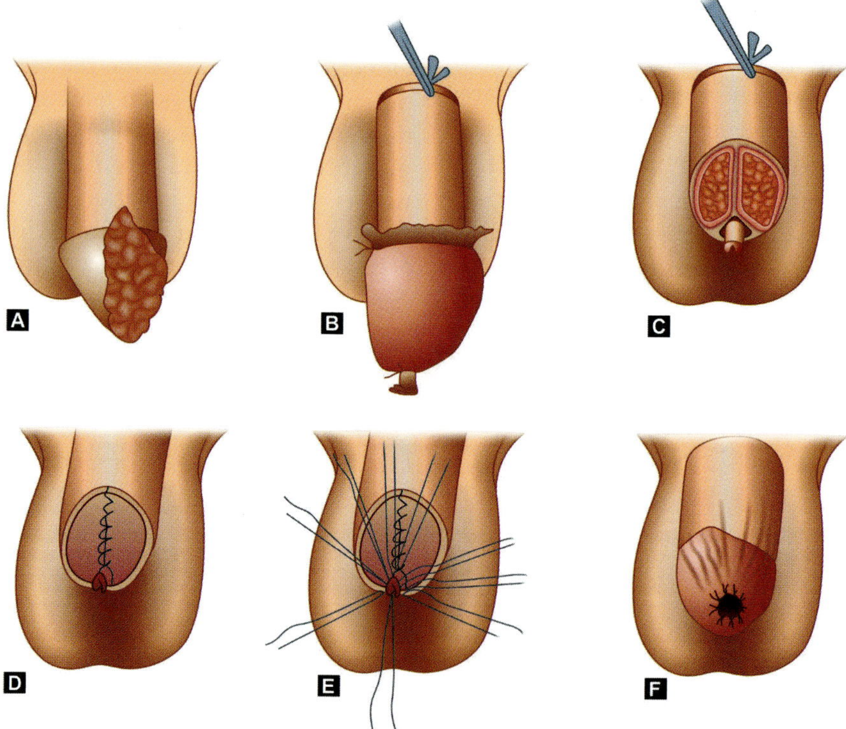

Figs 32.2A to F: Schematic drawing of parachute technique for partial penectomy. (A) Penile tumor elective for partial penectomy; (B) A surgical glove is secured distally to the proposed line of amputation and a tourniquet is applied at the base of the penis; (C) Skin is incised circumferentially around the penis, deepening to Buck's fascia, the urethra is isolated from the corpora cavernosa, divided and spatulated only ventrally; (D) Corpora cavernosa are closed with continuous sutures with Vicryl 2–0, the tourniquet is removed and adequate hemostasis is obtained; (E) Final suture is performed with Vicryl 4–0 in a "parachute" fashion, beginning from the ventral portion of the urethra and the "V" flap, followed by the "V" flap angles and than by the dorsal portion of the penis; (F) Final aspect

functional results in context to reduced neo-meatal strictures.

Similar to the conventional technique, patients are generally operated in the supine position, under spinal anesthetic block. After proper asepsis, a surgical glove or condom secured distally to the proposed line of amputation excludes the lesion. A tourniquet is applied at the base of the penis. The skin is incised circumferentially around the penis, deepening to Buck's fascia. The urethra is isolated from the corpora cavernosa and divided, aiming to obtain at least 1 cm distal redundancy, but without oncological compromise (at least 1–2 cm margin). Dorsal vein complex is ligated, corpora are divided, and the surgical specimen is sent to the laboratory for frozen section analysis. Corpora are secured with continuous sutures with Vicryl 2–0, opposing the margins of Buck's fascia. Tourniquet is removed and adequate hemostasis is obtained.

Different from classical technique, the urethra is spatulated only ventrally. An inverted "V" skin flap with 0.5 cm of extension is sectioned ventrally. The suture is performed with Vicryl 4–0 in a "parachute" fashion, beginning from the ventral portion of the urethra and the "V" flap, followed by the "V" flap angles and then by the dorsal portion of the penis. After completion of the suture, a Foley catheter and light dressing are placed for 24 hours **(Figs 32.2A to F)**.

Partial Penectomy Caveats

- Watch for infection, bleeding and meatal stenosis.
- The risk of local recurrence is 4–13%, nodal recurrence is 14–19%, cancer specific deaths 11–27% (EAU guidelines 2017).
- Local recurrence: A second organ preserving procedure can be performed if there is no corpus cavernosum invasion.
- Overall, only 33.3% maintained their preoperative frequency of sexual intercourse and were satisfied with their sex life.
- Regular self-examination of penis. Follow-up is more extensive for the initial 2 years: Every 3rd monthly up to 2 years, followed by 6th monthly up to completion of 5 years.

33
Troubleshooting during and after Partial Penectomy

Srivatsa N, Raghunath S Krishnappa, Nagaraja VH, Tejus C

MARGIN POSITIVITY

One of the most common issues after partial penectomy is a positive resection margin. Historically, the margins were recommended to have a 2 cm clearance from the proximal most point of induration to decrease the incidence of margin positivity. However, this precluded most of the patients from undergoing partial penectomy as a 2 cm margin would not provide an adequate residual stump sufficient to facilitate erect voiding.

In most of the old case series, margin positivity rates were close to 14%.[1] With the widespread availability of frozen section analysis, the rates steadily declined and recently is close to less than 1%.[2]

The application of frozen section analysis has also considerably reduced the margin length required for clearance from the conventional 2 cm to the present standard of a few millimeters.[2,3] It is now mandatory to attempt a penile preserving surgery only with the resource of frozen section analysis. One of the caveats of frozen section analysis is the "margin retraction phenomenon". In this, the frozen section report appears all clear but once the specimen is introduced into formalin, the tissues shrink and brings the positive edge of the disease closer to the final margin. To avoid this, the pathologist must be requested to mention the distance of presence of disease from the margin when the tissue is being reported on frozen section analysis.

INADEQUATE LENGTH OF URETHRAL STUMP

This is one of the most common issues encountered intraoperatively. A retracted urethral stump disfigures the penile stump and puckers the neomeatus which causes subsequent recurrent neomeatal stenosis or splaying of urine. Care should be exercised to maintain an additional urethral stump of 1 to 1.5 cm during partial penectomy. In cases where the urethral margin is positive for malignancy and/or the urethra is inadvertently cut proximally, neomeatus should be considered by developing a penile skin flap. The vascularity of the urethra is typically derived from vessels running at 3 and 9 o'clock positions and it is also possible to mobilize the urethra taking care to preserve the corpus spongiosum to protect the vessels. An additional length of up to 1 cm can be safely gained with this maneuver to provide an adequate urethral stump for closure using the parachute technique.[4]

Revision of the stump should generally be reserved as a last salvage as it would affect the functionality of the remnant penis.

However, it can be considered when the initial transection has been much distal, as in the situations of glansectomy.

POST-PROCEDURE BLEEDING

Post-procedure bleeding is a common occurrence and the best way to prevent the same is by individually identifying the vessels and either cauterizing them with bipolar cautery or by transfixing them. At a deeper level, it is important to identify and bipolarize the cavernosal vessels. A careful closure of the tunica albuginea is very important to prevent subsequent bleeding which occurs with penile stump tumescence. It is also prudent to release the tourniquet after closure of the tunica albuginea to ascertain adequate hemostasis. A pressure dressing applied on the stump over an urethral catheter, maintained for 48 hours will also be useful in achieving hemostasis. In most instances, the catheter can be removed along with the dressing if hemostasis is adequate and wound is clean and healthy, at the end of 48 hours.

Video endoscopic inguinal lymphadenectomy (VEIL) is a new minimally invasive procedure that can result in lower complication rates and shorter hospitalization stay without compromising oncologic results. Originally described by Tobias Machado in 2006 and subsequently published in 2007, he described the VEIL using laparoscopic instruments and the oncological outcomes on 10 patients so studied were similar to contemporary literature of open inguinal lymph node dissection (ILND). Subsequent observations from the same group and also by Sudhir Rawal et al in 2012 revealed that VEIL had a morbidity rate of only 15% while standard open ILND had a 70% morbidity rate. In addition, the number of nodes removed was the same for VEIL as it is for open ILND, while also showing no local or systemic relapse after a median follow-up of 33 months. However, long-term data is still lacking in this promising new treatment modality for ILND and would benefit from larger multicenter trials with an extensive follow-up period.

REFERENCES

1. Positive resection margins in partial penectomies: sites of involvement and proposal of local routes of spread of penile squamous cell carcinoma. Velazquez EF1, Soskin A, Bock A, Codas R, Barreto JE, Cubilla AL. Am J Surg Pathol. 2004;28(3):384–89.
2. Minhas S, Kayes O, Hegarty P, Kumar P, Freeman A, Ralph D. What surgical resection margins are required to achieve oncological control in men with primary penile cancer? BJU International. 2005;96:1040–43.
3. Penile preserving and reconstructive surgery in the management of penile cancer. Arthur L. Burnett. Nature Reviews Urology. 2016;13: 249–57.
4. Advances in Surgical Reconstructive Techniques in the Management of Penile, Urethral, and Scrotal Cancer. Michael Bickell et al. UCNA. 2016;43(4):545–55.

34

Surgical Technique of Video Endoscopic Inguinal Lymphadenectomy

Srivatsa N, Raghunath S Krishnappa, Nagaraja VH, Tejus C

All patients are thoroughly investigated pre-operatively and optimized. This procedure can be accomplished either under general anesthesia or under combined spinal and epidural block anesthesia. Surface marking: Markings are done for femoral triangle, inguinal ligament, anterior superior iliac spine, and saphenofemoral junction. Patient positioning: The lower limb is folded at knee and thigh externally rotated to make the femoral triangle more prominent. The limb fixed to the table. The video monitor is positioned at the contralateral side at the level of patient's pelvic waist. Port placement and gas insufflation: An incision of 1.5 cm in the skin and in the subcutaneous tissue is made 2 cm distal to the femoral triangle vertex. A plane developed deep to Scarpa's fascia with trocar and balloon and blunt finger dilatation. Thirty-degree camera is introduced through this 10 mm port, and CO_2 gas insufflation done at 14 cm of H_2O to create the space. Further, 10 mm and 5 mm ports are inserted under vision. Second port is inserted through a 1 cm incision at around 2 cm above and 6 cm medially to the first incision for a 10 mm port. A third 5 mm incision for 5 mm port is made laterally in symmetrical position on the opposite side for using graspers, scissors, or harmonic shears. The insufflations pressure is subsequently reduced to 8 cm of H_2O which should be sufficient to complete the procedure. Intermittent decompression of the flap is beneficial to prevent pressure ischemia of the flap.

DISSECTION AND IDENTIFICATION OF LANDMARKS

The dissection is carried out deep to the Scarpa's fascia and superiorly. The main landmarks of dissection are medially—the adductor longus muscle, laterally—the sartorius muscle, superiorly—the external oblique aponeurosis and inguinal ligament, and the inferior margins were the apex of the femoral triangle. Transillumination, external pressure on the skin by palpation and surface markings allow good orientation and monitoring of the progression of the dissection. The dissection is done with the help of harmonic scalpel in all cases. Identification of the important structures: The saphenous vein is identified medially, and the external oblique aponeurosis and inguinal ligament are dissected superomedially. The identified saphenous vein is dissected cranially up to the fossa ovalis. Saphenous vein need not be divided in all patients. If necessary, saphenous vein has to be divided using hem-o-loc clips. Dissection is started initially at the vertex of the femoral triangle. All the fatty and lymphatic tissue above the fascia covering the muscle is dissected. It is carried superiorly along the saphenous vein until femoral vessels are reached. The tributaries of saphenous vein are identified and ligated with the help of harmonic and vascular clips. The femoral artery is identified at femoral triangle. At this point, the fascia over the muscle is opened in all directions. The dissection is completed, and specimen consisting of all the fibrofatty tissue with deep and superficial inguinal lymph nodes will be taken out through the 10 mm port, if necessary with a slight expansion of the port site. Suction drain is placed through the lateral port and port incisions closed. Compression dressing is applied which prevents hematoma formation and the dressing is retained for 48–72 hours which usually results in good flap approximation. Elastic compression bandage was applied on the side of surgery. Early ambulation of the patient is allowed to prevent morbidity including deep venous thrombosis. Patients are usually fit for discharge in 24 hours duration. Drain is removed during follow-up once the output is less than 30 ml/day. Drains are usually retained for 10–12 days or sometimes furthermore. Drains are hence to be anchored well and longer retention of drains are to be counseled preoperatively to all patients.

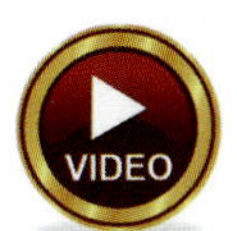

Scan QR Code for Video on
Robotic VEIL (Video-Endoscopic Inguinal Lymph Node Dissection) for Carcinoma Penis (Ca Penis)

35

Troubleshooting during and after VEIL

Raghunath S Krishnappa, Srivatsa N, Nagaraja VH, Tejus C

INJURY TO VASCULAR STRUCTURES

Injury is rare but can be a major complication. Careful identification of the tributaries of vessels, of the venous system in particular goes a long way in preventing inadvertent bleeding. Hook dissection near the insertion of veins into the great saphenous vein and skeletonization of the great saphenous vein at the level of insertion into the femoral vein subsequently helps prevent inadvertent injuries. It is prudent to clip these vessels rather than cauterize them. Small arterial branches can be avulsed during dissection and most of these branches are easily controllable with thermal vessel sealing devises. If the rent appears big, a rescue stitch can be handy to minimize blood loss and retain the endoscopic vision without flooding of operative field. An endoscopic repair may be attempted but often proves difficult due to limited availability of pneumo and space. It may be necessary to make a small opening at the site of vascular injury to gain access and control the bleeding. Larger injuries are extremely rare and may necessitate a more major vascular reconstruction.

INJURY OF FEMORAL NERVE

Injury is rare and encountered when excessive thermal dissection is carried out lateral to the femoral artery. Dissection lateral to the femoral artery is seldom necessary and not important. It is mandatory to delineate the complete artery just distal to the inguinal ligament and subsequently carry out the dissection. Even when fibrofatty tissue is being cleared lateral to the artery in select situations, it should be remembered that the femoral nerve is typically outside the sheath and the dissection should be limited to within the sheath. If the nerve injury is identified, an open repair may be necessary. Thermal nerve injuries tend to be wider than it appears and will in most instances require nerve grafting, typically with sural nerve.

FLAP NECROSIS

Scarpa's fascia is a well visible plane and a large breach in this fascia usually causes flap necrosis. VEIL was designed primarily to avoid flap necrosis and hence, it is imperative that the anterior flap dissection is always maintained in the sub-Scarpa's plane. Small defects are usually inconsequential and larger defects may need to be observed closely in the postoperative period. Necrosis in flaps may be dealt with either excision and primary repair if the area is small or with flaps or skin grafting if the resultant defects are wide.

4

Miscellaneous

CHAPTERS

36

Meatal Stenosis

Pavan Jain, Arvind P Ganpule, Vijay Victor

LEARNING OBJECTIVES AND SUMMARY

- Identify the symptoms and signs of meatal stenosis.
- Order appropriate investigation and explain their rationale.
- Interpret investigations and plan appropriate treatment.

"Non-therapeutic childhood circumcision, performed on about one-third of the world's men for cultural, religious, or other non-medical reasons, is arguably the most prevalent procedure worldwide. It is generally acknowledged that meatal stenosis, a pathological narrowing of the urethral aperture, is one of the more frequent late consequences after circumcision. Indeed, in 1881, the surgeon William M. Mastin noted that meatotomy, a procedure used to treat meatal stenosis, was so common among Jewish men that many referred to it as their "second circumcision" and that a "marked narrowing is believed to exist in, at least, 95% of all cases."

Paediatrician Joseph Brennemann noted in 1921 that his "attention was drawn with increasing frequency to a peculiar lesion of the meatus urinarius occurring only in circumcised male children" He spoke about meatal ulceration and its most likely aftereffect, meatal stenosis, which can cause symptoms like painful urination, spraying or diversion of the urine stream, urgency and frequency of the urge to urinate, hematuria, and enuresis.

Meatal stenosis is clinically defined as narrowing of the urethral orifice. Meatal stenosis occurs in children almost only after circumcision during infancy. It can either be congenital, occurring along with hypospadias or acquired. The incidence of congenital meatal abnormalities associated with hypospadias varies from 9.6% to 31%, of which meatal stenosis is the most common, affecting 9.1–16.7% of patients. Meatal stenosis, an abnormal narrowing of the urethral opening (meatus), is a common complication after circumcision occurring in 9–10% of males.

Case Capsule

A 45-year-old gentleman with past history of epididymo-orchits in the past one year, now presented with a poor stream of urine. He had two episodes of culture proven urinary tract infection (UTI) and was treated for the same. On examination, his urethral examination was normal and he had meatal stenosis. The rest of the systemic and local examination was normal.

Case Discussion

What are the causes of meatal stenosis?
Congenital causes, occurring in association with hypospadias complex 9.1–16.7%.[1,2]

Acquired causes: Post-circumcision.

The overall meatal stenosis prevalence in ethnic Danish and other non-Muslim males (uncircumcised) was 0.121% compared with 0.99% in Muslim males (circumcised).[3]

BXO is another cause of meatal stenosis.

Secondary to radiotherapy.

Changes in the meatus caused by radiation are the same as in the urinary bladder. Endarteritis and ischemia occur, which induces tissue fibrosis. Impaired tissue healing leads to atrophy and contraction in the meatal region and, as a result, meatal stenosis develops.

What is the normal urethral meatus size?

The normal urethral meatus is 10 Fr before 4 years of age, 12 Fr from 4 to 10 years of age, and 14 Fr after 10 years of age, this can be calibrated with a bougie à boule or sound.[4]

What is the theory or pathogenesis behind the meatal stenosis?

One theory purports that after disruption of the normal adhesions between the prepuce and glans and removal of the foreskin, a significant inflammatory reaction ensues, resulting in a severe meatal inflammation and cicatrix formation.

Other theories include frenular devascularization or chronic meatitis from diaper irritation of the exposed, unprotected meatus

What are the symptoms the patient presents with?

Symptoms include
- Urinary stream deviation in an upward direction resulting from a meatal baffle **(Figs 36.1A and B)** or ventral web located at the inferior of the meatus
- A narrow, high-velocity stream, and
- Penile pain at the initiation of micturition.

How does a clinician make a diagnosis of meatal stenosis?

The diagnosis can be made with the help of a good physical examination, and measuring the width of the meatus. In females a voiding cystourethrogram may also be done. Urine analysis and culture with ultrasonography

of the kidney and the bladder can also be performed. During urination physician observes whether stream of urine is straight or not. Measurement of rate of urine flow helps in making appropriate diagnosis.

Physical examination can be varied. Previous studies report a normal meatus size of 3.69 to 5.4 mm in average measured dorsoventraly.[6–7] On physical examination, stenosis of meatus could range from mild narrowing to pinpoint opening with obstructing ventral webbing tissue.[8] If a child is watched while urinating an upward, thin and forceful stream will be observed with possibly incomplete bladder emptying.[9]

What are the grades of meatal stenosis?

Three grades **(Figs 36.1A to C):** Grade 0 (wide open meatus, visible mucosa), Grade 1 (minimal mucous/fibrotic tissue visible), and Grade 2 (pinpoint meatus/no mucosa visible/ large fibrotic layer) **(Table 36.1).**[5]

Grade 0 – open meatus + mucosa seen + no web seen

Table 36.1: Grades of meatal stenosis			
Grade	**Meatus**	**Mucosa**	**Web**
0	Wide open	Seen	No
1	Open	Mild	Fibrotic tissue seen
2	Pinpoint	No mucosa visible	Large fibrotic layer

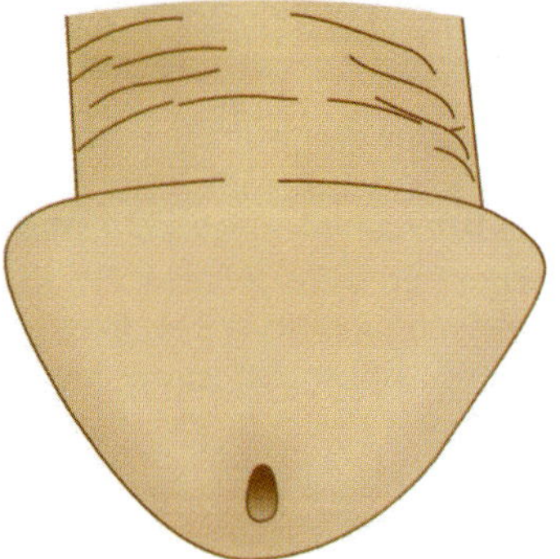

Fig. 36.1A: Grade 0: Wide open meatus and no web seen

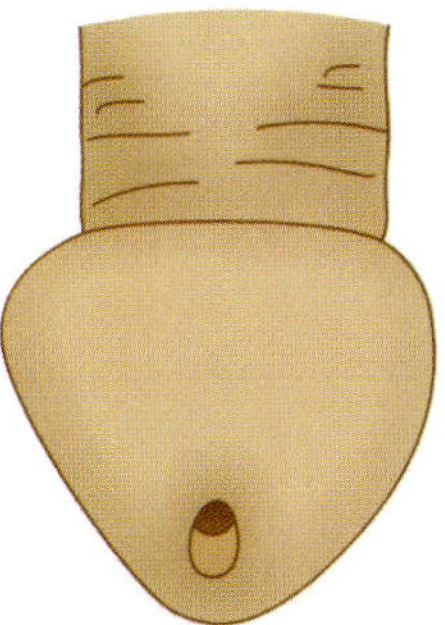

Fig. 36.1B: Grade 1: Open meatus + mild mucosa seen + web seen

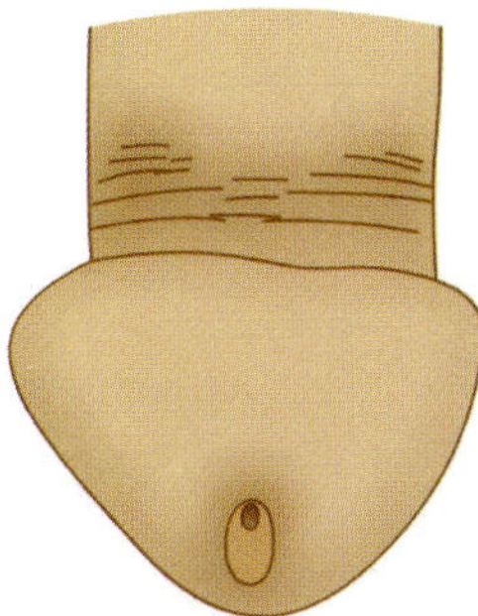

Fig. 36.1C: Grade 2: Pinpoint meatus + no mucosa seen + large web seen

What is the pathogenesis of meatal stenosis post-circumcision?

Symptomatic meatal stenosis is seen in 3–8% of boys after circumcision.[13] It is found in up to 20% of circumcised boys when defined anatomically as a meatal diameter less than 5 Fr between the ages of 5 and 10 years.[14] One proposed mechanism is trauma to the exposed urethral epithelium from clothing or exposure to feces. Application of ointment after each diaper change for 6 months has been shown to significantly decrease the incidence of meatal stenosis.[15]

Complications and natural outcome of meatal stenosis

The meatal stenosis severity grade is associated with narrow stream as reported by parent, prolonged urination, and upward deviation of urinary stream, with increasing severity with worsening stenosis. Meatal stenosis grade is also associated with significant worsening of uroflow measures: A lower Qmax, Qmean and a longer time-to-Q_{max} **(Fig. 36.2)**. Post-void residual volume is not significantly different between the different severity grades. The implementation of a grading system in clinics, may aid in decision making regarding surgical intervention in the appropriate patients, and avoid unnecessary procedures.

The severity of meatal stenosis seen on physical examination correlates well with obstructive symptoms and decrease of urine stream seen on uroflowmetry. These findings confirm the importance of the grading system in the evaluation of patients with meatal stenosis and may be additional measure that assist in consulting parents on the indications to meatotomy.[16]

In some case reports, meatal stenosis has also led to development of chronic kidney disease.

What are the relevant investigations necessary in arriving at a diagnosis of meatal stenosis?

Urinary tract imaging usually does not reveal any obstructive changes in the urinary tract without other urologic issues but may be indicated for associated UTI or urinary incontinence. A uroflowmetry can be done, which will demonstrate an obstructive pattern as depicted in the **Fig. 36.2**.

The most definite investigation for diagnosis of meatal stenosis is a voiding cystogram, descriptive image which is shown in **Fig. 36.3**.

Treatment options available?

Treatment is purely surgical either a meatotomy or a meatoplasty can be done.

Surgical Treatment

The literature supports meatotomy or meatoplasty in meatal stenosis since if left untreated, this condition may lead to recurrent urinary

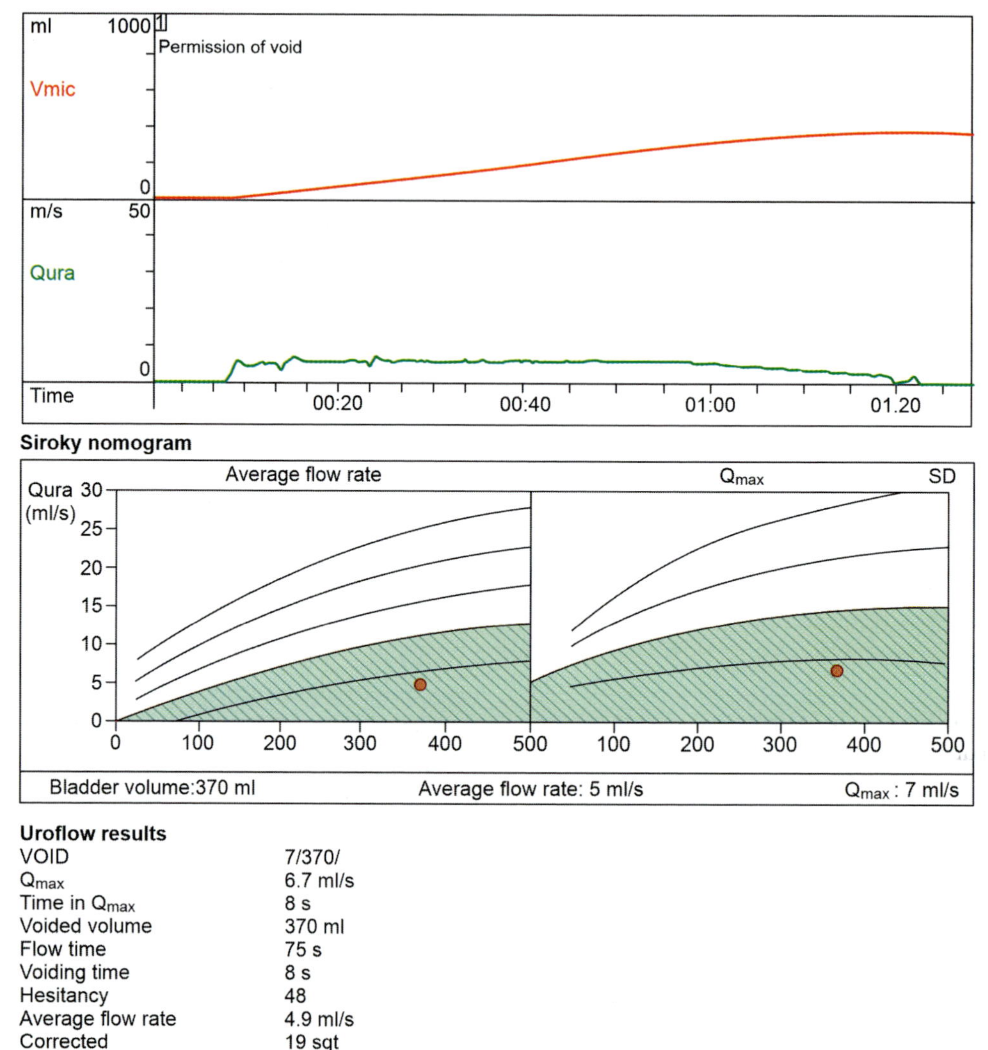

Uroflow results

VOID	7/370/
Q_{max}	6.7 ml/s
Time in Q_{max}	8 s
Voided volume	370 ml
Flow time	75 s
Voiding time	8 s
Hesitancy	48
Average flow rate	4.9 ml/s
Corrected	19 sqt
Residual urine	0 ml
Miction index	4.93 ml/s

Fig. 36.2: Plateau-shaped curve

tract infections and occasionally bladder complications.[10,11]

With the aid of topical lidocaine and prilocaine (EMLA) (Cartwright et al., 1996)[12] or under general anaesthesia, a ventral incision long enough to create a normal meatal calibre can be used to perform a meatotomy or meatoplasty to treat secondary meatal stenosis. The likelihood of recurrence is generally lower when the urethral mucosa is sutured to the glans with tiny, quickly dissolving sutures. Meatal tailoring utilising clamps without the use of sutures is an alternate but equally effective approach.[17]

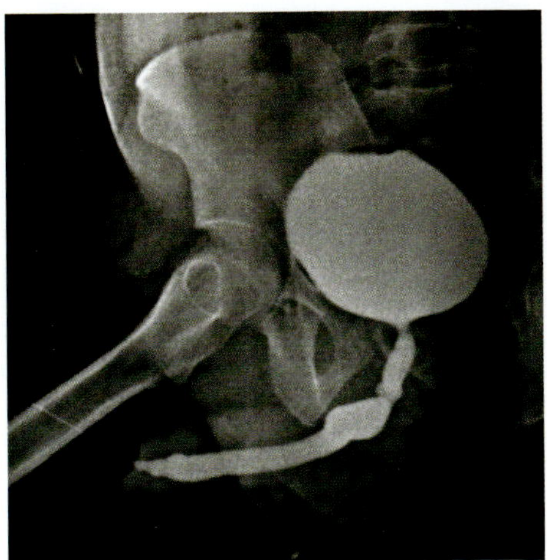

Fig. 36.3: Micturating cystourethrogram showing meatal stenosis

What are the Steps of the Operation?

Patient in place of child.

Minimal skin prep and drape of the genitalia. No prophylactic antibiotics needed.

Betadine povidone iodine solution is used to scrub the genital region, and allowed to remain for approximately 3 minutes prior to initial incision.

The penis should be draped off with sterile towels.

A right-handed surgeon will stand to the left side of the patient and one jaw of a well-lubricated mosquito hemostat is then introduced into the tip/ventral aspect of the urethral meatus to a depth of approximately 2–3 mm.

The ventral tissue is then crushed by closing the hemostat.

The crushed ventral tissue is incised sharply with microsurgical scissors and the inner urethral mucosa and glanular tissue are reapproximated using 7–0 vicryl sutures in an interrupted fashion.

What is Blandy's meatoplasty?

Blandy's meatoplasty: Creation of a midline flap **(Fig. 36.4)**. Urethrotomy is extended till normal urethral lumen. The flap is advanced into the urethrotomy defect.

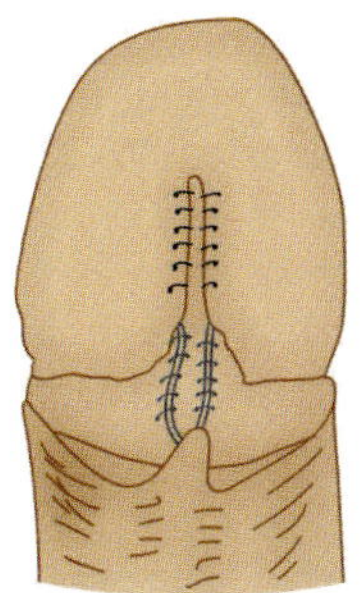

Fig. 36.4: Blandy's meatoplasty

Post-operative follow-up

One measure of a successful outcome of meatoplasty for symptomatic urethral meatal stenosis has traditionally been witnessed voiding and subjective assessment of urinary stream. This evaluation is flawed by nonobjective criteria and potential differing interpretations by different clinicians.

Summary

Meatal stenosis can be either congenital or acquired and can affect both children and adults.

The diagnosis can be made with the help of a thorough clinical examination.

A uroflowmetry done prior to surgical intervention and post-intervention, may help us document the improvement in the peak flow rates of the patient.

Treatment is carried out by performing either a meatotomy or meatoplasty as is documented in the attached video below.

REFERENCES

1. Khan M, Majeed A, Hayat W, et al. Hypospadias repair: a single centre experience. Plastic Surg Int. 2014;2014:7.
2. Pan P. Can grafted tubularized incised plate urethroplasty be used to repair narrow urethral plate hypospadias? Its functional evaluation using uroflowmetry. J Indian Assoc PediatrSurg. 2019;24:247–251.
3. Morris BJ, Krieger JN. Re: Cultural background, non-therapeutic circumcision and the risk of

meatal stenosis and other urethral stricture disease: Two nationwide register-based cohort studies in Denmark 1977–2013. Surgeon. 2018; 16(2):126–129

4. Austin S Litvak, John A Morris J. William Mcroberts, Normal Size of the Urethral Meatus in Boys. The Journal of Urology, Volume 115, Issue 6.

5. Mekayten M, Meir E, Jacob B-C, Landau EH, Khoury AE, Gofrit ON, duvdevani M, Hidas G, Formulation and validation of Meatal Stenosis Grading System, Journal of Pediatric Urology.

6. GS Bhat, M Shivalingiah, GG Nelivigi, C. Ratkal, "The size of external urethral meatus on maximum stretch in Indian adult males.," Indian J. Surg. 2014;76(1):85–89.

7. M Orkiszewski, J Madej, T Kilian. "How wide a urethra should we produce?," J. Pediatr. Urol., 2006;2(5):473–476.

8. BJ Morris, JN Krieger. "Re: Cultural background, non-therapeutic circumcision and the risk of meatal stenosis and other urethral stricture disease: Two nationwide register-based cohort studies in Denmark 1977–2013," The Surgeon, 2018;16(2):126–129.

9. MH Wang. "Surgical Management of Meatal Stenosis with Meatoplasty," J. Vis. Exp. JoVE, no. 45, Nov. 2010.

10. MF Campbell. "Stenosis of the External Urethral Meatus 11 Presented at annual meeting, American Association of Genito-Urinary Surgeons, Stockbridge Mass., June 11, 1943.," J Urol. Dec. 1943.

11. BJ Morris, JN Krieger. "Does Circumcision Increase Meatal Stenosis Risk?—A Systematic Review and Meta-analysis," Urology, 2017;110:16–26.

12. CM Fronczak, CA Villanueva, Clinic meatotomy under topical anesthesia, Journal of Pediatric Urology. 2017;13(5):499.e1-499.e3.

13. DP Smith, et al. The efficacy of LMX versus EMLA for pain relief in boys undergoing office meatotomy J Urol. (2004).

14. PC Cartwright, et al. Urethral meatotomy in the office using topical EMLA cream for anesthesia J Urol. (1996).

15. D Ben-Meir, et al. Meatotomy using local anesthesia and sedation or general anesthesia with or without penile block in children: a prospective randomized study.

16. Mekayten M, Meir E, Yutkin V, Gofrit ON, Duvdevani M, Landau EH, Hidas G. Is there a correlation between meatal stenosis severity, lower urinary tract symptoms and uroflowmetry? J Pediatr Urol. 2022;18(3):342.e1-342.e6.

17. Cubillos J, George A, Gitlin J, Palmer LS. Tailored sutureless meatoplasty: a new technique for correcting meatal stenosis. J Pediatr Urol. 2012;8(1):92-6. doi: 10.1016/j.jpurol.2010.10.002. Epub 2010 Oct 25.

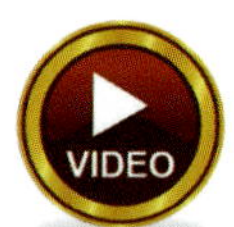

Scan QR Code for Video on
Meatoplasty

37

Shah Penile Prosthesis

Rohan Batra, Vineet Malhotra

CASE

A 65-year-old gentleman underwent robotic Radical prostatectomy 3 years back for localized Ca Prostate (3+4). His PSA on follow-up is 0.01 ng%. After the surgery, he complains of erectile dysfunction. He was advised 5 mg Tadalafil for the past one year. But there was no improvement. After that, he was started on intracavernosal injection (bimix). He got good response to injections but he is uncomfortable with injections.

Management

- The patient has undergone robotic radical prostatectomy (RP).
- The preoperative erectile function and documentation of IIEF scores are noted.
- Co-morbidity like diabetes mellitus, hypertension are noted.
- Check the previous operative notes, whether the patient has undergone a nerve sparing approach or a non-nerve sparing approach.
- Start penile rehabilitation in the form of low dose Tadalafil 5 mg.
- Initial treatment through intra cavernosal injections of bimix (papaverine + chlorpromazine).
- If the patient developed good erections on ICI (Bimix) injections, continue it.
- If patient is not comfortable in injections, the next option for the patient is vacuum erection device or penile prosthesis.
- At present, three types of prosthesis available, i.e. Shah prosthesis, semi rigid prosthesis or three-piece implants **(Fig. 37.1 and Table 37.1)**.

TABLE 37.1: Types of prosthesis		
Prosthesis type	**Name**	**Advantages**
Malleable	Boston scientific Tactra AMS Spectra Shah prosthesis Zephyr ZSI 100 Coloplast genesis	Easier to place Less expensive
Three-piece inflatable	AMS 700 CX AMS 700 CXR Coloplast Titan Zephyr ZSI 475	More natural erection and flaccidity Less chance of pain and erosion

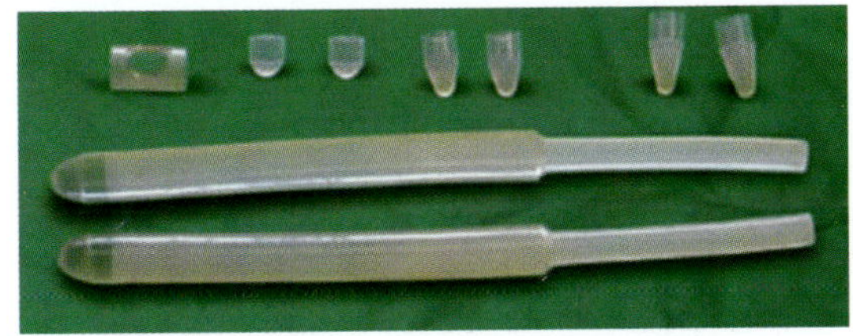

Fig. 37.1: Shah's prosthesis (semi-rigid)

- *Surgical steps:* The main techniques utilized include a penoscrotal approach or an infrapubic approach. The broad steps to insert a semi-rigid prosthesis are:
  - *Preoperative preparation:* Antibiotics such as Vancomycin and Gentamicin 1 hour prior to the procedure. After pubic hair shaving, five-minute wash with chlorhexidine/alcohol skin prep. Patient position is supine with slight frog leg with pubic symphysis at point of flexion so that it elevates the pubic rami up allowing more proximal crural exposure. Foley catheter insertion is done.

Features of Shah Penile Implant

Table 37.2: Features of Shah's penile prosthesis

The Shah penile implant is available in different diameters and lengths

Diameter (it has 2 removable sleeves)	Length of stiff anterior segment
09 mm (WH 09)	7 cm
11 mm (WH 11)	9 cm
13 mm (WH 13)	11 cm
15 mm (WH 15)	13 cm

The two removable sleeves (13—11—9) allows the adjustment of the prosthesis in narrow corpora so that it can snugly fit in the corpora. The prosthesis also contains rear tip extenders (RTE of 1, 2 and 3 cm) **(Table 37.2)**.

Firstly, stretched penile length is measured from pubic symphysis to tip of penis. This step holds significance to choose the correct length of prosthesis and also aids in counselling of the patient.

The initial incision can be placed at penoscrotal junction or infrapubic approach. However, we prefer the penoscrotal approach. A horizontal incision of around 3–4 cm is placed over the skin and deepened. The dissection is done till the exposure of the corporal bodies. It is important to identify the urethra at this point. The Foley's catheter aids in identification of urethra.

After exposure of corporal bodies on both sides, stay sutures are taken 5 mm away from the urethra on both sides with polyglactin 910 (vicryl 2-0). Another stay suture is taken over corporal bodies 5 mm away from the previous stay suture. This will be our corporotomy site.

The corporotomies are made through a stab knife incision on both the sides. The length of the corporotomy should be around 2–3 cm so that the prosthesis can easily go through it.

After the corporotomy, the dilatation of the corpora has to be done.

Dilate the corpora on one side distally first and then proximally. Distally, follow the dilators keeping the direction of dilators outwards. Dilate till the mid glans is reached. Do not force the dilators into the glans.

After the distal dilatation, the proximal dilatation is done till the bony eminence of pubic rami is felt. Thereafter the dilatation sequentially is done till 9, 11, 12, 13 Fr. During dilatation, measure the length of the distal and proximal dilatation. This aids in choosing the correct length of the prosthesis.

Keep flushing the corpora and dilators with antibiotic saline solution throughout the dilatation process.

Selection of the size of penile prosthesis will depend on the length counted during dilatation and the maximum size of dilator used.

The prosthesis are taken from the sterile packing and kept in betadine solution and rinsed with antibiotic saline solution. Cut the rear end according to the length of the dilatation. If required, the sleeve is also cut to reduce the diameter.

The prosthesis are inserted firstly distally and then proximally through the corporotomy incision. Both the prosthesis are inserted and then check whether the length is adequate and it reaches till mid glans.

After satisfactorily placing the prosthesis, the corporotomies are closed with vicry 2-0 which were already placed as stay sutures.

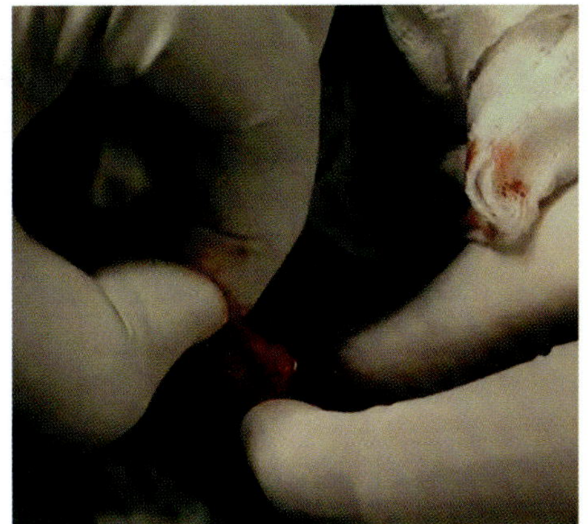

a. Peno scrotal incision

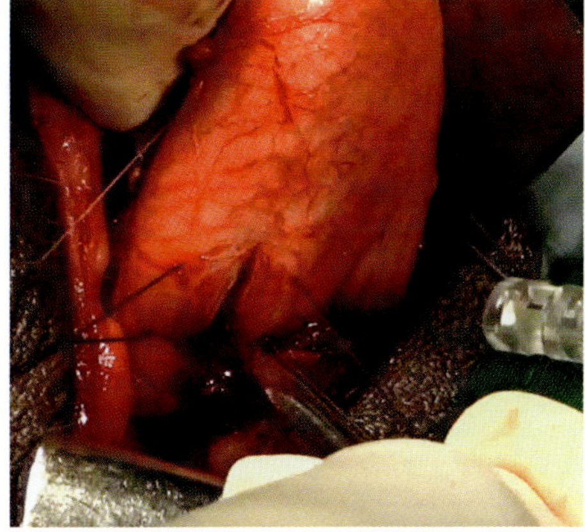

b. Incision on corporal bodies

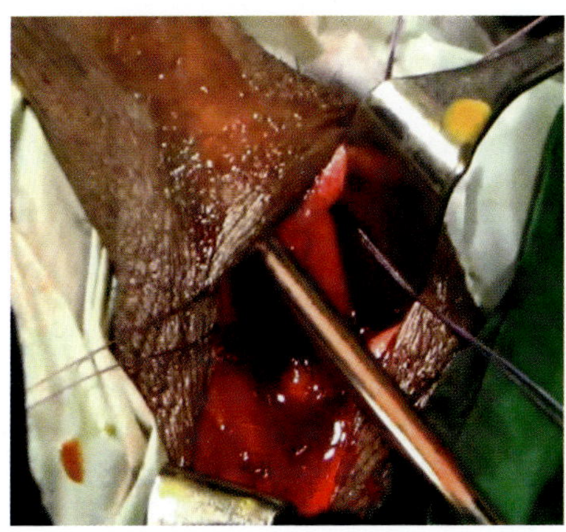

c. Corporal dilatation

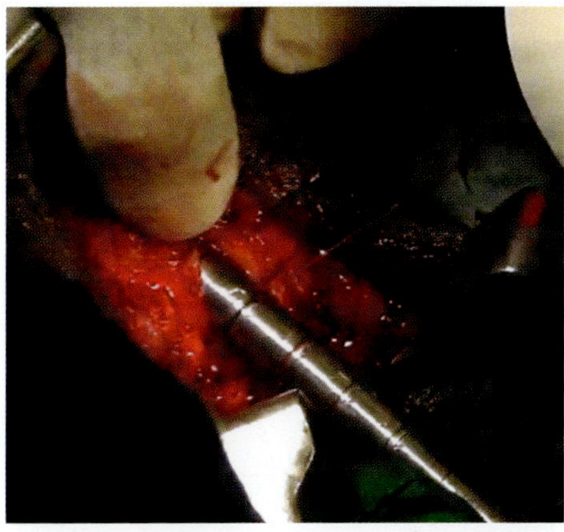

d. Measurement of corporal length

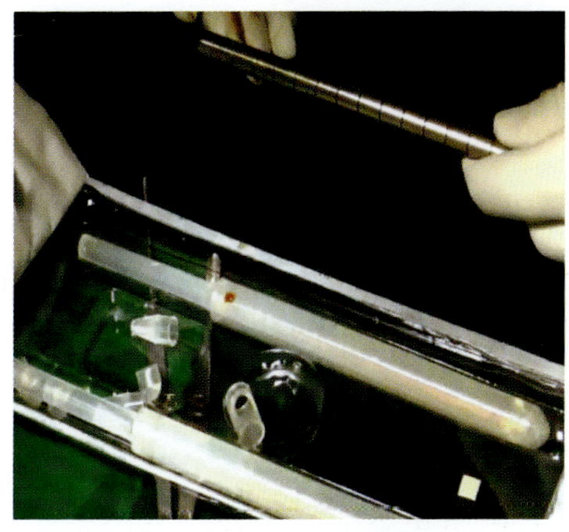

e. Selection of prosthesis

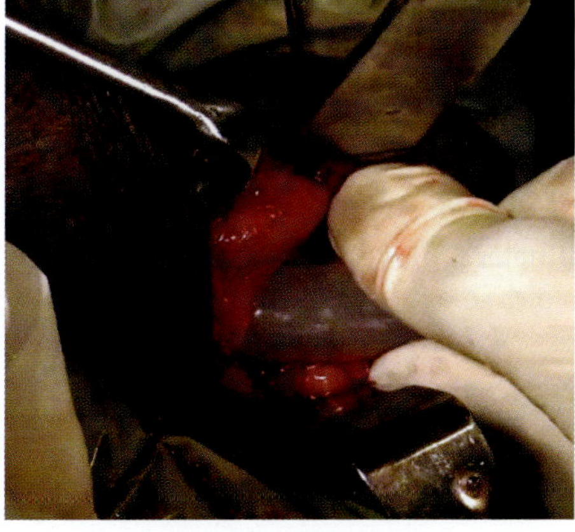

f. Insertion of prosthesis

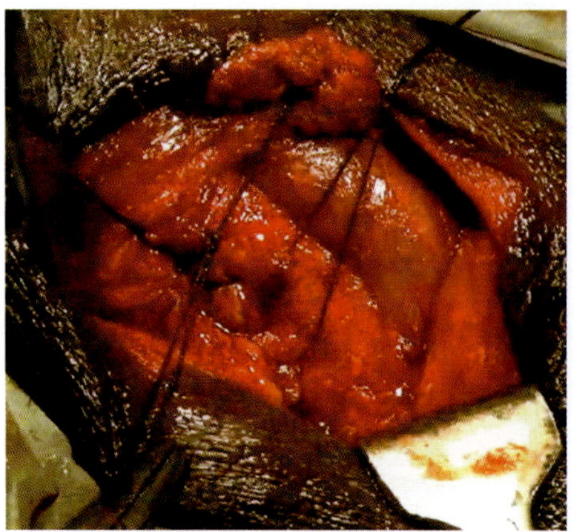

g. Closure of corporotomy

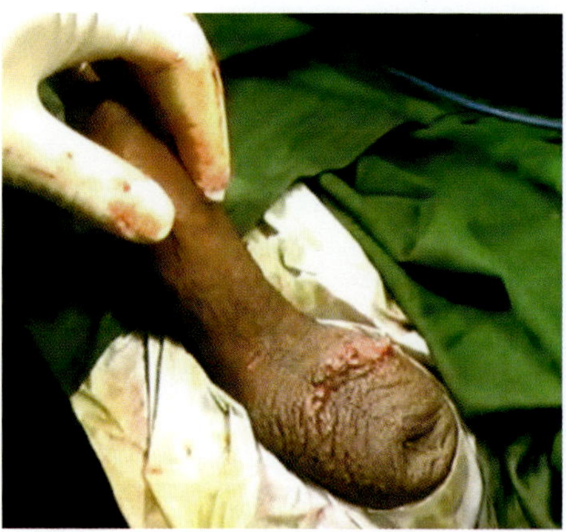

h. Final skin closure

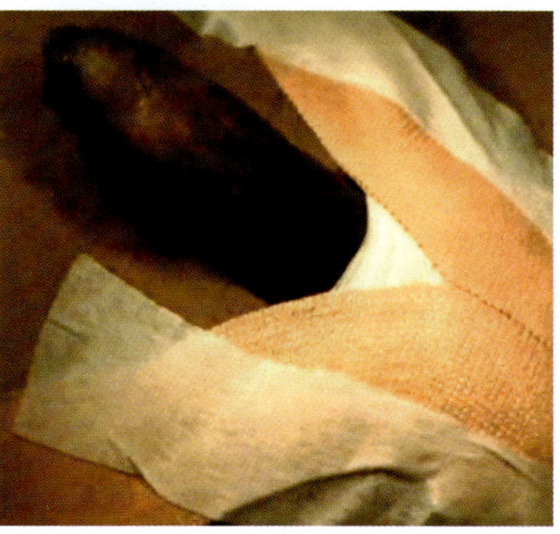

i. Final dressing

Closure: Wound is closed in 3 layers. Buck's fascia and scrotal pouch is closed with 3-0 vicryl and skin with 4-0 ethilon or rapid vicryl.

Postoperative care: Compression dressing for a day.

Catheter removed on 1st postoperative day.

Avoid sexual intercourse for six to eight weeks.

The following precautions can be taken to optimise the results:

The hinge has to be positioned correctly. For that, measure the stretched penile length and dilatation length correctly. The hinge segment will be positioned at the base of the penis with approximately 2 cm in front of the symphysis pubis.

The removable sleeves are an advantage and can be removed if dilatation is difficult.

The sleeves can also be removed in a segmental way if the corpora are tapering at tips or there is extensive fibrosis at tip.

Appropriate RTE may be added if the length cut has been made short.

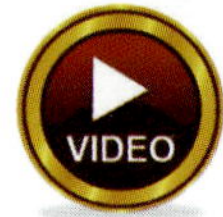

Scan QR Code for Video on
Shah Prosthesis Insertion for ED